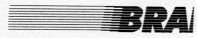

Introduction to
Air Medicine

Clyde Deschamp, Ph. D.
The University of Mississippi Medical Center, Jackson, MS

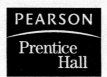

PEARSON
Prentice
Hall

Upper Saddle River, New Jersey 07458

Library of Congress Cataloging-in-Publication Data

Deschamp, Clyde.
 Introduction to air medicine/Clyde Deschamp.
   p. cm.
 Includes index.
 ISBN 0-13-113494-9
  1. Aviation medicine.   I. Title.

RC1062.D47 2006
616.9'80213—dc22

2005050966

Publisher: Julie Levin Alexander
Publisher's Assistant: Regina Bruno
Executive Editor: Marlene McHugh Pratt
Senior Acquisitions Editor: Stephen Smith
**Senior Managing Editor for
 Development:** Lois Berlowitz
Associate Editor: Monica Moosang
Editorial Assistant: Diane Edwards
Executive Marketing Manager: Katrin Beacom
Director of Marketing: Karen Allman
Marketing Coordinator: Michael Sirinides
Director of Production and Manufacturing: Bruce Johnson
Managing Production Editor: Patrick Walsh
Production Liaison: Julie Li
Production Editor: Lisa S. Garboski, bookworks
Manufacturing Manager: Ilene Sanford
Manufacturing Buyer: Pat Brown
Senior Design Coordinator: Cheryl Asherman
Interior Designer: Amy Rosen

Cover Designer: Michael Ginsberg
Cover Image: Joy Ferchaud/University
 of Mississippi Medical Center
Director, Image Resource Center: Melinda Reo
Manager, Rights and Permissions: Zina Arabia
Manager, Visual Research: Beth Brenzel
**Manager, Cover Visual Research
 and Permissions:** Karen Sanatar
Image Permission Coordinator: Joanne Dippel
Composition: The GTS Companies/York,
 PA Campus

Pearson Education Ltd.
Pearson Education Singapore, Pte. Ltd.
Pearson Education, Canada, Ltd.
Pearson Education—Japan
Pearson Education Australia Pty, Limited

Pearson Education North Asia Ltd.
Pearson Educación de Mexico, S.A. de C.V.
Pearson Education Malaysia, Pte. Ltd.
Pearson Education, Upper Saddle River, New Jersey

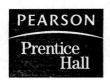

ISBN 0-13-113494-9

Contents

Chapter 14

Finance   217

Chapter 15

Benefits of an Air Medical Program   227

Chapter 16

Outreach and Promotional Activities   235

Chapter 17

Military Operations   247

Chapter 18

International Air Medicine   271

Chapter 19   Fixed-Wing Operations   293

Chapter 20   Starting a New Air Medical Program   309

Preface

This book began as a five-page outline for a two-hour orientation lecture for the employees of a newly created air medical program. Over time the lecture was expanded to be more comprehensive and a search was begun for a reference text. It was soon learned that no such text existed. There were books on aviation, flight physiology, prehospital medicine, flight nursing, and aviation communications. Each of these books focused narrowly on one aspect of air medicine. Several important components of air medicine were not mentioned at all or were given only superficial coverage in existing books. There was nothing available that presented an overview of air medicine and all its components. This book was written to help fill that void.

Air medicine combines the excitement, challenges and rewards of prehospital, critical care, and emergency medicine with the unique pleasure of flight. Fixed-wing and rotor-wing aircraft alike are wonders to behold. Their ability to soar above the clouds gives them an almost magical quality. The appearance of one of these craft often evokes high expectations. That is as it should be since the patients transported by these programs are often the sickest of the sick.

This book is introductory in that it assumes no previous knowledge of air medicine. It was designed to be read by anyone with an interest in the field. However, it does go into significant detail in some areas and a background in the medical field will aid in the understanding of some topics. Physicians with an interest in emergency or critical care medicine, paramedics, and emergency and critical care nurses will likely have the greatest appreciation for the content.

The following people were invaluable in helping put this book together: Attila Hertelendy, who wrote the majority of Chapter 18 (International Air Medicine) and Chapter 19 (Fixed-Wing Operations). Attila's international and fixed-wing experiences added a slightly different perspective to a book that was otherwise written from a U.S. perspective. Attila is a faculty member in the Department of Emergency Medical Technology at the University of Mississippi Medical Center in Jackson, Mississippi.

Carl Bottorf, RN, Flight Nurse, U.S. Air Force Reserves and Angelina R. Leve, RN, Flight Nurse, U.S. Air Force Reserves co-authored Chapter 17 (Military Operations). These two contributors have extensive experience with the military and added a perspective that was clearly beyond the scope of knowledge of the author.

Mark Galtelli, BS, NREMTP, CCEMTP, CF-P contributed a great deal to Chapter 16 (Outreach and Promotional Activities). He also provided several photos. Mark is Senior Paramedic for the AirCare program at the University of Mississippi Medical Center, Jackson, Mississippi. Duke Baker, an employee of Petroleum Helicopters, Incorporated and Lead Pilot for the AirCare program, provided material and advice for several chapters.

Donna Norris, BSN, CFRN, Chief Flight Nurse for the AirCare program provided suggestions and insight for several chapters. She was also instrumental in providing perspective in several areas. Others providing suggestions and data for the book include Mathew Zavarella, MS, RN, NREMTP, Chuck Carter, RN, NREMTP, and Dan Turner, RN, CFRN. A special thanks is offered to J. Maurice Mahan, Ph.D., Lu Harding, and F. B. Carlton, Jr., MD for their support.

Closer to home, I want to acknowledge the patience and support of my wife, Nancy, and our sons, Chris and David, who are a continual source of inspiration and motivation.

Reviewers

JOHN L. BECKMAN, FF/PM INSTRUCTOR
Affiliated with Addison Fire Protection District
EMS Instructor
Addison, IL

STEVEN DRALLE, EMT-P
South Texas CES Manager
American Medical Response
San Antonio, TX

BOB ELLING, MPA, REMT-P
Faculty American College of Prehospital Medicine
Schenectady, NY

PRESTON LOVE, RN, BSN, LP
Flight nurse/Paramedic
San Antonio Airlife
San Antonio, TX

RONALD W. WALTER, BS, NREMT-P, CCEMT-P
Base Coordinator
STAT MedEvac
West Mifflin, PA

TAMMY WETHERALL, CCEMT-P
Director of Training and Education
Meda-Care Ambulance
Milwaukee, WI

CHAPTER 1

Introduction

Objectives

Upon completing this chapter, the reader should have a better understanding of the following topics:

* The definition of air medicine

* The air medical program in the community

* Basic aircraft types

* Principles of flight

* Aircraft attitude and movements

KEY TERMS

air medicine (aeromedicine), p. 2

angle of attack, p. 6

drag, p. 6

Introduction

The purpose of this book is to introduce nurses, paramedics, physicians, and other members of the health care team to the concept of air medicine, including equipment, personnel, safety, and operations. This information may be of particular interest to newly hired flight team members and to emergency medicine and other medical residents preparing for an air medical rotation (Figure 1-1).

Paramedic and nursing students who have an opportunity to study air medicine in the classroom or as part of a preceptorship will also benefit from reading this book prior to or as a requirement of those courses. Hospital administrators may find sections of this book helpful when considering the addition or restructuring of a flight program. Firefighters and first responders may benefit from reading the chapters

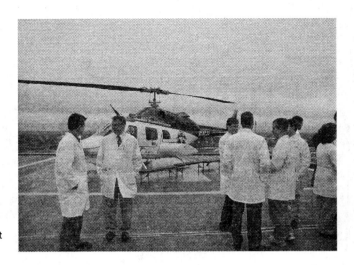

Group of students getting first look at medical helicopter

A medical subspecialty that incorporates elements of emergency medicine, critical-care medicine, paramedicine, nursing, and public safety into the treatment and transport of patients by air.

on safety and setting up a landing zone. The chapter on aircraft and equipment may be of interest not only to health care professionals but also to pilots and others with an interest in aircraft. **Air medicine** (AM) incorporates the use of an aircraft and other specialized equipment into the practice of emergency and/or critical-care medicine. Many consider it to be a subspecialty of emergency medicine. In some systems the air medical program is aligned with a department of surgery or critical-care medicine. In any case, air medicine is a unique field. While it incorporates elements from medicine, paramedicine, nursing, and public service areas, when taken as a whole it is very different from other medical disciplines. The knowledge and skills required to practice air medicine are unique, as are the equipment and machinery. The flight program is much more than an extension of an emergency or critical-care department, and it must be accepted as such.

From a more personal perspective, air medicine offers those individuals who are lucky enough to become a part of it a career that is exciting and rewarding. Most of the patients encountered by a flight team are acutely ill or injured, and the team's actions can make the difference between life and death or between debility and uneventful recovery.

Newly hired personnel are sometimes overwhelmed by the magnitude of responsibilities they take on when they join a flight team. For many it is the first time in their careers that their medical knowledge and skills are put to the test. The patient assessment performed by the flight team is sometimes the sole basis for complex medical decisions (Figure 1-2). The physical examination must incorporate much more than vital signs and auscultation of the lungs. The history has to be

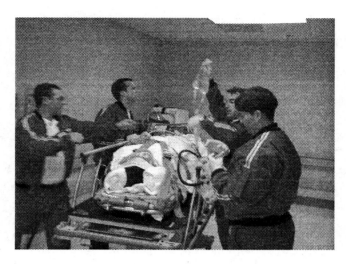

FIGURE 1-2
Action shot of flight team assessing
a patient

complete. There is no emergency medicine or critical-care physician standing in the background to detect subtle clues that may be overlooked. Flight team members must be competent, confident, and willing to accept complete responsibility for their actions.

Air medicine involves taking nursing and paramedicine to a new level. This challenge applies to physicians as well. Air medical crews often respond to complex motor vehicle crashes, industrial accidents, and other out-of-hospital emergencies that require knowledge and skills not taught in medical school or encountered in most residency programs. Medical extrication, crash scene triage, and functioning in unpredictable and uncontrolled environments are situations with which most physicians are unfamiliar. Patients may be difficult to isolate, bystanders may be threatening or even violent, and support staff is often limited to fellow team members. A temporary lapse of interpersonal skills may result in a verbal or physical confrontation. On the other hand, the AM experience offers the physician a unique opportunity to meet, assess, and treat emergency patients in a real-world environment. The air medical preceptorship may add a valuable new perspective to a residency program.

For medical residents, involvement in an air medical program may be voluntary or mandatory. In either case this involvement should be seen as a unique opportunity, one that is available to a select few. For those with an interest in research or publication, an air medical rotation presents a unique experience. Air medicine is still a relatively new field and one that has not been fully explored. There are numerous areas in which small research projects can be done with a moderate amount of effort.

Residents in emergency medicine and other critical-care areas should use this opportunity to gain knowledge and experience that may be of value later in their careers. Virtually all emergency medicine residencies eventually lead to employment opportunities in emergency departments or other critical care areas. These physicians may be called on to serve on advisory committees or as medical directors for air medical programs. Those with at least a fundamental knowledge and experience will be better equipped to make meaningful contributions to those programs.

Role of the Air Medical Program in the Community

An air medical program should be viewed as a resource for the entire community in which it operates. Due to the high cost of these programs, relatively few are available and they typically serve large geographic areas. These valuable resources should be made known to the medical community and should be made available for use by the medical community. These programs should be designed to link prehospital resources with in-hospital resources. They should also be used as a means to link resources at community hospitals with those at larger referral centers.

Competition between hospitals and hospital systems is a driving force in health care. However, there is a fine line between healthy competition and behavior that may negatively impact patient care. While hospitals may use air medical programs as marketing tools, the availability of these programs should never be withheld to the detriment of patient care, even if a patient is to be transported to a competing facility. Limiting access to select groups of hospitals, physicians, or patients is unethical.

Good faith efforts should be made by hospital administrators and others in positions of influence to ensure that the air medical program is integrated into the health care delivery system in a way that benefits both patients and the medical community. While many flight programs receive subsidies, those funds rarely cover more than a fraction of costs. Financial support from other hospitals in the area is an effective means of cost sharing. That may be in the form of a monthly or annual stipend or a service fee each time a patient is delivered. Financial issues can generally be resolved if everyone comes to the table with good intentions and negotiates in good faith. Patient care must always be the overriding concern.

Aircraft Types

Two basic types of aircraft are used as air ambulances: fixed-wing and rotor-wing (Figure 1-3). Fixed-wing aircraft (FWA) are exactly that: they have a large wing protruding from each side, firmly attached to the fuselage. These wings are rigid and provide the lift necessary to enable flight. Fixed-wing aircraft are generally capable of great speeds and of cruising at high altitudes. Their biggest shortcoming is that they require an airport for takeoff and landing, and airports are not always conveniently located.

Rotor-wing aircraft (RWA), on the other hand, have a smaller "wing" attached to a mast, which extends from the transmission on top of the aircraft. When the engine is started and the transmission engages, this wing, known as the main rotor, rotates, while the aircraft itself remains still. RWA are therefore capable of vertical takeoff and landing and do not require an airport. They can generally land in an open area not much larger than the diameter of the main rotor.

The Principles of Flight

The fact that a craft heavier than air, often weighing many tons, can leave the confines of Earth and soar with the birds is an awe-inspiring concept. It is essential for anyone planning to become a member of an AM flight team to have some understanding of the principles of flight.

Newton's Third Law of Motion, "For every action there is an equal and opposite reaction," is the basis for flight by heavier-than-air craft. The physics of flight are most easily explained through the use of a

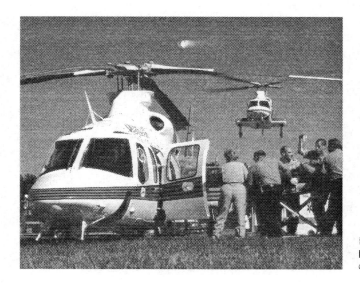

FIGURE 1-3
Rotor-wing aircraft
Courtesy of Sheldon Cohen/Bell Helicopter

Introduction 5

fixed-wing model. FWA have wings extending horizontally from each side of the craft. As the plane begins to move down the runway, air flows across the surface of the wings. The wings are curved so that the air is forced to curve downward as it approaches the rear. As the speed of this air increases, the airflow has a tendency to travel in a straight line. That tendency pulls the air away from the rear surface of the wings, creating a vacuum and lifting the wings upward. The amount of lift increases as airspeed increases. When there is enough lift to support the weight of the plane, it elevates above the runway and begins to fly.

There are four basic forces at work on an aircraft as it flies: thrust, lift, drag, and weight. *Thrust* is the force that propels the aircraft forward. In a propeller-driven aircraft, the propeller spins, increasing the pressure of the air behind it. That pressure in turn forces the aircraft forward. Jet aircraft produce thrust without the aid of a propeller. Air flows into the engine, where it is compressed, fuel is introduced, and the mixture is ignited. The air is then forced out the rear of the engine at high pressure, forcing the aircraft forward. Engine power in a propeller-driven engine is measured in horsepower, while that of a jet engine is measured in pounds of thrust.

Lift occurs when an aircraft's wing or airfoil is moved through the air. A wing can generate lift because its upper surface is more curved than its lower surface. As the oncoming air stream meets the leading edge of the wing, it divides. The air traveling over the wing must travel a greater distance than the air traveling under it. That forces the air moving over the wing to travel faster than the air underneath. This concept was first explained by Daniel Bernoulli, an eighteenth-century Swiss scientist who studied the relationship between velocity and pressure. According to Bernoulli, "An increase in velocity will result in a decrease in pressure." The pressure is greater over the underside of the wing than it is over the top. Basically, a vacuum is formed over the top of the wing, and that vacuum lifts the aircraft upward (Figure 1-4). The angle at which the wing contacts oncoming air is known as the **angle of attack**. The most efficient angle of attack for an airfoil is generally 4 or 5 degrees. Should the angle of attack be increased to 16 or 17 degrees, the airflow over the wing will become turbulent, resulting in a significant loss of lift. If the angle of attack is further increased, the wing will cease to produce lift and the aircraft will cease to fly. In order to climb, an aircraft must produce excess lift beyond what is required to support the weight of the aircraft. In a descent, the opposite occurs.

Drag acts opposite to thrust. It is simply the wind resistance to the passage of the wings, aircraft, and components through the air. As thrust and speed increase, so does drag. As speed continues to increase, more engine power is required to overcome drag. Since there is a limit to the amount of power an aircraft engine can generate, drag will eventually increase to a point where no further increase in speed is possible.

angle of attack
The angle between the direction of the cord of the blades and the relative direction of the wind.

drag
The wind force exerted against an aircraft as it attempts to move through the air.

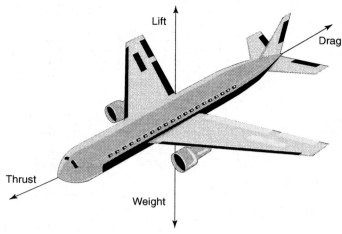

FIGURE 1-4

Illustration of the forces acting on an aircraft in flight

Aerospace engineers mitigate the forces of drag by designing aircraft wings with lower profiles and less surface area, which result in decreased drag and allow aircraft to fly faster. However, as wing size is decreased, greater speed is required to produce adequate lift, so these aircraft are generally unable to fly at slower airspeeds. Since they must take off and land at higher airspeeds, longer runways are often required.

Weight is the result of the gravitational pull of the earth on the aircraft in flight. This force directly opposes lift. The total weight of the aircraft includes the aircraft, fuel, passengers, and cargo. As aircraft weight increases, more lift is required to lift the craft from the ground and to maintain flight. More power is required to generate forward motion and to produce adequate lift. Weight is a concern for all types of aircraft, which have maximum weight limitations beyond which flight safety may be compromised.

Aircraft Attitude and Movements

Now that we have discussed how an aircraft flies, it is important to understand how it is controlled in the air (Figure 1-5). An aircraft has several movable surfaces that allow the pilot to change its attitude and direction. *Attitude* refers to an aircraft's orientation in relation to the horizon.

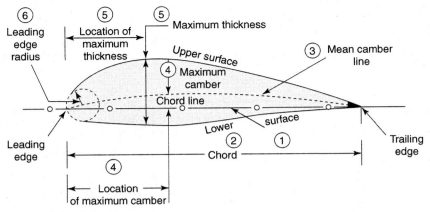

Illustration of aircraft control surfaces

Movements are relative to the pilot and aircraft, acting around a particular axis of the aircraft. Three types of movement are pitch, roll, and yaw.

Pitch is movement about the lateral axis (Figure 1-6). It is produced and controlled by the *elevator*, a horizontal surface attached to the tail of the aircraft that may be adjusted up or down. Back pressure on the

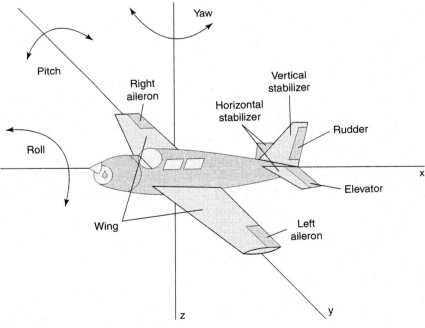

Illustration of pitch, roll, and yaw

control column causes the elevator to rise, producing a downward force on the tail and resulting in a nose-up attitude. When forward pressure is applied to the control column, the opposite occurs, resulting in a nose-down attitude.

Roll is movement about the longitudinal axis, which is produced and controlled by the ailerons. *Ailerons* are small, movable sections on the trailing surface of an aircraft's wings. They are moved to produce a banking motion. Turning the control column to the right causes the left aileron to drop, changing the shape of the wing and producing more lift. This increase in lift causes the wing to rise. Simultaneously the right aileron goes up, reducing lift and causing the wing to drop. The result is a roll to the right that establishes a banked attitude (Figure 1-6). When the controls are moved to the left, the opposite occurs. Movement of the ailerons is controlled by movement of the yoke, the steering-wheel-like device the pilot holds during flight.

Yaw is movement about the vertical axis, which is controlled by the rudder. The *rudder* is a movable vertical component of the aircraft tail. In fact, it usually comprises the rear section of the tail. It is controlled by foot pedals. Depressing the left rudder pedal causes the nose to move to the left, and depressing the right rudder pedal causes it to move to the right (Figure 1-6). Yaw, unlike pitch and roll, is not something the pilot normally produces but rather something to be controlled through proper use of the rudder.

Rotor-Wing Aircraft

While the basic principles discussed above also apply to RWA, there are some significant differences. An RWA's movable wings allow it a flexibility not possible with the FWA. The most significant advantage of the RWA is its ability to attain lift without having to move down a runway. The main rotor moves through the air in a circular pattern above the fuselage, allowing RWA to take off and land vertically.

Contrary to popular belief, it is not the speed of the main rotor that controls the amount of lift. Once the aircraft engine is started, it is set at a predetermined level of revolutions per minute (RPM) that is maintained during all phases of takeoff, cruise, and landing. The pilot controls the amount of lift by changing the pitch on the main rotor. When the aircraft is not in motion, the pitch on the main rotor is neutral so as to avoid producing lift. As the pilot prepares for takeoff, the pitch gradually increases until enough lift is achieved to move the aircraft into the air. Pitch is then adjusted periodically during flight to maintain the correct speed and altitude. An increase in pitch causes the aircraft to climb and/or move faster through the air. A decrease produces the opposite effect. Steering an RWA involves the same principles as steering an

FWA, but the process is somewhat different. The RWA has only two control surfaces, the main rotor and the tail rotor. As described above, the main rotor produces the lift necessary to attain and maintain flight. It is also used to control the direction and speed of the aircraft. A device known as a pitch plate, which is attached to the main rotor control head, allows the pilot to vary the pitch on the main rotor as it progresses through each revolution. For example, to move the aircraft forward, the pilot pushes the control stick forward, causing an increase in pitch when the rotor blade is near the rear of the aircraft. This results in increased lift on the aft side of the rotor and lifts the rear of the aircraft up. As the aircraft tilts forward, it moves forward. The same process is performed anytime the pilot wants to change the attitude or direction of the aircraft.

tail rotor
A small rotor generally located on the distal tail of the helicopter. It produces thrust to counteract the torque generated by the engine as it powers the main rotor.

The **tail rotor** is used primarily to keep the aircraft from spinning out of control. The forces generated by the engine and transmission produce torque. If left uncontrolled, torque would force the aircraft to spin in a direction opposite to the direction in which the main rotor is turning. The tail rotor is in effect an antitorque device. It is controlled by the pilot with foot pedals. The pilot also uses the tail rotor to change the direction in which the aircraft is heading. The technique and effect are very similar to those of the rudder in an FWA.

Piloting an RWA is much more difficult to master than flying a small FWA. There are more variables and more movements that must be conducted simultaneously to maintain flight. Takeoff and landing are the most difficult phases of rotor-wing (RW) flight, but controlling an RWA during hover is also challenging.

Summary

Air medicine is an exciting and rewarding field. Air medical teams are called out for the most acute and challenging patients and have a positive influence on many patient outcomes. Air medicine involves the incorporation of cutting edge technology and highly trained personnel in a challenging and exciting environment. Becoming part of a flight team requires a major change in orientation and responsibilities for medical personnel accustomed to the more controlled hospital environment. Medical extrication and dealing one on one with patients under stressful conditions are but a few of the challenges faced by members of the flight team.

Flight programs fall into two broad categories: fixed wing and rotor wing. Rotor-wing aircraft or helicopters are the most versatile and common form of the air ambulance. These aircraft are adaptable to a variety of flight and landing conditions and allow delivery of patients directly to a hospital. Fixed-wing aircraft on the other hand require an airport for takeoff and landing and are practical only for long-distance transports. Air medical programs have much to offer the medical community. They can play an important role in linking community and referral hospitals. Under certain circumstances they may improve outcomes for patients transported from the prehospital setting. These programs are valuable resources that must be shared with all hospitals in the community, and they must be operated in a responsible and ethical manner. Conversely, all hospitals in a community should contribute to the support of the program. An air medical program has much to contribute to the ill and injured in the community, and it can remain responsive to the community's needs while maintaining fiscal soundness.

REVIEW QUESTIONS

1. Air medicine may be defined as:
   a. The study of pathophysiology at elevations above sea level
   b. A specialty area of medicine practiced only by Air Force personnel
   c. A specialty area of medicine based on knowledge gained from the space program
   d. A medical specialty area that incorporates the use of aircraft and other specialized equipment into the practice of emergency and/or critical-care medicine

2. It is acceptable to limit availability of emergency air medical services under the following conditions:
   a. When a patient is unable to provide payment
   b. When a patient requires treatment available only at a competing hospital
   c. When a patient requires treatment at a hospital that does not provide financial support for the air medical program
   d. It is unethical for an air medical program to limit access to select groups of hospitals, physicians, or patients

3. The two basic types of aircraft utilized as air ambulances are:
   a. Fixed-wing and rotor-wing
   b. Turbine and reciprocating engine
   c. Retractable gear and nonretractable gear
   d. Visual flight rule and instrument flight rule

4. The force that propels an aircraft forward during flight is:
   a. Thrust
   b. Lift
   c. Drag
   d. Weight

5. The wind resistance to the passage of the wings, aircraft, and components through the air is called:
   a. Thrust
   b. Lift
   c. Drag
   d. Weight

6. Movement of an aircraft about the lateral axis that is produced and controlled by the elevator in a fixed-wing aircraft is called:
   a. Pitch
   b. Roll
   c. Yaw
   d. Acceleration

7. Movement about the vertical axis that is controlled by the rudder in a fixed-wing aircraft is called:
   a. Pitch
   b. Roll
   c. Yaw
   d. Acceleration

8. In a rotor-wing aircraft the _____ replaces the rudder of a fixed-wing aircraft:
   a. Cyclic
   b. Collective
   c. Main rotor
   d. Tail rotor

CHAPTER 2

Organizational Structure

Objectives

Upon completing this chapter, the reader should have a better understanding of the following topics:

* Organizational structures of typical flight programs

* Pros and cons of various organizational structures

* The priority of safety in the flight program

* Administrative and managerial positions in a flight program

* The four operational components of an air medical program

KEY TERMS

Federal Aviation
Administration (FAA),
p. 20

Federal Aviation
Regulations (FARs),
p. 20

instrument flight rule
(IFR), p. 21

visual flight rule (VFR),
p. 21

Introduction

Hospitals or hospital systems operate most air medical programs, which generally adopt the organizational structures of their sponsor hospital(s). However, AM programs are uniquely constructed and do not always mesh well with the hospital system. They incorporate personnel, machinery, regulatory requirements, safety requirements, and performance guidelines that are not duplicated elsewhere in the health care system. Any effort to fit a flight program into the mold used by other hospital departments may be problematic.

Table 2-1 Organizational Chart of a Typical Hospital-Based Air Medical Program

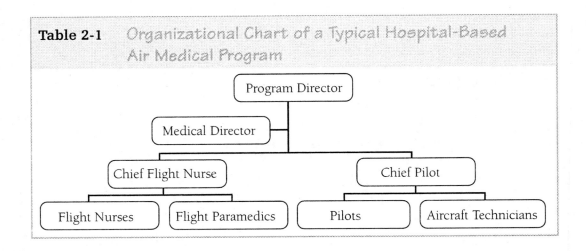

Hospital air medical programs may be set up as departments or as divisions of existing departments, such as emergency medicine or trauma services (Table 2-1). If they are set up as separate departments of air medicine, they generally have more autonomy and are less likely to be tampered with by those who may not have a complete understanding of their unique structure and requirements. Funding is also less likely to be diverted to other sources during times of financial hardship, and program personnel can focus all their energy on air medical issues.

Governmental entities, quasi-governmental entities, and public service agencies also occasionally operate air medical programs. These programs also adopt the organizational structure of their sponsoring organizations. For example, a flight program operated by a law enforcement agency may be organized in a militaristic fashion with a very strict chain of command and a tightly defined scope of operation. A program operated by a quasi-governmental agency may have a broader base of input and oversight and may be subject to political influences. (These are broad generalizations used to make a point. It is understood that these patterns may not apply in every situation.)

Organizational Structures

An air medical program may be organized in a variety of ways: as a freestanding entity, a department in a hospital, or a consortium. Freestanding entities may be classified as for-profit, not-for-profit, or quasi-governmental. Some programs may have characteristics of more than one organizational type.

For-Profit Organizations

It is unusual for stand-alone rotor-wing programs to be operated as for-profit entities. These programs are so expensive to operate that, in the absence of subsidies, they rarely make good financial investments. The exception is a program operated as part of a larger medical transportation program or as a department within a for-profit hospital. In that case the rotor-wing component may generate net income primarily as a result of its relation to other components or through its ability to expand the catchment area (the geographical area served by the program) and generate additional patients for its sponsor hospital.

The obvious benefit of establishing a for-profit air medical program is that the owner(s) may realize profits if the program does well. When profit is the primary motivation, owners generally operate a program in a cost-effective manner. But the desire for profits can be a double-edged sword. Financial incentives have tremendous potential to alter individual behavior. Managers have been known to pressure flight teams into accepting flights even when the weather is marginal or there are other safety concerns. Profit-taking may lead to a compromise in program quality. If funds are not poured back into the company in the form of maintenance and improvements, the quality of the operation is likely to deteriorate over time, and program safety may be compromised. However, if a for-profit organization is administered according to accepted business practices, it can be a very efficient means of offering a service.

Not-For-Profit Organizations

Not-for-profits are often created to meet a public need that is not otherwise being met. When all other variables are equal, a not-for-profit has the potential to operate more efficiently than a comparable for-profit organization. For one thing, no money is taken out of the company in the form of profits. For another, a not-for-profit is generally not required to pay taxes. All the money that would be taken out of a for-profit organization in the form of profits and taxes are retained by the not-for-profit and can be rolled back into the operation of the company.

Consortia

One way to lower the cost of operating a flight program is to spread expenses among two or more sponsoring institutions, typically hospitals, that form a consortium. Each member hospital receives the benefits without having to bear all the expenses. Members may pay a monthly and/or annual membership fee to support the program. Another option is for each member to reimburse the consortium for the cost of each patient delivered. Other programs use a combination of these two approaches.

In single-aircraft programs, the aircraft may be located at one of the participating hospitals or operated from a neutral location such as an airport. Another option is rotating the base of operation among participating hospitals, in which case the aircraft, flight team, and all support services move as a unit. This arrangement minimizes the possibility of preferential treatment for any one hospital, although it may disrupt normal operating procedures and raise safety issues.

Air Ambulance Districts

An air ambulance district is a quasi-governmental entity established specifically to support the operation of an air medical program. The district is usually empowered by state law to collect taxes for that purpose. Its members are typically counties, cities, or other government bodies. The funds collected are spent on aircraft, personnel, dispatch and communications equipment, and more. The district may be totally self-operated or may contract with an outside agency for communications, management, and aircraft operations.

An air ambulance district may encompass more than just an air medical program. It may serve as the foundation for a comprehensive emergency medical services system that includes everything from first response to ground and air critical-care transport services. It may incorporate operational and medical communications systems, medical control plans, and quality management programs. This comprehensive arrangement can be a cost-effective way to make these services available to all district members.

Importance of Safety

Because of the inherent dangers associated with flight, safety is a constant that must permeate every aspect of a flight program. Pilots, aviation technicians, medical team members, and program management must accept without reservation the principle that safety takes priority over all else. There can be *no* cutting corners where safety is concerned. That may be a difficult concept for hospital administrators or department heads to grasp. During tight budget times they are accustomed to making across-the-board cuts to conserve money and improve efficiency. Most of a flight program's budget is allocated to fixed costs, and any significant cut inevitably impacts safety.

The vast majority of injuries and fatalities in AM programs result from a combination of two errors: a breach in safety policy and tolerance of that breach by other team members. Often these errors are the result of poor communication among team members. Both can be addressed proactively through organizational design and administrative support. One solution has been the development of crew resource management (CRM) training programs. which are designed to prevent the development of conditions likely to result in safety lapses. The CRM program should be an integral part of recurrent training for all air medical programs. (CRM is addressed in more detail in Chapter 5.)

Operations

A typical AM program has four operational components: program administration, flight operations, medical operations, and communications.

Administration

Program administration involves planning, direction, and oversight. For an air medical program to function efficiently, it must be administered properly. Administration involves a number of different people and positions.

Upper-Level Management

As with any other program, the success of an air medical program ultimately depends on the degree of support it receives from those at the top. Upper-level administrators control the budget and determine if the program's needs are adequately met. In a hospital setting the hospital administrator has that authority. In not-for-profit organizations it may be an executive director or an officer of the board. In law enforcement organizations it may be the police chief or director of public safety. These administrators often determine the perceived value of the program and the institution's attitude toward the program. If they do not support the program, problems are inevitable.

Upper-level administrators often have little understanding of the complexity of an air medical program. In some large organizations top-level administrators do understand and support the program, but midlevel administrators do not. For a program to perform at maximum efficiency, there must be support from all levels of management. The program director should assume responsibility for educating administrative personnel.

The program director should also track all program activities, including financial performance. Gross income, net income, and direct and indirect operating costs should all be calculated and reviewed on a regular basis. That data may be used to gain support for the program from upper- and midlevel managers who may be concerned with financial performance to the near exclusion of other measures of success.

Program Director

Most programs (about 75 percent) have a dedicated program director who is responsible for coordination and administration of all aspects of the program. In hospital-based programs that person typically reports to a hospital administrator. In not-for-profit agencies the program director may report to a board of directors or a senior-level administrator. The program director determines the overall direction and quality of the air medical program. Responsibilities include short- and long-term planning, budgeting, and employee oversight and evaluation. Another key role is insulating the flight team from administrative decision-making, medical politics, and routine budget problems. Members of the flight team should be free to concentrate on aircraft operation and patient care and not be distracted by extraneous issues.

Chief/Lead Pilot

Virtually all programs have a chief or lead pilot, generally an experienced pilot with a significant amount of flight time and demonstrated leadership ability. This person serves as an important link between aircraft operations and medical operations and is responsible for scheduling, supervising other pilots, and making sure that FAA regulations are followed. In programs that contract with vendors, the lead pilot is generally the day-to-day link between program and vendor. The lead pilot must understand and appreciate the unique environment and expectations associated with a medical program. Interpersonal and communication skills are extremely important, particularly for the task of orienting new pilots. The program director should always consult the lead pilot when issues arise concerning the aircraft, aircraft technicians, and pilots.

Lead pilots should also play an active role in outreach and promotional activities. They should be one of the more visible representatives of the flight program. They are the ones who have time to talk with hospital personnel while waiting for the medical team to acquire a patient. They are also the ones often contacted when referring hospitals and EMS personnel have questions about issues related to the flight program, such as the location and design of landing zones, training of first responders, procurement of GPS units, and other procedures.

Chief Flight Nurse

Many programs (56 percent) have a chief flight nurse (CFN) who oversees day-to-day operations such as scheduling and handles personnel issues. Some programs may have a chief flight nurse in lieu of a program director. In those cases the responsibilities for administering the program are often divided between the CFN and a hospital administrator or other department head. One arrangement that works well is to have a program director to administer the program and a CFN to oversee day-to-day operations and quality management.

The chief flight nurse should be an experienced, well-respected, and approachable member of the program, a knowledgeable practitioner as well as a manager. Mentoring less experienced members of the flight team is an important responsibility. In many programs the CFN continues to work as a part-time member of the flight team and fills in when other regularly scheduled employees are out.

Since the CFN is generally responsible for quality management, a strong working medical knowledge is essential, as well as a solid relationship with the program medical director.

Medical Director(s)

Neither registered nurses nor paramedics, the two most commonly employed flight team members, are independent medical practitioners. State legislation requires physician involvement in EMS, including air medical programs. The medical director is the ultimate authority in matters concerning patient care. While this role is clear, the medical director's role in program administration is often less so. The medical director generally does not have the authority to discipline or terminate employees, even those who consistently fail to meet minimal patient care standards, but must work through the program director and human resources. It is essential that the program director, medical director, and chief flight nurse have close working relationships and support one another's efforts. (Medical direction is discussed in more detail in Chapter 12.)

Organizational Culture

Organizational culture consists of the values, beliefs, and expectations that members of an organization hold in common and use as behavior and problem-solving guides. Organizational culture includes the methods used to motivate employees and the degree to which employees are encouraged to participate in the planning and decision-making process. Pay and financial incentives are only a small part of this process. Other variables, such as input into planning and operations, recognition of achievement, and opportunity for advancement, play a greater role (Table 2-2). Air medical programs tend to employ intelligent and self-motivated people with a wealth of talent and experience. Involving them in planning and decision-making builds morale, brings different perspectives to the table, and often leads to innovative ideas and solutions. There are times when the program director, chief flight

Table 2-2   Chart of Employee Motivating Factors

Motivational Factors
- Employee opinions are valued by the organization
- Employees recognized for accomplishments
- Opportunity for advancement
- Organizational loyalty
- Safe and comfortable work environment
- Pay and benefits

nurse, or medical director must retain the right to make key decisions, but outside those rare cases, employee input should be regularly solicited and applied.

Flight Operations

Flight operations consist of all activities related to the aircraft and those personnel associated with its operation. Personnel include pilots, aviation technicians, and ground support personnel; their activities include preparation for flight, fueling, maintenance, loading, unloading, troubleshooting, repositioning, helipad/heliport design and maintenance, and the coordination and scheduling of these activities.

The **Federal Aviation Administration (FAA)** regulates aircraft operations very strictly. For example, **Federal Aviation Regulations (FARs)** dictate minimum training and experience requirements for pilots and aircraft technicians, time and stress limits for aircraft components, and minimum specifications for heliports. They limit duty time for pilots and prohibit the ingestion of mind-altering substances prior to and during duty time. They set limits on minimum visibility for both **visual flight rule (VFR)** and **instrument flight rule (IFR)** flight operations. These requirements are nonnegotiable and any violation may have severe consequences. The impact of FAA regulations must be taken into consideration during all phases of planning and operating an air medical program (Figure 2-1).

When starting a new program or significantly modifying an existing program, it is in the program's best interest to involve the FAA early in the planning process. Doing so may avoid having to make costly changes later. Local FAA agents are available in most urban areas to assist in all matters related to flight operations. They can also help new programs establish minimum flight standards, local operating areas, new helidecks, or approach and departure paths.

Federal Aviation Administration (FAA)
The federal agency charged with promulgating and enforcing rules and regulations concerning the operation of aircraft.

Federal Aviation Regulations (FARs)
The federal regulations governing the operation of aircraft in the United States.

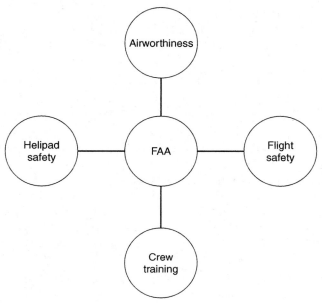

FIGURE 2-1
Illustration of the impact of the FAA on program activities

Medical Operations

Medical operations involve the personnel and physical components of the program related to patient care. These include the medical flight team, medical director(s), medical equipment, and the quality assurance/improvement process. In most programs, members of the medical flight team are dedicated solely to the flight program. In other programs they may be assigned additional responsibilities when not on flights. In a few programs, notably those staffed with resident physicians, personnel may be shared with other departments. In virtually all hospital-based programs, the hospital provides medical personnel and equipment. Medical direction is an important part of medical operations. Involvement of a medical director who is a physician knowledgeable about air medicine is essential for a high-quality program. (Medical direction is discussed further in Chapter 12.)

It is important to remember that an air medical program is a medical operation. While that sounds obvious, it may become less so for programs or personnel that are not hospital based, especially those that perform multiple roles. The standard of care must remain constant regardless of the base of operation. Personnel who do not have the benefit of frequent interaction with other medical personnel must find ways to keep their medical knowledge current. In these programs the roles of the quality management officer and the medical director become even more important, as they are responsible for keeping the medical program strong.

Communications

Communications involves receipt of medical information, dispatching, ongoing in-flight communications, and flight following. Communication is the glue that binds the air medical program together. Poor communication within any component of the program or between program divisions will compromise both efficiency and safety. It falls to the program director to ensure that vertical and lateral communication patterns are established and maintained. While it is easy to prescribe communications policies on paper, it is sometimes more difficult to keep those channels open as time passes. The communications technician or dispatcher is the hub for all activities occurring within the program. (Communications issues are discussed in Chapter 6.)

Summary

Air medical programs can be set up under a number of different for-profit and not-for-profit organizational structures. There are similarities in the ways these programs are operated, and pros and cons to each. The management is essentially the same. Personnel include administrators, a program director and/or a chief flight nurse, a medical director, pilots, and medical personnel. Operations are divided into communications, flight operations, medical operations, and program administration.

REVIEW QUESTIONS

1. Air medical programs may be operated by:

    a. Hospitals   **c.** Consortia

    b. Quasi-governmental entities   **d.** All of the above

2. Rotor-wing aircraft are typically operated by for-profit organizations only under the following circumstances:

    a. As part of a larger medical transportation program

    b. In cases where small and fuel-efficient aircraft are available

    c. The service area is very small so as to allow a low flight volume

    d. Rotor-wing aircraft can be operated profitably under nearly any circumstance

3. Air medical programs may be organized as:
   a. A free-standing entity
   b. A department in a hospital
   c. A consortium
   d. Any of the above

4. A not-for-profit air medical program may be able to operate more efficiently and with a greater reinvestment of funds due to the fact that not-for-profits:
   a. Are not required to pay taxes
   b. Are allowed to bill patients at higher rates
   c. Don't have to remove money from the organization to pay owner profits
   d. a and c

5. The most important single aspect of any air medical program is:
   a. Safety
   b. Patient care
   c. Employee benefits
   d. Size and speed of the aircraft

6. The four operational components of a typical air medical program are:
   a. Program administration, flight operations, medical operations, and communications
   b. Program administration, flight operations, medical operations, and flight following
   c. Program administration, flight operations, peer review, and communications
   d. Program administration, flight operations, peer review, and flight following

7. Responsibilities of this position include scheduling and supervising pilots, making sure that FAA regulations are followed, and playing an active role in the outreach program.
   a. Chief flight nurse
   b. Lead pilot
   c. Medical director
   d. Program director

8. This position serves as the hub of communications for all program activities:
   a. Lead pilot
   b. Medical director
   c. Communications technician/dispatcher
   d. Chief flight nurse

CHAPTER 3

History of Air Medicine

Objectives

Upon completing this chapter, the reader should have a better understanding of the following topics:

* The origins of air medicine

* Early development of the helicopter

* The role of the helicopter in the Korean and Vietnam Wars

* Early civilian uses of medical helicopters

* The future of air medicine

Introduction

Modern air medicine is a relatively recent phenomenon dating back only some 35 years. However, like most modern technologies, its roots may be traced back considerably farther. A discussion of air medicine would be incomplete and much less interesting without some understanding of its origins and evolution. This chapter will explore the ancestry of modern air medicine.

The Origins of Air Medical Transport

The first written record of the term *air ambulance* is in Jules Verne's *Robur le Conquérant* (1866), which describes the rescue of shipwrecked sailors by an airship (balloon) named the *Albatross*. The first documented use of an air ambulance occurred during the Siege of Paris in 1870. Balloons were used to evacuate more than 160 soldiers from the besieged city.

During the 1890s, M. de Mooy, chief of the Dutch Medical Service, suggested a system for evacuating the injured using litters suspended from balloons. Although government officials ultimately ruled this procedure too risky, de Mooy constructed several emergency balloons that were used quite successfully on the Amiens battlefront.

In 1903 the possibility of using combustion-driven vehicles to transport casualties from the battlefield was first raised. The idea was met with cynicism. One critic was heard to say, "Nothing has been found to equal the force of the horse for economy and safety. Patients, being probably in a nervous condition, will be alarmed at the idea of being taken off in a motor car." A similar statement was made when the French government was asked in 1917 to use biplanes as air ambulances. "Are there not enough dead in France today without killing the wounded in airplanes?"

French senator, pilot, and medical doctor Emile Raymond suggested aerial support for the military as early as 1912. In September of that year Raymond flew over a battlefield in a Bieroit airplane, reporting the location of injured soldiers for stretcher parties. In October 1913 another French doctor, M. Gautier, stated that surgery would be revolutionized if aeroplanes could be used to evacuate the injured. Later in 1913, two of his French compatriots, M. Uzac and Charles Julliot, suggested that air ambulance support during war be recognized and protected by the Geneva Convention. In 1923, during an International Red Cross meeting about the effectiveness of air ambulances, a supplement was written for inclusion in the Geneva Convention of 1906.

The first recorded attempt at designing an air ambulance in the United States occurred in 1909 in Pensacola, Florida. Representatives of the U.S. Army Medical Corps and Coast Artillery Corps engineered an airplane with provisions for a stretcher patient. The pilot would be a physician who would both fly the airplane and provide medical care. Unfortunately the aircraft crashed on the first test flight.

In 1931 Igor Sikorsky patented a design with a single large main rotor and a small antitorque tail rotor. In 1938 United Aircraft agreed to fund the development of the aircraft. The final product was an open-cockpit helicopter with a 65-horsepower engine that turned a three-blade main rotor. The VS-300 first flew in 1939. Although several models of the aircraft crashed, a determined Sikorsky continued to make modifications on the VS-300 and was ultimately successful in designing a practical rotor-wing aircraft. The S-47 was the prototype for the first helicopter produced in quantity for the U.S. Armed Forces. In World War II, the cabin of the S-47 was covered with fabric, allowing for flight in colder climates. Sikorsky continued to develop larger and more powerful helicopters. The S-51 and S-55 were first used for search and rescue and medical evacuation during the Korean War.

The Modern Era

If we had to trace the advent of modern air medicine to one point in time, it would have to be the beginning of the Korean conflict, when the potential of the helicopter as a medical tool was first fully appreciated. On August 4, 1950, just one month after the start of the Korean War, the first rotor-wing medical evacuation was performed with a bubble-fronted Bell 47 (as seen in the TV series *M*A*S*H*). The wounded were transported on basket stretchers attached to the top of the landing gear on the outside of the small helicopter (Figure 3-1). They were covered with blankets in a nearly futile effort to maintain body heat and prevent wound contamination.

It is estimated that more than 20,000 injured soldiers were evacuated by helicopter. The World War II casualty/death rate of 4.5 deaths per 100 casualties dropped to 2.5 per 100 casualties during the Korean War. While there were some technological advances in medicine during that period, the improvement is largely attributed to use of the helicopter to evacuate patients to definitive care more quickly. The external litter, however, did not allow for medical care during transport.

The next major advance in AM transport occurred during the Vietnam War, where the Bell UH-1 helicopter was placed into operation (Figure 3-2). Affectionately known as the Huey, this aircraft was large enough to

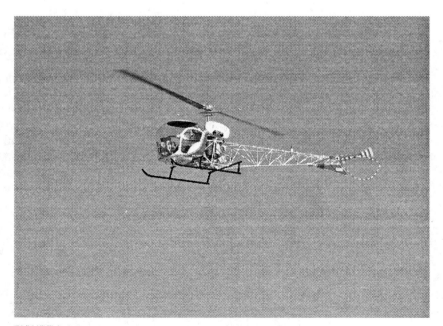

FIGURE 3-1
A Bell 47
Courtesy of Sheldon Cohen/Bell Helicopter

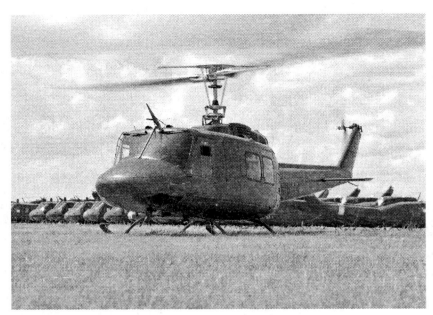

FIGURE 3-2
A UH-1
Courtesy of Sheldon Cohen/Bell Helicopter

hold patients inside, where medical personnel could begin treatment during the flight to a field hospital. The mass deployment of these aircraft as medivac units reduced the average delay until treatment to one hour. The ability to carry patients inside the aircraft was a key element in the reduction of mortality and morbidity. Military medics performed procedures previously done only by physicians: they started central lines, inserted chest tubes, and sutured bleeding wounds. This care, coupled with the initiation of specialty hospitals for the treatment of different types of injuries, resulted in a reduction in the mortality rate to 1 death per 100 casualties.

The success of the medivac helicopter in the military generated discussions about its potential in the civilian environment. The first known civilian application of a medical helicopter was in 1958 in Etna, California. Bill Mathews, a businessman, started a helicopter service to ferry patients for Dr. Granville Ashcraft, the town's only physician. The town druggist also used the helicopter to deliver drugs during emergencies.

Two programs were implemented in the United States to assess the impact of medical helicopters on mortality and morbidity in the civilian arena. Project CARESOM was established in Mississippi in 1969. Three helicopters were purchased through a federal grant and based in three small cities (Tupelo, Greenwood, and Hattiesburg). Operating expenses were paid from the grant for one year. Upon termination of the grant, Project CARESOM was deemed a success, and each of the three communities was given the chance to keep its helicopter in operation. Because of the high operating costs, the cities of Tupelo and Greenwood chose to discontinue their programs. In Hattiesburg an air ambulance district was formed and the program continued, supported by tax money paid by the residents of the seven participating counties. That program, named Rescue 7, has operated continuously ever since.

At roughly the same time the Military Assistance to Safety and Traffic (MAST) system was begun at Fort Sam Houston in San Antonio, Texas. MAST was started as an experiment by the Department of Transportation to study the feasibility of using military helicopters to augment existing emergency medical services. In its first 10 years of operation, MAST expanded nationally and transported more than 16,000 patients. Also, in 1969 the state of Maryland received a grant to purchase Bell Jet Ranger helicopters and started one of the nation's first medivac programs. The four helicopters, manned by paramedics, were strategically based throughout the state for quick response to emergency situations. When they were not carrying patients, the helicopters were used for law enforcement and traffic control.

Today there are over 220 rotor-wing flight programs operating in the United States, mostly hospital based. These modern aircraft represent a huge advance in technology over those used during the Korean War. Current models are larger, safer, quieter, and faster and incorporate modern medical technology (Figure 3-3). Many are configured as flying

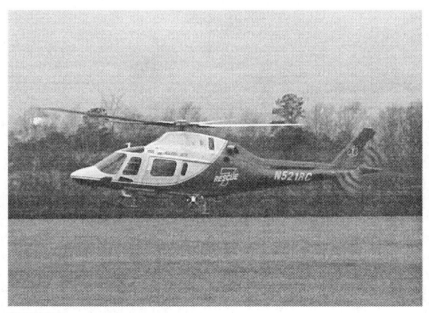

FIGURE 3-3
Modern RW air ambulance (Koala)
Courtesy of American Eurocopter

History of Air Medicine 29

critical-care units with all the necessary medical paraphernalia. Today's typical air medical program offers a turbine-powered aircraft with a cabin large enough to accommodate a patient and a medical team. The patient can be given advanced care before and during transport. Critical-care patients have access to ventilators, cardiac monitors, and a host of other equipment and supplies that were not available in hospitals even a decade ago.

A Look to the Future

Although no one knows for certain what the future holds, in air medicine a few things seem relatively certain. Turbine engines will continue to evolve, providing more power from lighter packages. These advances will allow for increased payload and additional range. Reliability will continue to improve, leading to even safer machines. Pilot support systems will advance, acting as backup for pilot decision-making and reducing the likelihood of accidents caused by pilot error. Flight following technology will continue to advance. The use of satellite tracking and communications systems will likely increase.

Tilt-rotor aircraft are currently in the test stage of development (Figure 3-4). As these machines gain acceptance in the aviation industry, they will almost certainly be adopted for air medical use and will offer significant benefits to air medical programs. A single craft that is capable of vertical takeoff and landing and has a cruise speed of 275 knots will become increasingly attractive to hospitals operating both rotor-wing and fixed-wing aircraft, especially in areas where long-distance flights

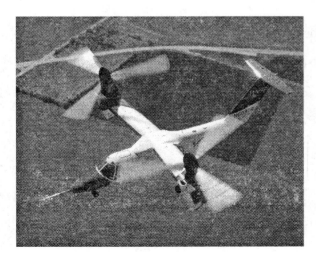

Figure 3-4
A tilt-rotor aircraft
Courtesy of Sheldon Cohen/
Bell Helicopter

are frequent. However, manufacturers will first have to demonstrate a record of safety and reliability at least equivalent to that of modern rotor-wing ships. The high price of tilt-rotor aircraft will also have to come down before they can be used by the medical community.

Health care reimbursement has been decreasing for the last decade. Some experts feel this will be a permanent condition of the health care system. Others believe that the current environment is so financially hostile that long-term survival is not possible and that major changes will have to take place in order for services to be continued. Yet others feel the pendulum will begin moving in the other direction, reimbursement dollars will flow more freely again, and air medicine may be able to attract some of them.

We will continue to see the formation of more partnerships and consortia as health care dollars become increasingly scarce. This arrangement will allow new, more cost-effective programs to be created and operated. It will also give struggling stand-alone programs a chance at survival. But future belt-tightening is inevitable. There will likely be a return to publicly funded emergency medical services, including air medical programs. Thinning profit margins are forcing many for-profit services to reconsider their operations.

Summary

Air medicine has an exciting history, extending from the first attempts in the early twentieth century to the independent civilian system that we know today. Modern air medicine came of age during the Korean and Vietnam wars. Civilian use of medical helicopters began experimentally in 1969 and has expanded in the decades since. The technology continues to advance, even as the financial climate becomes more constrained.

REVIEW QUESTIONS

1. The first functional helicopter was invented by:
   a. Alexander Graham Bell
   b. Igor Sikorsky
   c. Leonardo Aerospatiale
   d. John P. Vertol

2. The first widespread use of the rotor-wing air ambulance was during:
   a. World War I
   b. World War II
   c. The Korean Conflict
   d. The Vietnam War

3. This aircraft was widely used as an air ambulance during the Vietnam War:
   a. Bell 47
   b. Sikorsky S-76
   c. Bell 206-L4
   d. Bell UH-1

4. A government-funded program begun in Mississippi in 1969 to evaluate the practicality of rotor-wing air ambulance use in the civilian environment was called:
   a. Project CARESOM
   b. MAST
   c. MED Flight
   d. Stat Medivac

5. There are currently _____ rotor-wing air medical programs operating in the United States alone:
   a. 75
   b. 125
   c. 175
   d. More than 220

6. The tilt-rotor aircraft offers technological advancement over traditional air medical craft. Some advantages include that they are:
   a. Capable of service as both a fixed-wing and rotor-wing aircraft
   b. Capable of attaining speeds much greater than a typical rotor-wing aircraft
   c. Cheaper to operate than conventional rotor-wing aircraft
   d. a and b

Mission Types

Upon completing this chapter, the reader should have a better understanding of the following topics:

* The two major reasons for establishing an air medical program

* Types of air medical missions

* Types of scene responses

* The benefits of air medical programs in interfacility transports

* Other roles of air medical programs

* The importance of establishing appropriate launch criteria for a flight program

* The impact of over- and undertriage on patient care

* The role of the air medical program in the management of mass casualty incidents

KEY TERMS

critical-care transport,
p. 36

medivac (or medevac),
p. 34

Introduction

Civilian flight programs are generally established for one of two reasons. The first, to enhance patient care or to make medical resources more readily available to the residents of a given geographic or governmental area, has a humanitarian basis. Programs may be hospital-based, not-for-profit, or quasi-governmental entities. The emphasis is on service delivery and quality of patient care. These programs are often supported financially by a tax base or by government subsidies.

The second reason for setting up a program—and the driving force in modern health care—is the desire to generate income and remain competitive. Air medical programs are generally set up to expand a hospital's catchment area or to increase market share. That is not to say that a program set up primarily to generate profit cannot improve the quality of medical care and achieve the same goals as a not-for-profit program. However, it may be somewhat more difficult to maintain that focus when the driving force is profit, especially during tight budget times.

Regardless of the reasons for start-up, the operational aspects of air medical programs are generally similar. Missions consist of two basic types— scene responses and interfacility transports—as well as miscellaneous other activities such as delivery of medical supplies, blood, and donor organs. Programs operated by, or affiliated with, law enforcement agencies may also perform search-and-rescue and police functions in addition to medical activities.

medivac (or medevac)
Term sometimes applied to helicopters utilized for air medical purposes.

Military air medical programs, commonly referred to as **medivacs,** are set up primarily to provide medical support to battlefield personnel. Their first priority is evacuation from the battle zone. Their existence has little to do with finance, profit, or market share. They may also have a more complicated mission profile, especially during peacetime, when they spend more of their operating time on training exercises and less on actual patient transports. (Military operations are discussed in more detail in Chapter 17.)

Scene Responses

Scene responses involve flying directly to the site of an accident or illness (Figure 4-1). These flights may be triggered by automobile crashes, farm or industrial accidents, accidents at recreational areas, and medical or traumatic emergencies in rural areas. The percentage of scene flights made by a flight program varies, depending on its location and mission profile. Some programs do predominantly scene flights, others do few, and a small number do none at all. In remotely populated areas of the United States and Canada, some residents may be totally dependent on air medical programs for emergency medical care. In extreme cases, aircraft may require auxiliary fuel tanks or refueling stops to reach remote sites. Scene responses may also be justified in urban areas when traffic is heavy and movement of ground ambulances is impeded. Scene flights

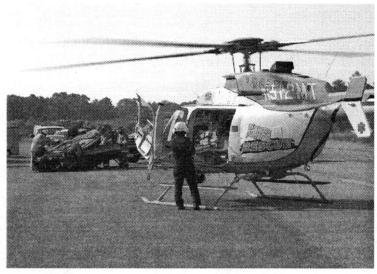

FIGURE 4-1
A helicopter landing at a motor vehicle accident
Courtesy of Sheldon Cohen/Bell Helicopter

often involve making landings in unimproved areas and are generally more complex and potentially hazardous than interfacility transports.

A scene response may be termed primary or secondary, depending on who is authorized to activate a launch and whether or not other agencies and personnel are on scene prior to arrival of the air medical team. A primary response is one in which the flight team is first on scene. A secondary response involves the flight team responding only after ground personnel have arrived on scene and determined a need for the flight team and/or aircraft. In the early years of civilian air medicine, primary responses were not uncommon, especially in rural areas. However, as the number of accidents and incidents mounted (and insurance rates began to escalate), many programs launched scene responses only when requested by first responders or EMS personnel and only when a landing area could be secured prior to arrival of the aircraft. This policy reduces the incidence of unexpected hazards and has contributed to a significant reduction in air medical incidents and accidents over the past 15 years.

Much has been written concerning the impact and appropriateness of using helicopters for scene responses. The consensus seems to be that it has a positive impact on outcomes for select patient types. For most patient types the rapid delivery of a highly trained and well-equipped medical team is the most significant contribution made by an on-scene response. (This is discussed in more detail in Chapter 15.)

Interfacility Transports

Caring for the critically ill or injured patient in an aeromedical environment. Critical-care transports often involve complex physiologic monitoring, the use of ventilators, and the administration of multiple medications.

Interfacility transports consist of moving a patient from one health care facility to another, generally from a hospital with limited capabilities to one offering more complex or specialized care (Figure 4-2). **Critical-care transports** often involve unstable emergency or high-maintenance patients, and they require a high level of medical expertise and the use of sophisticated medical equipment. Since air medical helicopters are commonly staffed and equipped as mobile critical-care units, this is a particularly appropriate role for them. Approximately 75 percent of all medical rotor-wing flights made in the United States are interfacility transports.

While generally not as hazardous as scene landings, the landing areas at some hospitals are less than ideal, and hazards do exist. Overeager medical personnel may approach the helicopter prematurely, exposing themselves to flying debris and possible contact with the main or tail rotors. Stretchers may be brought out with sheets that are not adequately secured, and items may be drawn into the rotor system. IV poles may extend to a height where they contact the main rotor. Unsecured items lying within the approach path may be disrupted by rotor wash and result in harm to bystanders or damage to the aircraft. Some hospital landing pads are located on rooftops or in close proximity to buildings or trees, and pilots must approach and depart these facilities with caution. Pilots should demonstrate familiarity with the landing zones at all frequently visited hospitals. One practice that has proved beneficial,

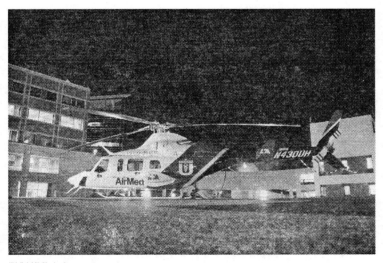

FIGURE 4-2
A helicopter landing at referring hospital
Courtesy of Sheldon Cohen/Bell Helicopter

especially for new pilots, is to keep a folder in the aircraft that contains pictures of all frequently used hospital landing areas, including the various approach paths. Notes may be attached to the pictures describing particular hazards and ways to avoid them. This practice allows new and experienced pilots to preview the landing zone and to prepare mentally prior to actual arrival.

Other Air Medical Missions

Organ Procurement/Delivery

Some programs allow their helicopters to be used to transport organ donors or organ recipients. Ordinarily, air transport of a patient who has a devastating head injury and has been pronounced clinically dead would be difficult to justify. However, if that patient were an organ donor and time-until-harvest were an issue, use of an aircraft may be warranted. The aircraft may either deliver the patient to the transplant team or deliver the transplant team to the patient. The most appropriate option often depends on the capabilities of the hospital where the donor is initially located and on the policies and procedures of the state or local organ recovery agency.

When resources at the local hospital are adequate, the preferred option is often to transport a surgical team to the remote site for organ harvest, then to fly the harvested organs back to a waiting transplant team. That option often allows the harvest team to accomplish its task more quickly and thereby improve organ viability.

In some programs the aircraft may be used to deliver organ recipients in a timely manner, which may be especially beneficial when a potential donor is not close to the transplant center. This option is generally used when the recipient and the flight program are both located in the same area and the transplant will take place at a distant site. However, emergency AM programs are rarely used for this purpose because of the risk that the aircraft may not be available at the time it is needed by the organ recipient.

Delivery of Pharmaceuticals

Another use for the air medical program is the delivery of blood, blood products, antivenin, and antidotes. This function is most common when the program is based at a tertiary-care facility that serves a number of smaller general hospitals. Here the program may play two roles. First, the flight team delivers the needed product to the smaller hospital, where

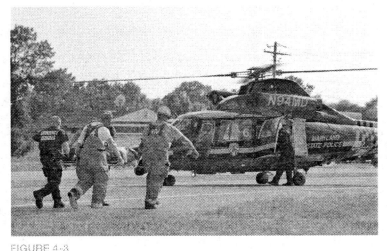

FIGURE 4-3
Maryland helicopter and crew
Courtesy of MIEMSS, Department of Public Information and Media Services

it may assist in the administration of the product. At that point the decision is often made to transfer the patient to the tertiary-care facility for definitive and long-term care, and the flight team transports the patient.

Law Enforcement

In some areas of the country, medical helicopters are staffed by law enforcement personnel. The most well known example is the state of Maryland, where seven state-operated helicopters perform both medical and law-enforcement functions, staffed by paramedics who are also sworn officers of the law (Figure 4-3). The flight team may be called on to transport a critical medical patient in one case and search for an escaped felon in the next. Using aircraft in dual roles has its pros and cons, and these arrangements are not common. It is difficult enough to master the knowledge and skills of an AM team member; staying current in both air medicine and law enforcement may be exceptionally difficult.

Launch Criteria

Each flight program should have a set of clearly defined launch policies that specify the circumstances under which the aircraft may be launched and the personnel authorized to make the launch decision. These policies should include examples of specific medical and traumatic conditions that may benefit from use of the aircraft. For many programs the costs of aircraft operation, the strict rules of reimbursement, and the inherent dangers of flight prohibit arbitrary use for lesser conditions. Written policies should be distributed to all EMS personnel, physicians, nurses, and hospitals that may be interested in using the aircraft for patient transport.

Matching patient care needs and use of the aircraft can be a difficult task, especially for new programs. Overtriage and undertriage are inevitable. The goal should be to control mismatches as much as possible. Undertriage occurs when the medical resources mobilized to care for a patient fail to meet the patient's medical needs in a timely manner. It is an indicator that those performing the initial assessment may not fully appreciate patient acuity levels. A recurring pattern of undertriage may indicate a lack of knowledge on the part of medical care providers, and recurrent training is often necessary. It may also indicate overly conservative EMS personnel who hesitate to launch the aircraft (or to mobilize other needed resources) for fear of reprisal. Undertriage may have a negative impact on patient outcomes and should rarely, if ever, be considered acceptable.

Overtriage is defined as the mobilization of excessive or unneeded medical resources for a given patient. Overtriage should be accepted as a necessary evil even in the best-run systems. It is not possible to match exactly patient care needs and medical resources in every situation, especially in the uncontrolled prehospital environment. For example, some patients with significant internal injuries may not present with a high acuity level until the condition has progressed to an advanced stage of decompensation. Waiting until that stage to mobilize resources may be too late and the patient may be lost as a result. The incidences of overtriage and undertriage are inversely proportional—as the incidence of one increases, the other will decrease. From a medical perspective, a certain amount of overtriage is necessary to prevent undertriage. According to the American College of Surgeons, overtriage of up to 30 percent is reasonable and should be considered acceptable. Beyond that point it is likely that a significant number of prehospital launches are not warranted, and corrective action may be needed.

A scene call where a patient is trapped in a car and inaccessible may be justification to launch an aircraft if prehospital personnel suspect serious injury based on vehicular damage or kinematics. Launch of the aircraft does not become a bad decision if at some later time the patient is found to have only minor injuries. While there must be accountability and aircraft launches should not be authorized arbitrarily, the process should not be overly restrictive.

Overtriage is best dealt with in a retrospective/prospective manner. Dispatch and patient care records should be reviewed and abuse should be addressed on a case-by-case basis. If patterns of abuse begin to emerge, there is likely an institutional problem, which should be brought to the attention of the performance improvement officer for the involved agency or agencies. Repetitive cases of prehospital overtriage are often associated with poor patient-assessment skills or overanxious EMS personnel. These problems can usually be dealt with effectively through the local EMS QA/QI officer or medical director. It must be understood that EMS personnel generally do not intentionally abuse flight programs. However, they are frequently in the position of having to make decisions with incomplete information. Emphasizing the need to perform a physical examination before requesting air backup is an effective way to deal with repetitive overtriage. An ongoing outreach program that addresses the criteria for requesting aircraft launch will generally keep misunderstandings to a minimum.

Scene Response

Launch criteria for scene responses may vary significantly by locale and program policy. Most programs launch their aircraft at the request of prehospital providers and/or when some minimum criteria for acuity level is demonstrated. This process of requesting the aircraft should not be laborious for prehospital providers. If it is, prehospital providers will become conservative in making requests or will stop making requests altogether. It is better to make aircraft launch a nearly automatic process. Generic criteria such as "The aircraft may be requested for any patient who, in the opinion of the paramedic, has an actual or potential life- or limb-threatening condition that may benefit from use of the aircraft and medical team" are generally adequate to convey the intended uses of the aircraft.

Some air medical programs perform primary scene responses in which they may be the first medical providers to arrive. This practice has been significantly curtailed over the past decade due to accident rates and insurance company requirements. Many programs now require trained responders to be on scene to direct the arrival and landing of the aircraft.

For various reasons, flight crews may not be able to fly directly to the scene of an illness or injury. There may be dangerous terrain or other hazards in the area, or the landing zone may be too restrictive. Some programs have policies against landing at unimproved sites. In those cases a viable option may be a predesignated landing area that flight personnel have previously determined to be safe for a helicopter landing. Landing areas may be constructed especially for this purpose. A more common approach is to use an existing area such as a fenced field near a volunteer fire department, a football field, or a fenced parking lot.

Interfacility Transport

Criteria for interfacility transports can be somewhat more specific since patients are already in a medical facility and undertriage is less likely to occur. However, even in these situations it must be accepted that occasionally the full implications of a patient's medical condition may not be fully appreciated because of limited diagnostic capability or expertise. This may be particularly true in rural areas where physicians not trained in emergency medicine as well as moonlighting residents and family practitioners provide emergency department coverage.

Below is an example of minimum criteria for determining if an AM aircraft should be used for an interfacility transport. It is not an exhaustive list but rather a guideline to help physicians determine if a request is in line with the intended use of the aircraft.

A. Trauma/surgical
   1. Airway:
      Tracheal or laryngeal disruption, expanding neck hematoma
   2. Shock:
      Hemodynamic instability not corrected by an IV fluid bolus
   3. CNS
      a. Head: Penetrating injury, open fracture, or depressed skull fracture(s) with lateralizing signs
      b. Spine: Unstable spine fractures without complete neurologic deficit
   4. Neck: Penetrating injuries with evidence of vascular or aerodigestive injuries
   5. Chest:
      Major chest wall injury (e.g., flail chest)
      Tension pneumothorax
      Massive hemothorax
      Wide mediastinum
      Cardiac injury
      Patients who may require prolonged ventilation
   6. Pelvis:
      Pelvic fractures with shock
   7. Extremities:
      Fracture/dislocation with loss of distal pulses
      Extremity ischemia
   8. Burns:
      Transfers to burn center
      Electrical burns
      >20% BSA burn
      Potential airway injury

9. Comorbid factors:
   Age >55
   Children
   Underlying cardiac or respiratory disease
   Morbid obesity (not to exceed weight limit of aircraft)
   Diabetes
   Pregnancy
   Immunosuppression
10. Surgery:
    Aortic rupture/dissection, etc.

B. Medical
   1. ICU candidates:
      Acute MI
      Severe poisonings
      Unstable GI bleeders
      Patients requiring ventilation, vasopressors, etc.

C. Neonates: As determined by neonatologist

D. Obstetrics: As determined by obstetrician; may include:
   1. High-risk pregnancy in labor
   2. Unstable mother
   3. Eclampsia

E. Organ donation: As determined by organ procurement program

The 90 Percent Rule

Inevitably there are times when an aircraft is launched to transport a patient and then has to abort the flight due to unanticipated weather conditions. However, it must be recognized that each aborted flight creates a potentially damaging ripple effect. In emergency situations, patients, family members, and treating medical personnel are often anxious about the patient's condition, and any complication makes them even more so. An aborted flight often forces medical personnel to hastily make alternative arrangements for transport. The patient may suffer as a result of delays.

If the flight program has done its homework and explained the possibility of aborted flights to referring medical personnel in advance, an occasional occurrence may be tolerable. If flights are aborted more than occasionally, irreparable damage will be done to the credibility of the flight program, and the number of referral requests will likely decrease. One effective method for preventing this outcome is known as the 90 Percent Rule. This rule simply requires that a pilot accept a flight only if he or she is at least 90 percent certain that all legs of the flight can be completed safely. While implementation of this rule may result in the loss of an occasional flight, its net impact is improved program reliability and enhanced credibility.

Mass Casualty Incidents (MCIs)

MCIs, also known as major incidents or multicasualty incidents, are events with patient numbers so large as to overwhelm existing EMS resources (Figure 4-4). The numbers required to meet these criteria may vary tremendously from one locale to another. In a remote rural area served by one ambulance team, a motor vehicle crash involving five or more patients may constitute an MCI. In a larger urban system, 10 to 15 patients can generally be handled without outside assistance.

There are generally three degrees of multicasualty assessment and response:

1. **Low-impact incidents** involve multiple patients but at a level that can be managed locally level. The number of patients may cause temporary disruption of normal response patterns, but all requests are responded to in a reasonable time frame. Any mutual aid performed at this level is generally for convenience only.

2. **High-impact incidents** involve more patients than can reasonably be handled by the primary EMS agency. There are not enough resources to respond to the MCI and to meet underlying system

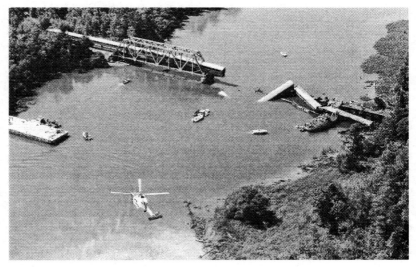

FIGURE 4-4
An MCI response
Corbis/Sygma

demands. At this level, mutual aid is required. The extent of mutual aid depends on the number of patients, accessibility, and underlying system demand.

3. **Disaster-level incidents** produce a number of patients that far exceeds the capabilities of the local EMS system, and extensive mutual aid is required. It is likely that the capabilities of local hospitals will also be overwhelmed and the patient load will overflow to hospitals in neighboring areas.

Most organized EMS systems have MCI/disaster plans that define the circumstances under which an MCI can be declared. These plans include variables such as the number of patients, location and accessibility of the event, underlying system status, hospital capabilities, and current hospital-bed capacity.

In any system, large-scale MCIs are rare. When they do occur, MCIs require the assistance of outside agencies. Air medical programs are frequently called on for assistance, particularly in rural or difficult-to-access areas where ground ambulances are less efficient. Hospitals may also require outside assistance. A small rural hospital may be overwhelmed by as few as two critical patients. Even a larger urban trauma center would have to retriage patients and change room assignments for as few as three critical patients presenting simultaneously. In the setting of an MCI the air medical program may be particularly beneficial in three areas: delivery of personnel, delivery of supplies and equipment, and transport of critical patients.

Delivery of Personnel

If an MCI occurs in a remote location, ground access may be limited and helicopters can play an important role in delivering personnel, equipment, and supplies to the scene. In very remote areas, helicopters may be the only mode of access until roads can be opened for rescue vehicles and ambulances.

In rare cases the air medical team may be first to arrive at the scene of an MCI. The team should perform a needs assessment, establish a command post, and begin the primary triage process. As other qualified personnel begin to arrive, they should be assigned responsibilities and directed to appropriate areas. At some point the triage function should be delegated to other qualified personnel and the flight team freed to transport critical patients and ferry personnel and equipment as necessary. In remote areas the aircraft may be most valuable in the role of ferry.

The prompt arrival of triage and treatment teams may have a significant impact on outcomes when there are large numbers of potentially salvageable patients. Some areas have a dedicated triage team that responds to MCIs, and team members may be delivered to the scene by air.

Delivery of Supplies and Equipment

A problem commonly associated with the management of multicasualty incidents is the exhaustion of personnel and supplies. Any incident lasting more than 1 or 2 hours requires replenishment of supplies for both medical personnel and patients. The aircraft may be used to transport critical patients from the scene of the disaster to an appropriate medical facility. On the return trip the aircraft can transport drinking water and snacks for rescue personnel and medical supplies for patients.

Transport of Critical Patients

This may be a primary or secondary role of the air medical team, depending on the availability of other medical personnel when the team arrives on scene. Early on, the triage function is of utmost importance and should be the first consideration. However, if adequate medical personnel are available to perform triage and treatment functions, the flight team may, at the direction of the transportation officer, begin transporting high-acuity patients. A frequent problem encountered during MCIs is the overcrowding of local emergency departments. The flight team may help alleviate that problem by transporting patients to more distant medical facilities. Due to the speed of the aircraft, that may be accomplished without significantly increasing out-of-service time.

Influence of Third-Party Payers

Health maintenance organizations, preferred provider organizations, and traditional insurance companies may influence which patients an air medical program transports and the hospitals they transport to and from. A program that has a contract with one of these payers may gain exclusive rights to transport their emergency or critical-care cases. Conversely, a program without a contract may be denied access to that population. Over the past decade the terms of insurance companies providing hull and liability insurance for aircraft have also become stricter. The insurance provider may offer coverage only if the aircraft operator agrees to adhere to the terms dictated by the insurance company. Those terms may stipulate the minimum conditions under which a program may operate, including launch criteria.

Summary

Rotor-wing air ambulances are used in two basic roles—scene responses and interfacility transports. They have demonstrated value in each of these roles. Scene flights involve responding directly to the site of an illness or injury. Most scene flights are made at the request of an EMS agency already on scene. These secondary responses are generally safer since personnel are already on scene who can locate a suitable landing area and clear bystanders from the area. The medical efficacy of aircraft scene flights has been hotly debated but there are circumstances when an on-scene landing is beneficial to patient care.

Interfacility transports involve transporting a patient from one hospital to another, generally from a smaller community hospital to a referral center. Interfacility transports are less risky and may offer enhancements in patient care during transport. They also may decrease out-of-hospital time by 50 percent or more. Some programs also utilize their flight programs for other medically related transports, such as organ recovery, pharmaceutical delivery and mass casualty incidents. The helicopter may be invaluable when managing a mass casualty incident.

Launch critera will determine the conditions under which a rotor-wing air ambulance may be used for scene responses and interfacility transports. These critera must be determined in advance so as to avoid unnecessary delays at the time a request is made. Launch criteria should be distributed to all potential users so as to avoid confusion and to minimize over- and undertriage.

REVIEW QUESTIONS

1. One of the major reasons for establishing an air medical program is:
   a. To create free advertising for the sponsor hospital
   b. To allow medical residents a new area in which to practice
   c. To make medical resources more readily available to the residents of a given geographic or governmental area
   d. To provide new jobs for hospital personnel

2. A type of air medical response that involves flying directly to the scene of an out-of-hospital emergency and arriving before or at the same time as ground EMS personnel is called:
   a. Primary scene response
   b. Secondary scene response
   c. Invited scene response
   d. Exclusive scene response

3. Under what circumstance might a scene response in an urban area be warranted?

4. Rotor-wing aircraft are particularly well suited for transporting critical-care patients between facilities due to their:
   a. Speed
   b. Expertise of staff
   c. Availability of critical-care equipment
   d. All of the above

5. The condition that occurs when the medical resources mobilized to care for a patient fail to meet the patient's needs in a timely manner is called:
   a. Overtriage
   b. Undertriage
   c. System overload
   d. Triage resistance

6. The incidences of overtriage and undertriage are:
   a. Similar; when one is high, the other is also usually high
   b. Similar; when one is low, the other is also usually low
   c. Unrelated
   d. Inversely related; when one is high the other is low

7. The 90 Percent Rule states that:
   a. Pilots should accept a flight only if they are 90 percent certain that all legs of the flight can be completed in a safe manner
   b. 90 percent of patients transported should be in critical condition
   c. A patient should be transported only if there is 90 percent certainty of payment
   d. VFR aircraft pilots should accept a flight only if there is 10 percent or less probability of rain

Safety and Risk
Management

Objectives

Upon completing this chapter, the reader should have a better understanding of the following topics:

* General safety guidelines for working near a helicopter

* Types of landing areas and characteristics of each

* Dangers associated with an aircraft in flight

* Management of in-flight emergencies

* Relative safety of single-engine versus twin-engine helicopters

* Crew resource management and its benefits

* Techniques of risk management

KEY TERMS

Introduction

Aircraft, especially rotor-wing aircraft, are inherently dangerous—especially while on the ground. Helicopters have large and rapidly moving parts that for the most part are uncovered and unguarded, making them extremely hazardous to the unwary. All flight programs must have in place a comprehensive and ongoing safety program. Safety awareness must permeate all aspects of the program, including administration, budget, and operations. Every potential hazard should be addressed and a plan devised to reduce risk.

Safety on the Ground

When the aircraft is on the ground, it is often the center of activity. Crew members may be loading and unloading patients, replacing supplies, performing maintenance, and other duties. EMS personnel may approach the aircraft during prehospital responses. All these activities bring people into close contact with the aircraft and expose them to a number of potential hazards.

Main Rotor

Each main rotor blade on a helicopter typically weighs more than 100 pounds and makes 300 to 400 rotations per minute (Figure 5-1). Any object (or person) struck by a turning rotor blade is likely to suffer significant trauma. Even if the object is insignificant, such as debris, extensive (and expensive) damage may be done to the rotor blade itself. Most mishaps involving the main rotor occur when something is moved or blown into the rotor's path. When a helicopter is approaching or departing the landing area, a revolving pattern of airflow known as rotor wash is created. A large aircraft can produce enough rotor wash to lift and toss items weighing 50 pounds or more. Landing areas must be kept clear of unsecured items. Stretcher mattresses, pads, and sheets are a particular problem, as they can easily be pulled off the stretcher and drawn into the rotor. Other loose items such as paper documents, gowns, and caps must be held tightly or bound to prevent them from being blown about. If the rotor makes contact with any object, the aircraft must be grounded until an aviation technician performs an inspection and declares it safe for flight, a process that can take hours.

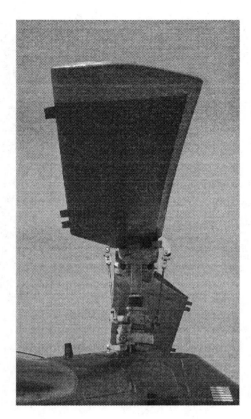

FIGURE 5-1
The main rotor

Tail Rotor

Most people who approach a helicopter are aware of the danger presented by the very obvious main rotor and are careful to avoid its path. It is the much smaller and less intimidating tail rotor that causes many of the injuries and deaths. Located near the distal end of the tail boom, the tail rotor is shorter and narrower than the main rotor (Figure 5-2). It spins so rapidly it is difficult to see at all times and virtually invisible at night. Adding to the danger is the fact that the tail rotor is located on the retreating blade side of the aircraft—the side on which the main rotor rotates toward the tail. This configuration produces a current of air that flows downward from the main rotor and rearward toward the tail and the tail rotor. Any loose items blown away from a passenger on that side of the aircraft will generally be blown in the direction of the tail rotor. A number of deaths have occurred when a disembarking passenger chased a loose hat or paper directly into the path of the tail rotor. The tail rotor is extremely dangerous, and the entire tail region should be considered off limits whenever the rotors are in motion.

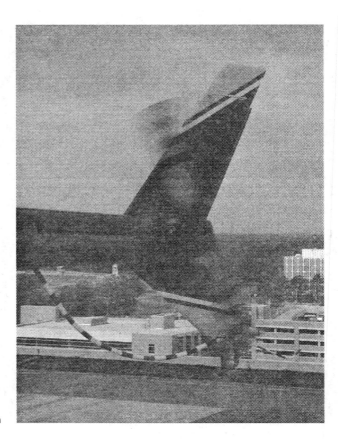

FIGURE 5-2
Tail rotor in motion

To load (or
unload) a patient
while the rotors
are turning.

There may be occasions when **hot loading** or unloading (the movement of a patient to or from the helicopter while the rotors are turning)
is necessary because of the urgency of a patient's condition. At least one
crew member (or other responsible party) should be assigned to keep
the tail rotor area secure. Some helicopters, such as the BO-105, EC-
135, and BK-117, are loaded from the rear, and crew members move
about under the tail boom much closer to the tail rotor than would otherwise be advisable. Extreme caution should be used when loading and
unloading those aircraft while the rotors are in motion.

Aircraft designers have long worked toward a safer tail rotor system. The first effort resulted in a traditional tail rotor located on an elevated tail boom, at a height where it was less likely to be a hazard. The
next development resulted in the enclosed ("fenestrated") tail rotor that
has become associated with the American Eurocopter Dauphine. The
most recent development is the "rotorless" tail boom (NOTAR) on the
McDonnell Douglas Explorer aircraft. Although each of these systems
has contributed to the evolution of tail-rotor safety, most air medical

helicopters still use a standard tail rotor, and the tail area of all rotor-craft should continue to be considered extremely dangerous and off limits regardless of aircraft type.

General safety guidelines for operating near a helicopter include the following:

* Avoid the tail of the helicopter anytime the rotors are in motion. The aircraft should be approached and exited only from the front, and only with the approval of the pilot or a member of the flight team.
* Do not wear hats or any loose item of clothing near a helicopter.
* Do not carry anything that extends above head level (e.g., IV pole, umbrella), as these items may contact the rotor blade.
* Do not carry any loose items such as sheets, pillowcases, newspaper, or loose sheets of paper near the helicopter. They can be blown about by rotor wash and sucked into the engine intakes or other vulnerable areas of the aircraft.
* Make sure there is no loose debris in the landing area. The rotor wash from a midsized or large helicopter can transform debris into dangerous projectiles.
* Keep all vehicles away from the aircraft. Ambulances in particular may be tall enough to make contact with the main rotor, and ambulances and law enforcement vehicles often have tall antennas. Vehicles should not be allowed closer than 50 feet to a stopped aircraft, and farther when the aircraft is in operation.

Landing Areas

The only real advantage that a helicopter has over a fixed-wing craft is its ability to take off and land vertically. But helicopters cannot land safely just anywhere. The landing area must be relatively level, free of obstructions, and capable of supporting the weight of the aircraft. The surface must also be free of loose dirt or sand so as not to be a risk for **brownout.** The ideal landing area is a large, clean, obstacle-free concrete pad that is used only for helicopter operations. Less ideal landing areas may also be acceptable as long as they are properly prepared.

Helicopter landing areas are classified into three categories:

1. Helispot (temporary landing zone): A **helispot** is a temporary or makeshift landing zone. It is an unimproved area that is free of obstacles and large enough to accommodate a given helicopter. It could be a field or pasture alongside a roadway or the backyard of a rural residence. A helispot is generally used only once or infrequently. It is the most uncontrolled and potentially unsafe type of landing area.

brownout
A condition that may occur when a pilot attempts to land a helicopter in an area of loose soil or sand, which mixes with the rotor wash and produces a dark cloud around the aircraft, reducing the pilot's visibility and potentially resulting in a crash.

helispot
An open area that has been cleared of obstacles on which a helicopter can land safely. Generally used for scene flights.

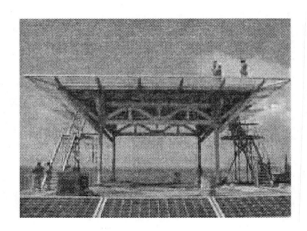

FIGURE 5-3
A helideck
Courtesy of Helidex

helipad

A temporary landing site, built to enable a helicopter to land safely. Generally not a permanent structure.

heliport (helideck)

A permanent helicopter landing site that conforms to FAA and other government regulations.

2. Helipad: A **helipad** is a semipermanent area where a helicopter can be safely landed. It may be a section of a parking lot, a field, or a street or highway that is blocked off as needed. In some cases it may be painted and have landing lights in place. Frequency of use can vary tremendously. Helipads are a common landing arrangement at many small hospitals.

3. Helideck (heliport): A **heliport** or **helideck** is the most permanent type of helicopter landing area (Figure 5-3). A helideck may be made of concrete, corrosion-resistant metal, or some combination thereof. The FAA has strict regulations regarding the dimensions, weight-bearing capacity, proximity of obstacles, maximum height of fences, size and types of lighting, and other considerations relating to helidecks. Experienced architects are often hired to oversee design and construction.

While the helideck is the safest, most advanced, and most desirable type of landing area, not all hospitals have one. Designing and building a helideck can be an expensive undertaking. A 50-foot-by-50-foot helideck can cost $100,000 or more. Rooftop helidecks may require modifications to structural support areas of the roof and can be even more expensive. FAA regulations stipulate minimum requirements for approach and departure paths, which may further increase the cost.

Safety in the Air

Most, but not all, of the dangers of the helicopter disappear once it is in flight. During flight, the crew and passengers are contained within the fuselage and are safely isolated from the main and tail rotors. Rotor wash also ceases to be a concern. However, there are potential dangers in the open sky, the most significant being other flying objects (human-made and naturally occurring) and mechanical failure.

A helicopter is only as safe as the pilot at the controls. **Pilot errors** are the most common cause of helicopter crashes, and any lapse in situational awareness or error in judgment may prove disastrous. Inadequate communication between the pilot and crew or between the pilot and ground personnel is frequently a contributing factor. Pilots and crew members must remain ever vigilant that they do not drift into complacency.

Weather

The safety of the environment in which aircraft operate is determined primarily by weather conditions, in particular, visibility, wind speed, and lightning. Poor visibility is frequently a contributing factor in helicopter crashes. It is essential that all AM programs adopt policies to minimize the probability of flight during such conditions. All crew members must be educated to the dangers that weather poses and should be empowered to decline or cancel any potentially dangerous flight. A good policy allows for any member of the crew to abort a flight at any time if there is concern about the weather.

Visibility

Visibility is the most common limiting factor for aircraft operators. Helicopters cannot take off or land without some degree of ground visibility. Even the most thoroughly equipped IFR-rated aircraft cannot operate safely in some low-visibility conditions. A pilot who attempts to depart or (especially) land without a safe cushion of visibility above the ground is operating the aircraft in an unsafe manner. Attempting to fly during poor visibility conditions has resulted in numerous accidents and fatalities. Even when flying under IFR rules, pilots must be able to break out of the clouds a safe distance above the ground. They must be able to see the ground in order to land the aircraft in the right attitude and in the right spot (for instance, not on top of a house or another aircraft).

The FAA mandates minimum visibility ranges for both VFR and IFR flight. In addition, many companies impose even stricter requirements on their personnel. Flight program personnel should never coerce or encourage a pilot to fly during marginal or unsafe weather conditions.

Thunderstorms

A thunderstorm is defined as a local storm that is produced by a cumulonimbus cloud and contains lightning and thunder. It usually produces gusty winds, heavy rain, and sometimes hail. Thunderstorms present a number of hazards to aircraft. First, lightning and hail can cause extensive damage to aircraft on the ground. Unless a hangar is available, this damage is largely unavoidable. Second, the winds associated with a thunderstorm may cause aircraft to lose altitude dramatically. A rapidly developing downdraft may cause an aircraft to drop 1000 feet or more in a matter of seconds. An aircraft at low altitude or in a takeoff or landing attitude may be slammed into the ground at a high rate of speed, with devastating results. A number of commercial airline crashes have been attributed to downdrafts and wind shear during thunderstorms.

Thunderstorms should always be avoided. Pilots should not attempt to take off or land during one. When in flight, pilots should maintain a safe distance from thunderstorms; they should never venture closer than 5 miles to any visible storm cloud. That range should be extended to as much as 20 miles for very large storms. Pilots should be wary of flying beneath thunderstorms, even when visibility is good, because of the destructive potential of shear turbulence and downdrafts. If a pilot inadvertently flies into the vicinity of a thunderstorm, he should reduce airspeed immediately to the manufacturer's recommended airspeed for rough flying conditions, and maintain a straight and level altitude on a heading that will escape the storm area in the least amount of time.

Turbulence

Turbulence refers to irregular airflow patterns that may be encountered by an aircraft during flight. These disruptions range from slight bumps to major alterations in altitude. Turbulence is rarely a threat to aircraft integrity, but it can cause items within the aircraft, including passengers, to be thrown about violently and may result in serious injuries. Turbulence can generally be anticipated when the weather is bad. However, it may also occur without warning, even during calm weather. The possibility of turbulence is the primary reason seat belts should be kept on and all equipment must be safely secured to the interior of the aircraft during flight.

Head Strike Envelope

head strike envelope
Inside the aircraft, the area within which the head may contact structures and equipment in the event of turbulence or a hard landing.

The **head strike envelope** is the area surrounding a passenger or crew member's head that could potentially be impacted during a sudden or violent movement of the aircraft. Steps should be taken to either remove potential head strike items or to render them relatively safe. Since most of the items in a helicopter are not easily movable, the latter approach is more commonly used. Padding an item or erecting a padded barrier between personnel and the item are two ways to reduce the danger.

Requiring crew members to wear helmets accomplishes the same goal without modifying the interior of the aircraft.

Other Aircraft

One of the primary responsibilities of a pilot is to maintain a safe distance between his aircraft and others. That can be more difficult than it sounds. A corporate jet at cruise speed can travel 8 miles in 60 seconds. It could be invisible to the naked eye one moment and dangerously close a minute later. While detecting other aircraft is largely the pilot's responsibility, two (or more) sets of eyes are better than one, and medical crew members should be on the lookout when they are not busy providing patient care. They should never assume that the pilot sees other aircraft until it is verbally confirmed.

Some helicopters are equipped with a traffic collision avoidance system (TCAS), a type of radar that warns the pilot when other aircraft are approaching. A TCAS is a valuable asset for medical helicopters, especially those operating in high-traffic areas. However, even that system is not foolproof, and vigilance is essential whenever the aircraft is in flight.

AM Safety in Perspective

Mechanical failures have become less common over the past two decades as FAA guidelines have become increasingly strict in regard to maintenance and safety. Modern turbine-engine helicopters have a safety record comparable to that of commercial airlines. Only 20 percent of AM accidents are caused by mechanical failure; the other 80 percent are attributed to pilot error. However, the risk associated with modern helicopter flight is slightly higher than that of automobile transportation.

A comparison of accidents and fatalities per 100 million miles traveled helps to put aircraft safety into perspective. During the period from 1995 to 1998, the fatality rate for passengers aboard commercial aircraft was 2.39 per 100 million miles flown. The fatality rate for automobile passengers was 1.8 per 100 million miles driven. Mile for mile, the risk of being killed in an aircraft crash is roughly 30 percent greater than being killed in an automobile crash. However, the risk is extremely low in either case.

The aircraft used for AM transport have a relatively good safety record. Since the accident rate for twin-turbine-engine helicopters is very near that of the commercial airlines, the following example helps put things into perspective. Professor Arnold Barnett of the Massachusetts Institute of Technology, using data from 1990 to 2000, has calculated that an airline passenger faces a death risk of one in 8 million on each flight. Statistically, if a given person made one airline flight every day, it would be 21,000 years before that person would be involved in a fatal crash.

According to a report prepared by the Air Medical Physician Association, over a 10-year period ending with 2001, AM programs were involved in 3.78 accidents per 100,000 flight hours. At that rate a program flying 60 hours per month would statistically be involved in one accident every 37 years.

More recently, however, the accident and fatality rate has begun to rise again. Over the 5-year period ending with 2001, there were 47 accidents involving AM programs, resulting in 40 fatalities and 36 injuries. Of the aircraft involved, 32 were twin-engine and 15 were single-engine.

In-Flight Emergencies

Although the modern turbine-powered helicopter is a safe mode of transportation, mechanical failure and/or pilot error does occur (Table 5-1). A significant equipment failure at altitude can prove disastrous. Crew members must be knowledgeable about potential mechanical failures and have a plan of action for each type. Overtraining in matters of safety should be the norm. It is far better to have a plan of action for even the most remote emergency and never have to use it than to have even a small incident and not know what to do.

Table 5-1	A Comparison of Accident Causes in Single-Engine and Twin-Engine Turbine Aircraft	
Primary Event	Single-Turbine	Twin-Turbine
Loss of engine power	31%	13%
In-flight collision with object	13%	14%
Loss of control	13%	13%
Airframe/component/system failure or malfunction	13%	30%
Hard landing	6%	3%
In-flight collision with terrain/water	6%	5%
Rollover	5%	1%
Weather	4%	4%
Other	9%	17%
Total	100%	100%

Loss of an Engine

Generally speaking, the seriousness of engine loss depends on the number of engines available and the speed and altitude of the aircraft. In all three categories, more is better.

In a single-engine aircraft, loss of the engine requires an immediate landing without power (**autorotation**). Contrary to popular belief, a helicopter will glide. While the glide ratio is not as good as that of a fixed-wing aircraft, a helicopter at cruise altitude allows the pilot a relatively large ground area from which to select a landing site. An engine failure occurring at night may be particularly problematic, however, especially in rural areas where there is little light and the ground is difficult to see. In some cases landing in the trees may be inevitable (Figure 5-4).

Loss of one engine in a twin-engine aircraft is generally less dangerous. An engine failure during the cruise phase of flight will result in a notable loss of power, but the aircraft will generally continue to fly until the pilot identifies a safe landing area. There is always a danger that failure of one engine may lead to failure of the second, so the pilot will want to land as soon as possible. Twin-engine helicopters are generally not capable of sustained long-distance flight following the loss of one engine.

An engine failure during takeoff or landing is a pilot's worst-case scenario. That is the most vulnerable phase of helicopter flight. There is little to no forward airspeed and the engines have little reserve capacity. Generally, if an engine fails, a pilot would prefer to be either very close

autorotation
The process of landing a helicopter without engine power. As the helicopter glides toward the ground, the movement of air across the rotor disk maintains rotor speed.

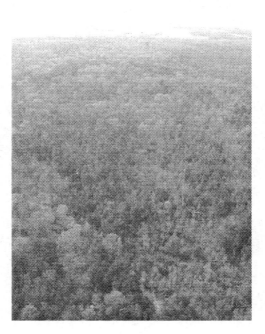

FIGURE 5-4
Aerial view of dense forest

to the ground or very far from it. Following liftoff, a helicopter is very vulnerable until a minimum speed and altitude have been reached. At that point an autorotation can be performed if an engine fails. If a single-engine aircraft loses an engine before the minimum altitude and speed have been reached, it will immediately cease to fly and will fall. If the helicopter is within 20 to 30 feet of the ground, the rotor speed may cushion the impact slightly; at more than 30 or 40 feet above the ground, it will generally free-fall. For this reason the pilot is eager to gain speed and altitude as soon as possible after liftoff.

Engine failure in a twin-engine aircraft during takeoff or landing will likely result in a hasty landing, but the aircraft will still be under the pilot's control. The second engine may be stressed beyond its limits and require major maintenance before being returned to service. Some later-model twin-turbine aircraft are designed with enough power to continue flying, even during takeoff or landing, if one engine fails. This capacity is called category A performance capability.

A general rule: During engine failure, any landing is a good landing.

Fire

A cockpit fire at altitude can be disastrous. The fire itself may cause mechanical disruptions that result in engine, transmission, or avionics failure. Smoke in the cockpit may decrease visibility and compromise the pilot's control of the aircraft. Smoke contains compounds that may affect the pilot's level of consciousness and mental status. Ideally, the aircraft is landed promptly and the cause of the smoke determined and corrected on the ground. In some cases an emergency situation may develop before there is time to make a safe landing.

Some modern aircraft have a fire suppression system with nozzles in the engine and baggage compartments. When activated by the pilot, a fire-suppressing foam is sprayed into these areas. Helicopters also have a portable fire extinguisher mounted in the cockpit. Crew members should know how to find and operate the extinguisher even in zero-visibility conditions.

Bird Strike

While low-flying aircraft commonly encounter birds, strikes are uncommon. When strikes do occur, damage is generally minimal. However, high-speed impact with a large bird such as a duck or goose may result in significant aircraft damage (Figure 5-5). In rare cases a bird has penetrated the windshield canopy and caused injury to the pilot or passengers. Some air medical programs require that their pilots wear helmets

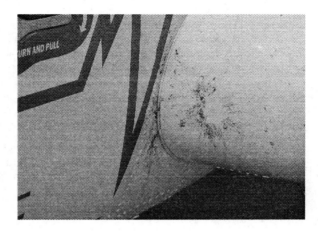

FIGURE 5-5
Canopy damaged by
bird strike

for this reason alone. Unfortunately, there is no warning system for birds. When flying in daylight hours the pilot can often spot birds and change course to avoid them. Crew members who are not occupied with patient care should also be alert for birds. Bird strikes are uncommon at night.

Flameout

flameout
Occurs when fuel ignition ceases during flight. It may be caused by flying in air with low oxygen concentration (e.g., over a forest fire) or by flying in very heavy rain.

Flameout is the loss of fuel ignition (the flame goes out) during flight. In turbine engines, a flame burns continuously within the fuel combustion chamber. That flame ignites incoming fuel and allows the engine to function as it was designed to. Flameout may occur as a helicopter flies through an area of low oxygen concentration such as heavy rain, over a large forest fire, or above industrial smokestacks. Whatever the cause, if the flame goes out, the engine immediately stops producing power. In a single-engine aircraft the pilot is forced into an autorotation. In a twin-engine aircraft the flameout may occur in one or both engines. Some aircraft have auto reignition, in which the engine senses the flameout and attempts to relight. Relighting may be virtually instantaneous and the pilot may not notice any loss of power.

Pilot Incapacitation

The possibility of a pilot becoming incapacitated during flight is something that medical crew members often joke about. But the joking masks a very real concern. Should this be something that air medical teams train for? No one seems to have an answer to that question. The consensus seems to be that if the pilot (in a single-pilot aircraft) goes, so does the crew, so it's probably not worth worrying about. Prevention is clearly the best option, but, as with any other type of flight emergency, some degree of preparation is clearly indicated.

Over the years a number of solutions have been proposed for managing such a situation. Unfortunately, most of these are unrealistic. Unless the autopilot is engaged, sudden pilot incapacitation will likely result in loss of control of the aircraft and a crash. If a member of the medical crew can maintain control of the aircraft, the chances of survival may increase somewhat. A helicopter is not difficult to maintain while in level cruise, although terminating cruise and attempting to land are another matter. As the aircraft enters the **in-ground effect (IGE)** phase of flight, it becomes difficult to control even for an experienced pilot and virtually impossible for a novice. However, a crash landing from 25 feet is preferable to one from 1500 feet.

Again, prevention is the best option. Ensuring that pilots are healthy does not eliminate all risks, but it does reduce them.

There is a strong link between a person's health status and the probability that that person will develop an acute medical emergency. For our purposes, *underlying health status* refers primarily to cardiovascular health and is the sum of a person's physical conditioning, diet, and genetic predisposition. Pilots are required to undergo an annual physical examination (**flight physical**) performed by an **aviation medical examiner (AME),** also referred to as a **flight surgeon.** Manifest medical conditions are sometimes detected during these routine exams, and pilots may be temporarily or permanently grounded as a result. However, this physical exam rarely includes any type of evaluation for subclinical disease processes. Currently, no FAA standards exist for lipid levels. In 1996 the FAA raised concern about cholesterol as a cardiovascular risk factor and proposed mandatory cholesterol testing in airman medical examinations. The proposal was withdrawn after objections from pilot advocacy groups.

Given their responsibility for the safety of patients and other crew members, it seems reasonable to require that pilots be periodically screened for conditions that may result in unexpected incapacitation. Screening should include an assessment of pulmonary and cardiovascular function and of risk factors. Pilots should be strongly encouraged to control modifiable risk factors such as smoking and diet. Genetic tendencies can be offset somewhat by exercise and a balanced diet. Individual flight programs should consider mandating these practices for their pilots.

Partial Incapacitation

A pilot is more likely to become partially incapacitated than totally incapacitated. Rapid onset of nausea, vomiting, severe headache, near syncope,

In-ground effect (IGE)
Apparent increase in aerodynamic lift experienced by an aircraft flying close to the ground.

flight physical
Periodic physical examination by a physician. All pilots are required by the FAA to undergo flight physicals to maintain their pilot certificate.

aviation medical examiner (AME)
A physician who is designated by the FAA to examine and certify airworthiness for pilots.

flight surgeon
Generally, the equivalent of a military aviation medical examiner. Flight surgeons often have more extensive training than do civilian AMEs.

and other conditions may all compromise a pilot's ability to operate the aircraft safely. The best course of action is generally for the pilot to land the aircraft as quickly as possible, even if that means landing in a remote field or a parking lot.

Towers and Utility Lines

Radio and television antennas may extend more than 2000 feet above ground level (Figure 5-6). Medical helicopters generally cruise at 1500 to 2500 feet, so these towers present a very real danger. Towers taller than 200 feet must be equipped with strobe or flashing beacon lights, but they may be obscured by low-visibility conditions. Towers lower than 200 feet are not required to have warning lights and may be nearly impossible to see at night. Cell phone towers, often less than 200 feet tall, are of particular concern as they multiply across the landscape. Most flight programs mark these towers on their aeronautical maps. It should be routine practice to maintain a safe distance from all towers, whether or not they are immediately visible. Medical team members should assist with identifying towers when not occupied with patient care. Pilots should be particularly cautious when approaching a new landing area, especially at night.

Utility lines can also be extremely hazardous, especially during scene flights. These reinforced metal cables have great tensile strength

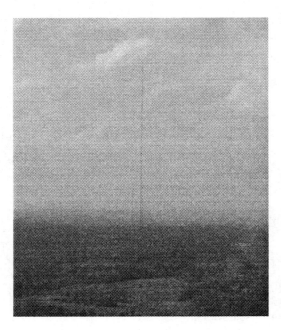

FIGURE 5-6
The WLBT tower in Jackson, Mississippi

Safety and Risk Management   63

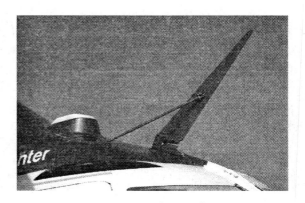

FIGURE 5-7
Helicopter with cable
cutters

and can cause significant damage to a helicopter. In numerous cases pilots have lost control of their aircraft and crashed following contact with power lines. Although these lines are readily visible from the ground, they are far less so from above. Thus pilots look first for utility poles and then for the wires running between them. Even small wires such as clotheslines may cause extensive damage to a helicopter. Here again, two or more sets of eyes are better than one in locating these hazards.

Some air medical operators equip their aircraft with "cable cutters." These knifelike devices extend upward and downward from the front of the fuselage and are intended to "catch and cut" any wire or cable inadvertently struck by the aircraft while in flight (Figure 5-7). Cable cutters are not 100 percent effective, however, and serious aircraft damage may result even when they work properly. They are of little help if the helicopter lands on top of a cable or if the rotors contact a cable. They are simply one more safety component that a program can add.

Lightning

Lightning is rarely a factor in aircraft accidents. The last accident attributed to lightning occurred in 1967. Commercial aircraft are often struck by lightning but rarely damaged. Modern aircraft are designed to conduct the current through the skin of the craft and away from the interior and avionics.

Lightning poses a greater threat to aircraft and crew members on the ground. Heliports are often located in open areas or on rooftops, both common targets for lightning strikes. It has been theorized that a turning helicopter produces an electrical field that may increase the likelihood of a strike. Rooftop heliports should be considered off-limits during thunderstorms.

Trees and Other Obstacles Near the Ground

Trees are occasionally cited as factors in aircraft accidents. From the air, trees are generally easy to see and easy to avoid. They are a greater hazard near the ground. Landing in a tight spot close to trees may result in contact with a limb. Even when clearance seems adequate, rotor wash may cause limbs to swing violently and strike the rotor. The aircraft should always be positioned a safe distance from trees and other obstacles.

In an unimproved area, obstacles near the ground may pose a hazard. On many helicopters the tail rotor comes very close to the ground as the pilot flares the aircraft to decrease forward motion in preparation for landing. At that point an obstacle 2 or 3 feet high—such as tree stumps, bushes, and debris—may contact the tail rotor and cause serious damage. This is another reason first responders should be on scene beforehand. They can identify the most desirable landing area and remove potential hazards before the flight team arrives.

Crash Survival

Although the likelihood of a crash is extremely low, it is essential that the flight team be adequately prepared should one occur. Since the vast majority of flight programs use a flight following system, the probability of being declared overdue or missing in a timely manner is good. In most cases fire and EMS teams are dispatched within 30 to 45 minutes of an aircraft's disappearance. However, in rural, heavily wooded, mountainous, or swampy areas it may take much more time (hours to days) for rescuers to locate and reach a crash site.

Flight crew personnel should have some training for survival under adverse conditions, including a course in wilderness survival and first aid. Programs that operate near large bodies of water should receive special training in water egress and survival.

Every aircraft should carry a survival kit containing at least the following items:

* Flashlight
* Compass
* Blanket
* Matches (in a sealed and waterproof container)
* Flares
* Candles
* Knife

Safety and Risk Management 65

- Fishing supplies (hooks and line)
- Water container or bottled water
- Safety pins

Other Safety-Related Issues

The Federal Aviation Act

Most of the safety-related issues discussed in this chapter are addressed by the FAA Act. The FAA certification process ensures that a program is set up and administered in a safe and orderly manner. Before it can begin operation, a new program must either complete a lengthy application and certification process or operate under the certificate of a vendor who has already completed the process. Certification involves ensuring that the program is in compliance with a long list of safety-related requirements.

Terrorism

In the post-9/11 era, terrorism must be considered a potential threat for anyone operating any type of aircraft. While statistically the probability of a medical aircraft being stolen or hijacked is low, every aircraft must be considered a potential terrorist target.

Aircraft should be routinely secured after each flight. Doors should be locked and keys removed. Helicopters should be kept in a secure area with controlled entry. It is against FAA regulations to erect tall fences close to a heliport, but even a very short fence is better than nothing. Frequent patrolling by security personnel and continual video monitoring minimize the risk of tampering. A rooftop heliport can be the most secure location for an aircraft as long as access to the rooftop is strictly limited. Using cards or keypads is a fairly secure method of limiting access. The best method that is currently available and also affordable is the employee identification badge with a magnetic strip.

Single Versus Twin

There continues to be a lack of consensus among air medical operators as to whether a twin-engine helicopter is necessary for air medical operation. In the early days of air medicine, virtually all helicopters were small, single-engine turbine aircraft. As the industry grew and matured, more programs started using twins, and in 1987 the number of twins surpassed the number of singles in operation. Today the medium-duty twin is the most commonly used air medical helicopter. The twin offers the power and safety of two engines and in recent years has had a slightly better safety record than the single. It must be noted, however, that when a twin is involved in an accident, fatalities are more likely to occur.

However, that is not to say that single-engine aircraft are unsafe. In fact, several single-engine models are among those with the lowest accident rates. In certain situations a single-engine turbine may be the best choice for an air medical program, as it is cheaper to purchase and maintain. Single-engine are a safe mode of transportation and continue to play an important role in air medical transport.

The single-versus-twin argument cannot be based solely on safety. A twin-engine aircraft has more power and a larger cabin. For many programs that attribute alone is reason to choose a twin over a single. Twins are also more likely to be instrument-equipped and rated for IFR flight, which reduces the number of flights lost due to marginal weather and may increase census for sponsoring hospitals.

Fire-Resistant Flight Suits

A number of manufacturers offer flight suits constructed of fire-resistant materials designed to protect wearers from high-intensity flames for a brief period of time, 20 to 30 seconds. These suits offer crash survivors a chance to escape a burning aircraft with a lower risk of being burned (Figure 5-8).

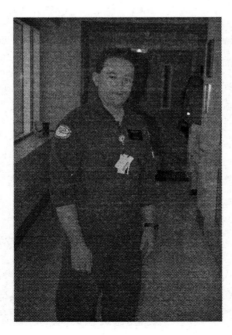

FIGURE 5-8
Nomex flight suit

They protect only those areas that are covered by the material and should therefore cover the entire body from neck to ankles. Protective gloves may also be worn, although few programs use fire-resistant gloves because they hinder access and are a contamination risk.

Flight Helmets

The use of helmets in air medical programs is a controversial topic. Some programs require them; others do not. Proponents argue that helmets may be beneficial during a potentially survivable crash because they may reduce the incidence of traumatic brain injury, facial injuries, and burns (Figure 5-9). Helmets complement fire-resistant flight suits by protecting the head and face from burns.

Opponents argue that the probability of a "real" crash is so low that helmets are nothing more than a nuisance. They are heavy and uncomfortable. One argument (with some logic) is that if helmets are warranted while flying in a modern turbine-engine helicopter with its impressive safety record, they are certainly warranted while driving in the family sedan, where the risk of head injury is at least as great. Yet we don't see many people wearing helmets on the freeway.

While an impact significant enough to benefit the wearer of a helmet is unlikely, the helmet provides an added safety measure. It is true they are hot and bothersome for the new user, but with continued use they are more easily tolerated. They do have some beneficial features as well. Better models provide two different face shields, one clear and one shaded. The clear shield acts as a biological barrier when providing patient care in the aircraft. The shaded shield protects the wearer's face and eyes from the sun. Face shields also provide some protection in case of fire or if a bird or other foreign object should penetrate the canopy.

The Committee on Accreditation of Medical Transport Systems (CAMTS) lists helmets as one of the options for minimizing the risk of

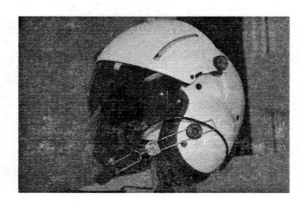

FIGURE 5-9
Flight helmet

head strikes. Statistically a helmet is much more likely to protect the user from a head bump caused by turbulence than from a head injury during a crash. Any added safety precaution is difficult to argue against, and the use of helmets is recommended.

Risk Management

Injury Reduction

Most of the injuries encountered in flight programs occur during the lifting and moving of patients—strains and sprains to the neck, back, and shoulder areas, and crushing injuries to the hands and fingers. The incidence of these injuries is often related to the type of patient loading/unloading system incorporated into the aircraft. Systems requiring the manual placement of patients into the aircraft are more likely to cause injuries than those that use articulating devices that extend outside the aircraft to accept the patient. Similarly, systems requiring employees to lean over or twist during the loading process are more likely to cause injury. The loading system should be a major consideration when considering the medical interior for a new aircraft. Educating new employees on proper lifting technique and requiring adequate lifting assistance for heavier patients may also reduce the incidence of injuries.

Crew Resource Management

crew resource management (CRM)
A comprehensive plan whereby human resources are used effectively and efficiently during all phases of flight. Its intended purpose is to reduce the probability of human error.

The concept of **crew resource management (CRM)** originated in response to a NASA workshop that examined the role that human error plays in air crashes. The basic principle is that human factors are important causes of flight-related incidents and accidents. Generally, a catastrophic event involving an aircraft is preceded by a series of errors in judgment; if any one of those errors had not been committed, the accident could have been prevented. CRM emphasizes the importance of making use of all available resources—information, equipment, and people—to achieve safe and efficient flight operations. It encompasses team training, simulation of potential safety breaches, interactive group debriefings, and measurement and improvement of aircrew performance. The three primary components of effective crew management are safety, efficiency, and morale.

The goals of crew resource management are to:

* Maximize human performance in an aviation setting
* Understand and maximize use of the various facets of group dynamics

* Recognize the beneficial and detrimental effects of stress and coping techniques
* Plan and critique flying operations more effectively
* Assess, mitigate, and manage risk inherent to current flying operations
* Utilize all resources in making better-informed decisions that consider the full range of options
* Manage workload to avoid task saturation or complacency
* Better communicate mission-essential information both inside and outside the cockpit
* Maintain or restore situational awareness for self and other aircrew members

A mnemonic that is often used to help learners remember the basic concept of CRM is:

D Detect: The pilot or other crew member detects that a change has occurred that requires attention.

E Estimate: The significance of the change is quickly estimated.

C Choose: Given the new circumstances, the crewmember chooses an outcome.

I Identify: The crewmember identifies feasible and practical responses to the event.

D Do: The best option is implemented.

E Evaluate: The crewmember evaluates the impact of the action taken.

Debriefing

Debriefing is the process of reviewing and analyzing key events that occurred during the course of a flight, in particular any nonroutine event that could have potentially (or actually) led to an incident or accident. In air medicine the event may be related to the aircraft and flight, or to a patient or patient care activity. Debriefing serves three purposes:

1. It provides a forum for analyzing immediate past performance in an objective and nonthreatening environment.
2. In cases involving human error or equipment failure, it should lead to the formulation of a plan to minimize the risk of recurrence.
3. It offers crew members the opportunity to openly discuss their concerns and anxieties. Talking about experiences and feelings is often the first step toward recovery from stress-induced trauma.

All flight programs should have a debriefing policy that specifies which situations mandate debriefing and which person is responsible for convening the group in those situations. Beyond those defined situations, crew members should be granted the authority to convene a debriefing session at their discretion. It is important to acknowledge the fact that different crew members have different thresholds for emotional trauma and encourage self-recognition of that threshold.

Subtle Stressors of Flight

Beyond the hazards noted above, other, more mundane factors may have a negative impact on crew performance. Even these subtle stressors have the potential to compromise safety and have contributed to many aircraft incidents and accidents.

Emotional Trauma

The acuity level of patients transported by air medical programs is very high. Many patients either die or survive with major disabilities. Patients may have compromised mental status and may be agitated or violent. Family members and friends of patients may try to pressure the medical team to provide treatment that is not appropriate or to transport prematurely. Medical personnel in referring facilities may be overbearing and confrontational. In short, air medical team members are typically subjected to high levels of emotional stress. This stress will exact a high price if it is not recognized and managed properly.

Vibration

Prolonged exposure to low-frequency noise and vibration has been shown to cause fatigue in flight crew members. Even noise below the range of human hearing may have adverse effects. Little can be done to diminish low-frequency sound waves, but it is important to recognize that they are a stressor.

Extremes of Temperature and Humidity

Exposure to temperature and humidity extremes may contribute to mental and physical fatigue. The body consumes energy in its efforts to regulate body temperature. Prolonged exposure to low-humidity conditions dries the mucosa and may cause the loss of significant quantities of fluid from the body, dehydration, and electrolyte disturbances. Similarly, high-humidity conditions may result in the body's inability to release excess heat and hyperthermia. In hot and moist environments, profuse sweating is common, adding to the probability of dehydration and electrolyte disturbances.

Circadian Dysrhythmia

The human body is strongly influenced by circadian rhythms, which are predictable physiological and behavioral patterns that are linked to time of day. Sleep and wakefulness, digestive activity, body temperature, and mental alertness are all influenced by circadian rhythms. The human body seems to be programmed to sleep at night and to be alert and active during the day. But flight personnel often work rotating shifts or cross time zones during work shifts, disrupting their natural patterns of sleep. The result may be fatigue and sleepiness during waking hours and insomnia during sleep hours, which may lead further to mental sluggishness, loss of motivation, and compromised job performance. In air medicine, compromised job performance may mean compromised patient care or compromised ability to operate the aircraft safely. Either of these is unacceptable.

There may also be long-term health implications of circadian dysrhythmia. Studies suggest that shift workers have a higher incidence of a number of diseases, including gastrointestinal disturbances, mental illness, and heart disease. In particular, the Helsinki Heart Study, an ongoing study of the Finnish population, found that over a 5-year period, rotating-shift workers had a 40 to 50 percent greater risk of coronary heart disease (CHD) compared to day-shift workers. Compared to white-collar workers, the increased risk was 70 percent.

Certain steps can be taken to minimize the effects of circadian rhythms. The best solution is to simply eliminate rotating shift work. Those who work the same shift on a long-term basis are more likely to become accustomed to that shift and to "reset" their circadian rhythms. If this is not an option, rotating shifts as infrequently as possible may help. It generally takes 3 to 5 days for the body to become accustomed to a change in work times. After that the trauma associated with the change decreases.

Jet Lag

jet lag
A form of circadian dysrhythmia caused by moving from one time zone to another.

Because of the limited range of travel, **jet lag** is rarely a problem for personnel traveling by helicopter. However, those who perform longer-distance fixed-wing transports may experience its effects. Jet lag is a form of circadian dysrhythmia that occurs because changing time zones confuse the body's inner clock. Moving from one time zone to another throws the body out of sync with surrounding activities. Trying to adapt to the predominant schedule may result in mental and physical symptoms such as fatigue, insomnia, disorientation, edema, allergies, headaches, bowel irregularity, and lightheadedness. It can take up to several days to adjust fully to a new time zone.

Several activities have been shown to contribute to jet lag. Drinking alcohol or other substances with diuretic properties tends to make symptoms worse, as does remaining in one position during a long flight.

Conversely, keeping hydrated, stretching, walking about during long flights, and eating small meals at times compatible with the new time zone can minimize the effects of jet lag.

Infection Control

Air medical programs are often called on to transport patients with communicable diseases. In some patients the disease has been diagnosed. In others the transport is arranged because of some other illness or injury and the communicable disease is in a subclinical stage and not yet recognized. In the former case, the risk is obvious and all necessary precautions are taken. In the latter case, the risk is less obvious and the flight team may be less diligent about following infectious-disease precautions.

With the growing number of antibiotic-resistant bacteria and other microorganisms for which there are no effective treatments, the risk of contracting an infectious disease is a constant, and diligence is essential. High-acuity patients often have active bleeding or other conditions involving the shedding of body fluids. Built-in blood dams help control the spread of large quantities of fluid. However, smaller quantities inevitably find their way into areas of the aircraft that are difficult to access. When allowed to sit, these fluids form an ideal growth media for pathogenic microorganisms.

Aircraft Disinfection

The aircraft should be thoroughly cleaned at the end of each patient transport. This is one area in which crew members tend to become complacent over time. They should be reminded frequently of the potential implications of not disinfecting the aircraft, namely the risk of cross-contaminating other patients and even members of their own families.

Disinfecting agents should be readily available at each patient destination site. Generally this is not a problem for programs that transport patients to only a few hospitals. If multiple hospitals are involved and access to disinfectants is a problem, small supplies should be kept aboard the aircraft. Using disinfectant wipes for the hands during flight may also minimize the risk of cross-contamination.

Summary

Aircraft, especially rotor wing aircraft, are inherently dangerous. When on the ground the main and tail rotors present the greatest danger. Contact with either if these may result in serious injury or death. During flight, trees, radio towers, and other aircraft are potential hazards. Poor visibility may compromise the pilot's ability to detect hazards and is often a complicating factor in aircraft accidents. The risk of contacting trees, poles, wires and debris is increased in those aircraft with blind spots. In such cases a spotter should be used to make sure that all hazards are identified.

A comprehensive safety program is necessary to ensure the safety of equipment and personnel. Each member of the flight team must be educated regarding the hazards associated with aircraft operations and how to perform around those hazards in a safe manner. Safety must permeate every aspect of the program and take priority over everything else, including patient care. Assuming that safety precautions are in place and all potential hazards can be avoided, the helicopter is a very safe mode of transportation.

Accidents most often occur when some member of the flight team becomes complacent and fails to follow the established safety standard. The danger rate increases dramatically when other members of the flight team follow suit or allow the behavior to continue. Vigilance, self-discipline, and effective communication are essential components of a safe program. So long as all personnel adhere strictly to established safety standards, the likelihood of suffering an injury or being killed in a helicopter is relatively small.

REVIEW QUESTIONS

1. The most dangerous part of a helicopter is the:
   a. Main rotor
   b. Tail rotor
   c. Engine exhaust
   d. Pitot tube

2. A common cause of passenger contact with a moving tail rotor is:
   a. Crew members who direct passengers to approach and depart the aircraft from the rear
   b. Standing in the landing zone as the aircraft lands
   c. Being stationed near the tail of the aircraft in order to keep others away
   d. Chasing a personal item that has been blown toward the rear of the craft by rotor wash

3. Explain why hot loading/unloading may occasionally be justified.

4. All the following are good safety practices EXCEPT:
   a. Direct ambulance personnel to wait as near the helipad as possible when approaching so as to facilitate prompt movement of patients
   b. Avoid the tail of the helicopter anytime the rotors are in motion
   c. Do not carry loose items such as sheets, pillow cases, papers, etc. near the helicopter when the rotors are in motion
   d. Do not carry anything that extends above head level as those items may contact the main rotor blade

5. A temporary or makeshift landing zone often in an unimproved area is called a:
   a. Helideck   c. Helispot
   b. Helipad   d. Helizone

6. The most common cause of helicopter crashes is:
   a. Mechanical failures   c. Rapid changes in weather conditions
   b. Instrument failure   d. Pilot error

7. Define "head strike envelope."

8. A twin-engine helicopter is much safer than a single-engine helicopter
   a. True
   b. False

9. Items that should be included in a crash survival kit include all the following EXCEPT:
   a. Blanket   c. Tylenol
   b. Flashlight   d. Compass

Communications

Objectives

Upon completing this chapter, the reader should have a better understanding of the following topics:

* Communications equipment typically used aboard an air ambulance

* The three categories of communications

* The role of the dispatcher in the safety and operation of the flight program

* The flight-following process and its importance

* Basic aviation language

KEY TERMS

Introduction

Communications is an integral component of all air medical programs. Functional equipment and communications knowledge and skill are prerequisites for a safe and efficient operation. The Federal Communications Commission (FCC), an independent government agency directly responsible to Congress, is charged with regulating interstate and international communications by radio, television, wire, satellite, and cable. All communications equipment typically used in the operation of an air medical program falls under the jurisdiction of the FCC.

Equipment

When it comes to communications equipment, air medical helicopters are somewhat more complicated than four-wheeled ambulances are. The pilot must be able to communicate with air traffic controllers, weather stations, and other aircraft. Each aircraft must have frequencies for plotting location and course. The medical team must be able to communicate with its dispatch center, hospitals, first responders, paramedics, rescue teams, and law enforcement personnel. Aircraft radios are typically multiple-band programmable devices that allow flexibility in communication.

In medium-size and larger helicopters, there are typically two different receive-and-transmit units (R/Ts), one in the cockpit for the pilot and another in the patient compartment for the medical team. Having two separate units allows for independent communications activities. The pilot can communicate with the control tower while the medical team is discussing a patient with a receiving hospital or physician. In smaller aircraft, where the pilot and medical team are in close quarters, this may not be practical and both parties may use the same R/T.

Many flight programs cover large geographical areas, and maintaining contact with a communications center on the ground can be difficult. Radio transmission **towers** on the ground transmit radio frequencies in a straight line. If a target aircraft is so far away from the tower that the curve of the earth blocks the transmission, communications will be difficult. Air medical programs typically deal with this problem in one of three ways.

1. Radio transmission towers: Generally, a tower's effective range is proportional to its height. The higher the tower, the greater its range. In relatively flat areas, towers can be an excellent mode of communication. An R/T with an antenna at 500 feet above ground level (**AGL**) should enable effective communication with an aircraft at 75-plus miles in any direction. An antenna placed at 1000 feet should provide a range of greater than 100 miles when the aircraft is at cruise altitude. Radio technicians can modify the pattern of radio waves being emitted from a transmitter. This is known as adjusting the gain. In normal mode, radio waves are transmitted vertically and horizontally in a 360-degree pattern from the antenna. As gain is increased, the transmission pattern becomes flatter and more parallel to the ground. This increases the intensity of the radio waves being transmitted and increases the effective range of the radio. The downside to adding gain

tower (TWR)
Generally refers to a control tower in the context of contact with an air traffic controller. May also refer to a privately owned radio antennae tower.

AGL
Above ground level. Vertical elevation above the ground.

to a transmitter is the loss of the vertical 360-degree transmission pattern, which may decrease the transmitter's ability to communicate with radios working in close proximity that fall under the modified transmission pattern.

2. Multiple towers: A single tower may be ineffective in hilly or mountainous areas where there are many "dead spots." One solution is the use of multiple towers strategically located throughout the service area. The goal is for the aircraft to have access to a tower from any location in the service area. Transmissions from the aircraft are received by the nearest tower and forwarded to the dispatch center through telephone lines or repeaters. If repeaters are used, the signal is relayed to the dispatch center through a series of adjacent towers. When the dispatcher transmits to the aircraft, the process is reversed. Towers should be placed in areas of high elevation where transmissions are least affected by terrain. In certain problematic areas even multiple towers may not be enough for reliable communications.

3. Satellite communications: This is a newer mode of communication that is unaffected by terrain. Satellite communications have become more user-friendly over the past several years. The communications devices are slightly larger than a conventional cell phone but small enough to be easily transported. One company offers a unit that is mounted in the aircraft and links to the intracabin communications system. The device may also be unplugged from the aircraft system and used as a stand-alone unit outside the aircraft. Satellite communications systems are not cellular phones. They have idiosyncrasies that take some getting used to. In addition to the larger size, there may be lag time between transmission and reception, and thick cloud cover may cause interference.

Communication Bands/Frequencies

There are a large number of radio frequencies that may be used for operational and medical communication. These frequencies are grouped into ranges of bandwidths known as bands. The FCC dictates the appropriate uses for each of these bands. For example, very high frequencies (VHF) may be assigned to law enforcement and public service agencies. Ultra high frequencies (UHF) are often assigned to ambulance services for medical communications and for the transmission of biomedical information. A typical aircraft radio transmits and receives on frequencies between 118.000 and 136.975 MHz (megahertz).

Because they need to communicate with a variety of agencies, air medical helicopters are generally equipped with programmable multi-band radios. These devices allow users to program in the frequencies of any agency they may need to communicate with. A typical air medical radio has frequencies for law enforcement, hospitals, ambulances, rescue personnel, and fire departments. These radios are often very complicated and must be programmed by an experienced person.

Types of Communication

Communication can be divided into three categories: operational, medical, and intracabin.

Operational Communication

Operational communication is divided into two distinct areas: communication with air traffic control and communication with a dispatch center.

Air Traffic Control

ATC

Air traffic control or air traffic controller.

Air traffic control (**ATC**) refers to the monitoring and regulation of aircraft movements through different segments of air space. *Air traffic controllers* (ATCs) are employed by the FAA to monitor and direct the position and movements of aircraft and to ensure that they move about in a safe and coordinated manner (Figure 6-1). Their primary concern is to keep all aircraft a safe distance from one another. They enforce the primary rule of aviation: No two objects (aircraft) can occupy the same point in space and time. In busy metropolitan areas there are large numbers of aircraft operating in a relatively small space. Simultaneously monitoring all these aircraft and keeping them separated by altitude and direction of movement can be a difficult task.

ATCs have broad authority to regulate airspace. However, their numbers are small and safe aircraft operation requires the cooperation of aircraft operators. Severe penalties, up to loss of license and criminal prosecution, may be levied against those who violate ATC directives.

Dispatch (Communications) Centers

Virtually all rotor-wing flight programs have a dispatch center that coordinates the receipt of flight requests and all operational communications. The dispatch center is a program-specific entity that coordinates all communications to and from the flight crew. Dispatchers are employees of either the program or a vendor contracted to provide the service. The dispatcher receives the flight request and other pertinent information, typically from a physician, nurse, or emergency medical technician, sometimes from a law enforcement officer, firefighter, or other

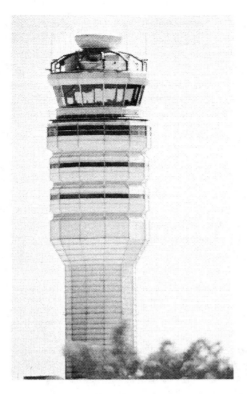

An air traffic control tower
Getty Images, Inc.-Taxi

first responder. Occasionally a launch may be triggered by a call from a citizen in the community. In any case, the dispatcher processes the request according to a predetermined protocol, collects the necessary information, and forwards it to the pilot and medical crew via pager, radio, cell phone, or standard telephone. A number of programs use alphanumeric pagers to transmit patient information and other specifics that may not be practical via voice pagers or radios.

At that point the pilot determines whether or not the flight can be safely attempted based on weather conditions, flight distance, safety of the proposed landing zone, weight and girth of the patient, and other factors. In reality much of this decision making is done in advance through ongoing communication between the pilot and the dispatch center. Once the decision has been made to accept a flight, the pilot and medical team prepare for departure. That process generally involves a series of prescribed, systematic preflight activities. For the pilot, those include completing a checklist that ensures all aircraft systems are checked and readied for flight. The medical team may assist the pilot by removing electrical cords, checking for obstructions, looking for other air traffic, communicating with the operations center, and preparing patients and other passengers. The first few minutes

traffic
A term used by air traffic control (ATC) to refer to one or more aircraft.

after liftoff are the most crucial part of a helicopter flight. The pilot communicates with the control tower and other aircraft **traffic** that may be operating in the area. The FAA has in place what is known as the "sterile cockpit rule," which states that the pilot is the only one routinely allowed to communicate during the liftoff phase of flight. This helps to minimize distractions for the pilot. As the aircraft gains speed and altitude and enters the cruise phase, normal intracabin communications are allowed to resume.

In many systems the pilot receives information separately from the medical team. This practice is intended to prevent the pilot from learning the age and medical condition of the patient and making launch decisions affected by emotion. For example, a pilot with a two-year-old child at home may decide to fly during marginal weather conditions if he knows that the patient is also a two-year-old.

flight following
The process of maintaining constant or intermittent contact with an aircraft for the purpose of tracking its location and condition.

Flight following is the continual monitoring and recording of an aircraft's position during flight by a remote party on the ground. Flight following is an essential part of the safety program and is required by the FAA. In its most basic form, flight following involves the use of a transponder. A transponder unit, consisting of a receiver and a transmitter, serves as a radar marker for the aircraft. Each time the transponder receives an inquiry from air traffic control radar on the ground, it blinks and sends out a coded reply. With each response, the aircraft appears as an anonymous data block on the radar screen. An air traffic controller who wants to identify a particular aircraft on the radar screen simply asks the pilot to push the IDENT button. That increases the intensity of the signal transmitted and identifies the aircraft.

position report
An exact description of an aircraft's location as transmitted to the ATC or other flight following center (see *flight following*).

AM programs generally use a more program-specific form of flight following. The dispatching agency usually performs this function. The aircraft makes contact with the dispatcher every 10 to 15 minutes and provides a **position report** that includes longitude, latitude, altitude, fuel status, number of persons aboard the aircraft, and **estimated time of arrival (ETA)** at destination. In case of emergency, the dispatcher can transfer these coordinates to a map and identify the approximate position of the aircraft. When the aircraft is flying under instrument flight rules (IFR), flight following can be done directly by an FAA flight service center.

Another option for flight following uses a satellite transmitting and receiving system. A transmitter in the aircraft sends a signal to several satellite receivers at predetermined time intervals. The satellite receivers triangulate the signal and transform it into a set of longitude and latitude coordinates that are downloaded to an Internet server and forwarded to the dispatch center or elsewhere. The data appears in the form of a vehicle on a map. As the vehicle moves, the image on the map also moves, giving the dispatcher real-time tracking ability. These systems are expensive and are currently in limited use but have tremendous potential for future application.

estimated time of arrival (ETA)
Approximate time at which an aircraft will reach an intermediary point or final destination.

Ground operations communication is essential for safely performing scene flights. The pilot and medical team may be in contact with primary responders (fire, EMS, law enforcement) prior to arrival on scene and during approach, landing, and departure. In well-developed systems, ground personnel secure and mark the landing area, coordinate aircraft arrival with other ground activities, and direct the incoming aircraft to the landing zone.

The advent of **global position satellite (GPS)** technology has made scene response more precise and efficient. Prior to GPS the pilot often had to make an educated guess at the exact location of the scene. Now first responders can determine their longitude and latitude with a portable GPS unit and provide those coordinates to the dispatch center. Once airborne, the pilot programs the coordinates into the aircraft GPS and flies directly to the location. GPS coordinates also allow the aircraft to fly in a straight line between hospitals during interhospital transports. In instrument-rated aircraft, the GPS links directly to the autopilot, which then plots the exact course.

global positioning satellite (GPS)
An electronic device that receives signals from orbiting satellites. It uses an advanced form of triangulation to calculate and display an exact location in the form of numbers indicating latitude and longitude. Some more advanced units also display location on a map display.

Medical Communications

Medical communications refers to the transmitting or receiving of patient information. Medical and operational information is generally transmitted over different radios or frequencies. As with ground ambulances, there is generally a radio frequency in the aircraft that is reserved for the medical crew to communicate with the on-line medical director (Figure 6-2). This is generally a private frequency that cannot easily be monitored

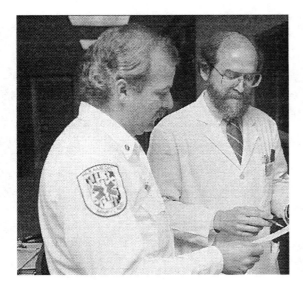

FIGURE 6-2
Medical director reviewing information received from flight team

by outsiders. The FCC has allocated a segment of UHF frequencies specifically for medical communications. However, VHF or 800-MHz radios, cell phones, flight phones, and other devices may also be used to transmit medical information. In some systems a FliteFone or similar radio-telephone switching system may be used. (Use of standard cell phones while in flight is prohibited by the FCC.)

Medical communications may be for consultation or for informational purposes only. The flight team generally notifies the receiving hospital 5 to 10 minutes before landing. That gives the hospital time to prepare for the patient's arrival and have a stretcher waiting at the landing area.

Medical communications should be limited to frequencies that are reasonably secure from eavesdropping. Patient confidentiality must always be a concern when discussing patient information by radio. Personal information—a patient's name, home address, and social security number—should never be provided by radio unless there is some overwhelming clinical reason to do so.

Intracabin Communications

Intracabin communications take place among crew members within the aircraft. Personnel are typically required to wear either a headset or a flight helmet containing an integrated headset whenever the aircraft is in operation (Figure 6-3). The headset suppresses aircraft noise and allows wearers to hear each other via small speakers mounted in the ear cups. A small microphone in front of the lips transmits the speaker's voice. The headset must be attached and worn properly for the wearer to

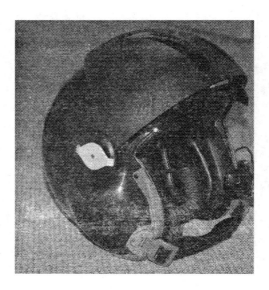

FIGURE 6-3
Close-up of medical helmet
with in-line controls

communicate effectively with other crew members. Ear cups should be seated snugly over the ears. The microphone should be adjusted so that it is directly in front of, and lightly touching, the bottom lip. The microphone may be activated by pressing a transmit button/switch located on the cord or, if set properly, voice activated each time the wearer speaks directly into the microphone.

The same microphone is used for communicating with others outside the aircraft. The handheld transmit housing contains two separate buttons/switches, one for intracabin communications and the other for out-of-cabin communications. Crew members should be certain that the correct button/switch has been selected before beginning a transmission. Air medical helicopters generally have programmable radios capable of communicating with hospitals, law enforcement, fire, public safety, game and wildlife, and many other agencies. When flying at 2000 feet and transmitting externally, the speaker's voice may be carried hundreds of miles and anyone monitoring the frequency will hear every word.

Communications Failure

Radio communications systems are notorious for their unpredictability. When a system fails, it may take days or longer to identify and correct the problem. For that reason there should be a plan for managing both operational and medical communications during outages. A backup plan may include the use of a secondary radio transmitter, a handheld unit, or, in emergency cases, a cellular telephone.

An aircraft operating under IFR conditions that experiences radio failure may have a particularly serious problem. Loss of contact with air traffic controllers could rapidly deteriorate into an emergency situation. Having radar and GPS systems on board may reduce the risks of such a failure.

Loss of medical communications capabilities must also be anticipated and planned for. Most air medical programs operate relatively autonomously and patient care should not be adversely affected by lack of communication. Each program should have a section in its protocol manual covering communication failure. In most cases a general statement allowing the medical team freedom to perform treatments that may otherwise require a verbal order for the management of life- or limb-threatening conditions is adequate.

The dispatch center should also have a contingency plan in case of lost communications. If the dispatcher is unable to raise the aircraft at the designated check-in time, there should be a protocol prescribing action to be taken. Generally, if the dispatcher cannot raise the AM team by radio, attempts should be made by other means such as pager or radio-telephone. If that fails, the dispatcher should contact the planned landing site to see if the aircraft has arrived. If these efforts fail to locate the aircraft, it must be assumed that an accident has occurred. At this stage the dispatcher should not hesitate to activate the program's overdue-aircraft plan.

Communication During an Emergency Situation

If an in-flight emergency should develop, there is a chance that the pilot may be too busy trying to control the aircraft or looking for a safe landing area to operate the radio. All core crew members should be capable of selecting the appropriate channel and communicating an emergency situation to someone on the ground. If flight following is being performed by a communications center, that is who should be contacted.

The flight following agency should have a **post-accident/incident plan (PAIP)** readily accessible to each air medical dispatcher. The PAIP outlines a course of action for the dispatcher in the event that a pilot declares an emergency. It addresses every potential emergency situation and contains instructions concerning notification of the appropriate emergency and rescue services and administrative personnel. It even includes prescribed statements to be made to the news media should they become involved.

If the aircraft is flying under IFR conditions and being tracked by a flight controller when an emergency situation develops, the reporting may be done somewhat differently. The pilot reports the emergency to the flight controller, who then contacts the appropriate emergency response agencies.

Cellular telephones are now in widespread use. They are basically handheld radios that transmit and receive from one tower (cell) at a time. On the ground that is generally what happens. From the air, however, a cell phone may activate multiple towers at once. For this reason the FCC has banned the airborne use of cell phones, with one exception: they may be used during an emergency if no other form of communication is available or effective.

A number of companies now have special licenses for offering a variant of cellular service for airborne use. These devices work off special frequencies and towers and do not interfere with standard cellular service. One variety transmits first to a satellite and is then routed to a receiving station on the ground. Both devices work well, although they are relatively expensive compared to standard cellular service.

post-accident/
incident plan (PAIP)
An action guide
for dispatchers
outlining a course
of action in the
event that a pilot
declares an in-
flight emergency
or fails to provide
a position report at
the designated
time.

The Language of Flight Communications

As with most specialty areas, flight operations have a language of their own. In fact, in air medicine, two specialty languages are involved. The first involves communications with the air traffic controller (ATC). A novice flight team member will likely have difficulty following a conversation between a pilot and an ATC. While it is very unlikely that a team member will have reason to speak with ATC directly, the intracabin communications system allows the medical team to monitor conversations between the pilot and the ATC. Often these discussions involve matters related to safety, and it may benefit the crew to listen in so they can help spot other aircraft or obstacles being discussed. Some programs have policies that the medical team monitor these communications anytime a patient is not on board. Obviously, when a patient is on board the medical team should be focused on patient care. In most modern AM helicopters the pilot can flip a switch that disables the intracabin communication system.

While the language used when communicating with ATC is not very different from everyday language, it may be delivered very differently. The goal is to be clear but brief. One controller may be responsible for multiple aircraft and there is no time for idle chatter. Single words and phrases are commonly used to convey information. Some of the key phrases used during radio transmissions to and from the ATC include:

Affirmative	Yes, or yes I will comply.
Approach control	Position at a terminal radar facility responsible for handling IFR flights to the primary airport.
Climb and maintain (or descend and maintain)	Climb (or descend) to an altitude of x and maintain that altitude.
ETA	Estimated time of arrival.
Heading	Compass direction. For example, "Turn to heading 180."
Lifeguard	Any air medical aircraft. Aircraft with these call signs are given priority.
Local traffic	Aircraft operating in the traffic pattern or within sight of the tower; aircraft operating within the immediate airport area.
Over	I am done with my transmission.

Position report	A report over a known location that is transmitted to the ATC.
Radar contact lost	The aircraft is no longer visible on the ATC radar screen. Indicates a need for an immediate verbal reply.
Radar contact	An indicator that the ATC has identified your aircraft on radar.
Roger	I received your transmission.
Say again	Please repeat your last transmission.
Souls	People. For example, "We are en route to Regional Medical Center. We have four souls on board."
Squawk	Change your radio frequency to . . . For example, "Radar termination approved . . . squawk 1200."
Stand by	I am busy, wait. Usually means that a controller or pilot must pause for a few seconds to attend to other higher-priority issues.
Terminating radar service	An indicator that an aircraft wishes to terminate ATC radar monitoring. Terminating radar service without ATC approval may result in the assumption that you have crashed.
Traffic	A term used by ATC to indicate one or more aircraft. For example, "Lifeguard 6, you have traffic at three o'clock, three miles."
Unable	Pilot response when an ATC directive cannot be complied with.
Unfamiliar	Pilot is not familiar with a directive given.
Wilco	I have received your message, understand it, and will comply.

Summary

An air medical helicopter is a hotbed of communications activity. The pilot communicates with air traffic control, the flight dispatcher, and personnel on the ground at the planned landing area. Medical personnel may communicate with ground ambulance personnel, the referring hospital, the medical director, and the receiving hospital. In addition members of the flight team must use the intracabin communications to communicate with each other. The aircraft radio is generally equipped with multiple frequencies to facilitate contact with any necessary agency.

In smaller aircraft there may be one radio and only one type of communication may take place at any given time. Larger aircraft will have two independent radio systems so that the pilot and medical team may communicate independently with their respective parties of interest. The coordination of communication activity is important for operational and safety reasons. Crew members should be intimately familiar with communications protocols. The pilot should always have radio priority and should be allowed to communicate with air traffic control and other aircraft without being interrupted.

Due to the critical role that communications plays during aeromedical operation, equipment failure may create significant problems. Loss of communication may lead to loss of operational efficiency and may compromise safety. A specialized language is required when communicating by radio. The use of a specialized language of phrases, numbers, and words that may seem foreign to the inexperienced. All members of the air medical team should be familiar with this language.

A special protocol may be implemented in the event of an inflight emergency and each member of the flight team will have specific communications responsibilities. Similarly, special actions may be required in the event of communications failure. All phases of flight are coordinated through communication with various entities in the air and on the ground. This process must be well understood and adhered to by all members of the flight team.

REVIEW QUESTIONS

1. The three basic types of aircraft communication are:
   a. Operational, medical, and intracabin
   b. Operational, medical and cellular
   c. Operational, cellular, and infrared
   d. Operational, cellular and intracabin

2. The term that refers to the monitoring and regulation of aircraft movements through different segments of air space is:
   a. Aerospace regulation
   b. Federal aerospace regulation
   c. Air medical monitoring
   d. Air traffic control

3. Explain the role of the dispatch (communications) center.

4. From a safety perspective the most crucial part of a helicopter flight is:
   a. Cruise
   b. High-altitude cruise
   c. The first few minutes after liftoff
   d. Landing

5. The rationale for transmitting potential flight information to the pilot separate from the medical team is:
   a. To encourage the pilot to take flights that the medical team may discourage
   b. So that the medical team can have more time to prepare for flight
   c. To allow the pilot time to eat before the flight is officially dispatched
   d. To prevent the pilot from learning the age and medical condition of the patient so as to eliminate emotion from the decision making process

6. Communications failure:
   a. Is extremely rare and does not require a backup plan
   b. Must be anticipated and a contingency plan must be in place
   c. Requires notification of the FAA
   d. Requires initiation of the post accident/incident plan (PAIP)

CHAPTER 7

Personnel

Objectives

Upon completing this chapter, the reader should have a better understanding of the following topics:

* Roles and responsibilities of various air medical personnel

* Orientation of newly hired personnel

* The role of duty time in program safety

KEY TERMS

pilot in command (PIC), p. 92

Introduction

Job titles and organizational structure differ among air medical programs, but there are also commonalties. Virtually all programs employ six categories of personnel. Pilots, aviation technicians, and communications specialists are considered operational personnel. Medical care providers and medical directors comprise medical personnel. Administrators/managers are the sixth category.

Pilots

Pilots are highly trained professionals who fly airplanes and helicopters to carry out a wide variety of tasks. Pilots must be licensed by the Federal Aviation Administration (FAA). Applicants for licensure must be at least 18 years old, have 250 hours of flying time, have vision correctable to 20/20, pass a physical examination, and demonstrate their flying ability

pilot in command (PIC) The pilot responsible for the operation and safety of an aircraft during flight. The PIC is the ultimate authority concerning all activities occurring within the aircraft during flight.

to an FAA examiner. The pilot's role extends well beyond operation of the aircraft itself. The unique hazards of flight require the pilot to be a communicator, safety expert, and team leader.

According to FAA directives, the **pilot in command (PIC)** is responsible for all aspects of aircraft operation and is ultimately responsible for the safety and well-being of all other crew members while the aircraft is in flight. However, the pilot's responsibilities begin long before the aircraft is in the air. He must check the aircraft thoroughly prior to each flight. Weight and balance calculations must be done to ensure that the load is safely distributed throughout the aircraft. The pilot confers with flight dispatchers and weather stations about weather conditions likely to be present during each flight. Based on this information they choose the fastest and safest route.

The pilot is also responsible for seeing that anyone who flies aboard the aircraft other than the flight crew receives a flight briefing prior to flight. The briefing must include operation of doors, emergency egress, restraint requirements, and operation of restraint systems. It may also include other components not required by the FAA, such as operation of headsets/helmets or use of the communication system. Patients who are unconscious or who have altered mental status are obviously exempt from this policy.

Smaller helicopters are generally flown by one pilot. Midsize twins may be flown by one or two pilots, larger twins by two. Some aircraft are single-pilot IFR certified, meaning that a single appropriately trained and experienced pilot may fly the aircraft in limited-visibility conditions that would be unsafe for flying under visual flight rules. Flying single-pilot IFR can be very demanding for a pilot, who must not only fly the aircraft but also continually monitor a vast array of indicators, communicate with flight controllers, and make course and altitude adjustments.

EMS pilots often have additional responsibilities, such as removing and refilling oxygen tanks, making public relations flights, and interacting with medical personnel. Helicopters generally fly at relatively low altitude, and pilots must be on the lookout for trees, power lines, radio transmission towers, and other potential hazards. Helicopter pilots may also be required to land at unimproved landing sites that may be unlevel and close to potentially dangerous obstructions. EMS flight programs are typically very selective about the pilots they hire.

With the depth and breadth of their military experience, military pilots are heavily recruited for civilian pilot jobs. From the late 1970s through the 1990s, there was a steady supply of ex-military personnel to fill civilian pilot positions. That began to change, however, as the 1990s came to an end and the size of the pool began to shrink. Civilian flight services suddenly had to begin recruiting and paying more competitively to retain their pilots.

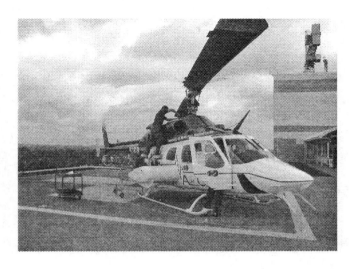

FIGURE 7-1
Aviation technician working on aircraft

Aviation Technicians

Aviation technicians, sometimes referred to as aircraft mechanics, are responsible for maintaining and repairing the aircraft (Figure 7-1). Although a few people become aviation technicians through on-the-job training, most become qualified by attending a vocational program certified by the FAA. Many of these schools offer two- and four-year degrees in avionics, aviation technology, or aviation maintenance management. The FAA requires at least 18 months of work experience for an airframe or power plant license. For a combined license, at least 30 months of experience working with both engines and airframes is required. Applicants for all licenses must also pass written and oral tests and demonstrate that they are competent to do the work authorized by the license.

Responsibilities of the aviation technician include ongoing maintenance of the aircraft, airframe systems, and engines; aircraft oxygen replenishment; inspection, removal, and installation of aircraft components; preparation and use of aircraft support equipment; and inspection, maintenance, servicing, repair, and fault diagnosis of all aircraft systems.

Highly qualified aviation technicians are an essential element of the flight program. The quality of their work is reflected in the airworthiness of the aircraft.

Communications Specialists

Communications specialists (also known as dispatchers) coordinate all communications-related activities of the flight program (Figure 7-2). They receive the initial call for assistance, dispatch the flight crew, perform flight

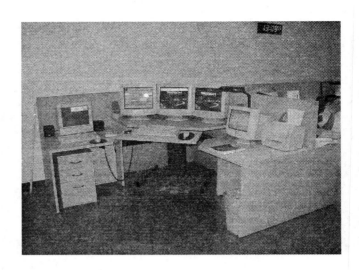

FIGURE 7-2
Modern communications center

following activities, and maintain records of these activities. Training ranges from that provided on the job to extensive formal training with certification. Many flight programs require that their personnel complete the National Highway and Traffic Safety Administration's Emergency Medical Dispatch (EMD) course. EMD is a three-day program designed for experienced communications personnel with an aptitude and desire to process emergency medical calls. The course meets the academic requirements for EMD certification in all states. While this certification is not specifically designed for air medical operations, much of the material is pertinent.

The National Association of Air Medical Communications Specialists (NAACS) recently developed a course specifically for communications specialists employed by air medical programs. The 10-hour course, known as the NAACS Training Course, includes call taking, dispatching, flight following, course plotting, and coordinate location.

In order for communications personnel to understand the importance of their jobs, it is essential that they go through an air medical orientation program. Orientation should include spending time with pilots, aviation technicians, and medical personnel, and at least one flight, preferably over a rural area that gives them an idea of the hazards of making an emergency landing in a dense forest or on a mountainside. This experience helps them to better appreciate the importance of their role.

Communications personnel must be well prepared to respond to in-flight urgencies and emergencies. The post-accident/incident plan (PAIP) is a desktop action plan for such situations. When a request for emergency assistance is received, the dispatcher need only flip to the appropriate page in the PAIP for concise instructions on what to do. (The PAIP is discussed in more detail in Chapter 6.)

Medical Care Providers

Medical care providers are responsible for assessing, treating, and otherwise dealing with patients who are managed by the air medical program. The patients transported by air are generally of high acuity, and the demands placed on medical caregivers are of similar magnitude. In the aircraft the medical crew is essentially doing the work that a team of physicians, nurses, and support staff would be doing in the emergency department or critical-care unit (Figure 7-3).

Aircraft size often limits the size of the medical team. Small helicopters may be staffed by a medical crew of one. Programs with medium and larger aircraft typically employ a medical crew of two (occasionally three), consisting of registered nurses, paramedics, physicians, respiratory therapists, and various combinations thereof. Most programs include a flight nurse with a background in emergency and/or critical care. In some programs the composition of the medical team varies by patient type. Personnel from different programs may have different opinions regarding the optimum composition of an AM team. Their opinions often are based more on personal experience and familiarity than on objective data. A number of studies have assessed the pros and cons of staffing with physicians, and findings have been mixed. Over the past decade, a majority of U.S. flight programs—70 percent in 2000—have moved to a registered nurse/paramedic team. The in-hospital emergency and critical-care experience of the nurse, combined with the prehospital emergency experience and more independent practice experience of the paramedic, make a nearly ideal team composition.

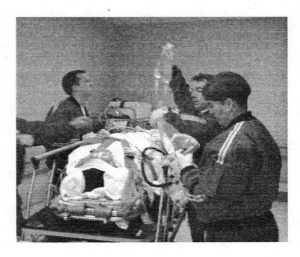

FIGURE 7-3
Flight team treating patient

Minimum Qualifications of the Medical Team

Although minimum requirements vary by profession and by program, the following are generally applicable.

Nurses should be graduates of an accredited school of nursing and should have passed the National League of Nursing Boards examination. A degree at the associate or bachelor's level indicates completion of a well-rounded curriculum and is preferred. Many programs also require two years of experience in an emergency department or critical-care area as a prerequisite for application. Completion of Advanced Cardiac Life Support (ACLS), Pediatric Advanced Life Support (PALS), and a trauma course such as Trauma Nurse Core Curriculum (TNCC), Basic Trauma Life Support (BTLS), or Prehospital Trauma Life Support (PHTLS) is often required. For programs that transport pediatric patients, Pediatric Advanced Life Support (PALS) and a Neonatal Resuscitation course may be required as well.

Paramedics should be graduates of a CAHEP-accredited school of emergency medical technology and should have passed the National Registry of Emergency Medical Technicians Board examination. In states not requiring the National Registry examination, passage of a designated state examination may demonstrate equivalent knowledge. Most institutions offering paramedic education have adopted the 1999 version of the DOT curriculum, which significantly increases the breadth and depth of required material. As a result, many institutions have begun offering associate degrees. These programs are generally similar to associate degree programs in nursing but with an emphasis on high-acuity patients. Graduates of programs of less than 1000 to 1200 hours may have significant gaps in knowledge.

A few programs around the country now offer bachelor's and master's degrees in emergency health sciences. These programs provide a solid basic education but also prepare their graduates to assume positions of leadership in the EMS community. Some curricula include a Critical Care Paramedic course. When combined with a clinical rotation or internship, that course prepares the paramedic to provide advanced and critical-care assessments and treatments during patient transports. It also provides classes in education and management.

Standard of Care

Members of the medical flight team should be held to a very high standard. The responsibility for setting standards and making sure personnel meet those standards falls to both the medical director and the program director.

The medical flight team is often called on to manage difficult patients who have not yet been stabilized by other medical personnel. This may mean managing patients with difficult airways, starting IVs on patients with whom others have been unsuccessful, and stabilizing patients who have been refractor to prior attempts. This level of performance requires high-quality personnel with high-quality training.

Flight nursing and flight paramedicine are beginning to be recognized as specialty practice areas that are very different from emergency nursing and field paramedicine. As a result, specialty certification examinations have been written for these two fields. These exams test knowledge in flight physiology, emergency medicine, and critical-care medicine.

The Core Medical Team

The core medical team is the group of medical care providers who consistently fly aboard the aircraft. They are the heart of the flight program. As time aboard the aircraft increases, so does familiarity with both routine and nonroutine procedures. There should be at least one member of the core medical team aboard each flight. Having someone who is thoroughly familiar with the aircraft and with safety procedures adds a measure of consistency and minimizes the risk of safety violations and equipment mishandling.

Specialty Care Teams

Some programs employ a fixed combination of personnel for all patient types, and others vary crew composition when specialty-care patients are being transported. For example, there may be a neonatal transport team, a pediatric transport team, an adult transport team, and a balloon pump transport team (Figure 7-4). The use of specialty teams ensures

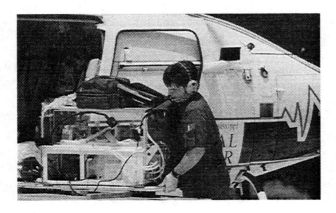

FIGURE 7-4
Neonatal transport team with isolette

that personnel are familiar with the patient type being transported and with any specialty care equipment that may be associated with that patient type.

However, care should be exercised when considering specialty care staffing, which has disadvantages as well as advantages. The foremost concern is lack of familiarity with safety procedures and equipment. In the aircraft environment everyone has two roles, patient care and safety. New people cannot perform the safety function because they are unfamiliar with it. Worse, those who fly only occasionally may be distracted by the aircraft and scenery and have difficulty concentrating on patient assessment and care. The background noise produced by the aircraft and the headset/helmets are also impediments for those unaccustomed to their use.

Specialty care teams may not fully appreciate the public relations and marketing role played by the flight program. Occasional fliers may not be as concerned with maintaining good relations and may inadvertently compromise a relationship that has taken the core team a long time to develop.

Members of specialty care teams should be required to undergo a thorough orientation before being allowed to fly in a recurring role. This orientation should be similar to that required of the core medical team and should include the complete safety training program.

Specialty care teams that fly frequently will overcome these weaknesses and concerns, while those that fly only occasionally may not. In any case there should always be one member of the core team aboard the aircraft during any patient transport to ensure consistency, proper operation of equipment, and adherence to safety procedures.

Medical Directors

Medical directors are the physicians who provide medical insight and oversight to the program. Their input may be in the form of planning, direct involvement, radio or telephone consultation, and retrospective analysis. Medical direction is covered in more detail in Chapter 12.

Administrators/Managers

Administrators/managers are responsible for goal setting, planning, operation, and oversight. Most flight programs employ a program director who oversees all aspects of the program. That person is typically the link between the air medical program and outside entities, including upper-level administration, the news media, outreach groups, and so on. An important role of the program director is to insulate the flight team from nonmedical distractions such as budget woes and medical politics. Administration is covered more thoroughly in Chapter 2.

Recruiting and Hiring

There is a relatively small pool of experienced air medical personnel, both medical and operational, from which to hire. When a program needs new or replacement team members, the program director must decide the value of experience. Recruiting seasoned personnel may require advertising regionally or nationally, paying travel expenses, and in some cases paying relocation expenses. The other option is to hire local people who may lack flight experience but may otherwise be well qualified. The best option may depend on the stage of development of the program. Programs just getting established would be wise to recruit at least a few key people in both operational and medical areas who have air medical experience. Those employees can provide valuable insight as the program develops and be available to mentor other less experienced personnel.

Well-established programs, on the other hand, may prefer to hire local people with more generic experience. There is generally a large pool of eager applicants, typically high achievers who are ambitious and looking for more autonomy. New hires can be put through an in-depth orientation program that includes ride-along time with experienced personnel. At the end of the orientation the program has employees who have been trained to meet the specific needs of the program. However, even in well-established programs the occasional hiring of an experienced outsider can "shake things up" and bring new ideas and new options that can lead to improvements.

Pilots and Aviation Technicians

Pilots may be required to attend ground and simulator training to orient them to the specific aircraft. They must also accumulate a specified number of flight hours in that aircraft type and in the local flying area. Even pilots with prior air medical experience should go through a program-specific air medicine orientation program before being placed on shift.

Aviation technicians should be similarly prepared. They are generally required to attend a lengthy program to orient them to the specific aircraft for which they will be responsible. The value of this training cannot be overemphasized. It is essential that technicians are qualified and confident in their own abilities.

Medical Personnel

Once hired, air medical team members are typically required to complete an extensive orientation program that includes didactic and clinical components and introduces the specialized skills necessary to meet the needs of the high-acuity and complex medical patients routinely encountered by the flight team. Since most programs do not include a physician in the crew, this training may include expanded-scope knowledge and skills and is a crucial step in the preparation of a credible team member. When nonphysician personnel become proficient in performing complex medical procedures, the distinction between physician and nonphysician crew members diminishes significantly.

The orientation program should be tailored to match the role of the flight team. If a big part of program activities involves scene flights, the orientation should include an overview of prehospital operations. Nursing personnel may have little or no experience with out-of-hospital medicine and may require a significant amount of instruction and ride-along time before they can function as independent team members.

Paramedics, on the other hand, generally have little critical-care experience and require extensive orientation in assessing and managing those types of patients. Rotations through the cardiac, medical, surgical, pediatric, and neonatal intensive care units may provide necessary hands-on experience. All medical personnel, regardless of background or experience, should be required to spend time in the operating room performing difficult intubations, an important role in almost all flight programs.

Part-Time Personnel

The use of part-time personnel is a common practice in business and industry, especially where there is a shortage of qualified personnel. It is also a common practice in the health care setting. Many air medical programs employ part-time pilots, aircraft technicians, and medical providers. As long as part-time people can work often enough to maintain their skills, this is an acceptable practice. However, in many AM programs the volume is barely adequate to maintain proficiency in full-time personnel and generally inadequate for part-time personnel. In those cases either the use of part-time people should be discouraged or there should be a mandatory recurrent training program for infrequent fliers.

How many flights does one need to make to gain and maintain an adequate experience and competence level? While the number may vary depending on the experience and retention capabilities of the individual, eight flights spread over a month is a reasonable minimum number.

Less than that and procedures will be forgotten and skills will erode. If part-time or full-time personnel do not make at least that many flights each month, they should be encouraged (or required) to participate in a skills maintenance program.

Technical Standards

Flight personnel must work in an environment that is sometimes very demanding. Patients range in size and weight from small and light to large and very heavy. Regardless of size and weight, they must be efficiently loaded and unloaded, sometimes in aircraft that are small and cramped. Patients sometimes become violent and must be restrained. The performance of medical techniques such as endotracheal intubation requires a certain amount of forearm strength. To ensure that employees are capable of performing these tasks, many programs set technical standards that applicants must meet to be considered for employment. These standards may include lifting strength, visual and hearing acuity, and the ability to perform complex tasks in limited spaces.

For safety reasons, all helicopters have maximum gross weight limitations and aircraft components have structural limits. Exceeding those limits may result in component failure and loss of control, which may lead to a crash. The FAA prohibits pilots from operating an aircraft that exceeds its rated maximum gross weight.

Many programs limit the quantity of supplies and equipment carried aboard the aircraft. Medical crew members may add an extra bag of IV fluid or an extra splint. After all, one little bag of fluid is of little significance. However, over time other crew members add items of their own, and the cumulative weight can become significant. Since the pilot is not aware of the gradual weight increase, weight and balance calculations may be erroneous and the aircraft may exceed maximum gross weight limitations. All crew members should take the beginning-of-shift check sheets seriously and adhere strictly to the requirements.

Another common practice for controlling total weight is to establish maximum body weight limits for crew members. This practice has nothing to do with discrimination against heavy applicants. It is necessary to allow a margin of safety so that the aircraft can transport one or more heavy patients without exceeding weight limitations and compromising safety. For a program with one pilot and a medical crew of two, reducing body weight by 10 pounds per person results in a 30-pound increase in payload. That could mean the difference between being able to transport a large patient and having to decline the flight because of the weight limitation. (Even when personnel weight limits are implemented, some patients must be transported by ground because they are too heavy or too large to transport by air.) The desire to join an air medical team has provided many nurses and paramedics with the motivation to lose weight.

Duty Time

Pilots

In the early days of air medicine, rotor-wing pilots commonly worked shifts of 24 or more hours. Following a rash of incidents and accidents caused by judgment errors resulting from pilot fatigue, the FAA set strict regulations limiting pilot duty times. These regulations address both shift length and the number of hours that a pilot may actually fly during each shift. A pilot may be on duty for up to 14 hours—not 14 hours of continuous flying, but 14 hours of being on duty and available for a flight. Actual flight time is limited to 8 hours per shift. If a pilot reaches the maximum number of hours, he is required to ground himself. The regulation also requires a minimum of 8 hours of uninterrupted rest between shifts.

This regulation has serious implications for air medical operations, especially those operating only one aircraft. It requires a backup plan for relieving a pilot who reaches the maximum number of hours during a shift. For example, a pilot who is working a 12-hour day shift is dispatched on several flights and accumulates 7 hours of flight time by midafternoon. At that point he is limited to 1 more hour of flight time for the remainder of the shift. If a flight is dispatched that is longer than an hour, the pilot has no choice but to decline the flight. Most programs handle the situation by having a relief pilot come in early. Occasionally the relief pilot also has a busy shift and requires relief. Although that rarely occurs, it does happen. In that case a third pilot must be called on to prevent the primary pilots from violating FAA regulations.

Another potential problem area involves the 14-hour limit on shift length. A pilot who reaches that limit is expected to ground the aircraft at the time the limit is met. For example, a pilot who is working an 07:00 to 19:00 shift is dispatched on a long-distance neonatal flight at 17:30. According to the FAA regulation the pilot must complete the flight by 21:00. If the medical team takes longer than anticipated to stabilize the patient and prepare for transport and the pilot is unable to complete the flight by 21:00, he is expected to decline the flight and wait for a relief pilot to come and retrieve the aircraft.

There is one way to legally avoid this problem, but the FAA frowns upon it and it should rarely, if ever, be used. The *sliding shift method* allows the pilot to push shift times forward by up to 2 hours, thereby allowing rest time to be uninterrupted and minimizing the number of hours worked during the next shift. This practice requires extensive paperwork and can cause problems if the next shift is also busy and requires pilot relief. Most programs prefer to avoid this option except in exceptional circumstances.

Aviation Technicians

The important role aviation technicians play in an air medical program cannot be overstated. They are responsible for the mechanical integrity and safety of the aircraft. They literally disassemble and reassemble much of the aircraft as they go through repair and maintenance procedures. Taking an aircraft out of operation for an extended period of time can cost a program significant income, so technicians are often under pressure to complete their work quickly. That pressure may be externally applied or self-imposed and can mean working for long periods of time without rest. Mental acuity is just as important for aviation technicians as it is for pilots. A single mistake may compromise the aircraft's operating capability or make it unsafe.

The FAA does not regulate the shift and duty time of aircraft technicians, although such an action appears to be on the horizon. The CAMTS recently endorsed a proposal that would limit shift time to 14 hours. While that is a reasonable first step, the regulation should also factor in activity level and mandatory rest periods as the FAA has with pilots. A technician who is on duty for 14 hours performing light maintenance or paperwork may be safe to complete an additional procedure. However, a technician who has been struggling with a difficult engine change for 8 hours may be fatigued both mentally and physically to the point where work quality may suffer.

One solution to this problem is to require an informal evaluation of the technician's fatigue level after 12 hours of duty time. The pilot meets with the technician to determine his general mental status. The pilot then communicates with the program director, and the two decide whether the technician is able to continue working. While this may not be scientifically based, it does serve to make the technician evaluate his fatigue level and allows someone not immediately involved with the work to give an opinion.

Medical Team

Duty time may also be a factor for the medical team. Evidence suggests that judgment and skills begin to deteriorate after 10 or 12 hours of work time. However, the degree of degradation depends on workload and whether or not team members rest during the course of the shift.

Many programs have abandoned 24-hour work shifts in favor of shorter 8- or 12-hour shifts. While this may add to personnel costs, it may reduce fatigue-induced errors.

Continuing Education

Continuing education is important for all health care providers, but especially for members of a flight team, who deal with the sickest patients under less than ideal conditions. Their assessment and management skills must be up to date and well honed. Hospital-based flight programs are generally associated with larger, more progressive medical institutions, teaching institutions, and tertiary care facilities. These institutions are often hubs for the proliferation of new medical information, and keeping current is relatively easy. Health care providers at referring hospitals and prehospital personnel look to AM teams for new knowledge and skills. It is essential that they are active in teaching, research, and other activities that keep them on the front lines of emergency and critical-care medicine.

Summary

Personnel associated with an air medical program include pilots, aviation technicians, and various medical personnel. The quality of the program is directly linked to the quality and development of the personnel it employs. Demand for flight positions is generally very high, and those doing the hiring can afford to be very selective. Pilots are responsible for aircraft operation and for the safety of the aircraft and all passengers during flight. Pilots are required to gain proficiency in a number of skills as part of their education/training process. Aviation technicians perform all maintenance and repair activities on the aircraft. To be licensed these individuals are required to complete extensive education and work-related requirements.

Composition of the medical team may vary among programs. Physicians, registered nurses, EMT-Paramedics, and respiratory therapists are all commonly utilized by air medical programs. Programs utilizing smaller aircraft may staff only one medical caregiver. However, programs utilizing midsized and larger aircraft typically operate with a team of two. The most common configuration is registered nurse/EMT-Paramedic. Some programs vary team composition according to the type of patient being transported. For example, a specialty team my be used for neonatal, pediatric, or obstetric patients. Regardless of team composition, the medical flight team must be highly motivated and highly trained. Training must include aircraft operation, safety, and all other activities specific to the aircraft environment.

REVIEW QUESTIONS

1. Highly trained professionals who operate airplanes and helicopters to carry out a wide variety of tasks.
   - **a.** Pilots
   - **b.** Paramedics
   - **c.** Nurses
   - **d.** Aviation technicians

2. Those persons who are responsible for maintaining and making repairs to aircraft.
   - **a.** Pilots
   - **b.** Paramedics
   - **c.** Nurses
   - **d.** Aviation technicians

3. Discuss education and certification options that may be required when hiring individuals to become part of the air medical team.

4. When hiring part-time personnel it is important that the individuals hired:
   - **a.** Work frequently enough to maintain their knowledge and skills
   - **b.** Work only infrequently so as not to take time away from full-time personnel
   - **c.** Be hired only if members of the local union
   - **d.** Are not employed elsewhere so they can be avilable at all times

5. What type of orientation should be provided when hiring a new flight nurse or flight paramedic?
   - **a.** These people have completed a comprehensive education program and no additional orientation is required
   - **b.** An extensive orientation program that includes didactic and clinical components and introduces the specialized skills necessary to meet the needs of the high-acuity and complex medical patients routinely encountered by the flight team
   - **c.** A brief orientation to cover aircraft operations
   - **d.** A brief orientation to FAA rules and regulations

Aircraft and
Equipment

Upon completing this chapter, the reader should have a better understanding of the following topics:

* Desirable characteristics of a rotor-wing air ambulance

* Different types of aircraft and the pros and cons of each

* Rotor-wing aircraft most commonly used for air medical transport

* Equipment commonly carried aboard the rotor-wing air ambulance

KEY TERMS

avionics, p. 110

night vision, p. 111

night vision goggles (NVG), p. 111

Introduction

The most visible and important component of an air medical program is the aircraft itself. All other program activities center around it. The capabilities and reliability of the aircraft determine the capabilities and reliability of the entire program. Selection of a new aircraft should be done in a deliberate and systematic manner. Not only the long-term viability of the flight program but the very lives of crew members depend on the reliability of this piece of equipment.

The ideal medical helicopter has a large cabin, minimal maintenance requirements, a fast cruise speed, and a range of more than 350 miles. It produces minimal noise, has a very high useful load, is economical to operate, and is absolutely safe. Unfortunately, the ideal helicopter has not yet been developed. While a number of commercially available aircraft meet some of these criteria, none meets them all. For that reason each AM program should carefully select its aircraft according to its own specific needs.

- Programs operating in areas where low visibility is a problem should choose IFR-equipped aircraft.
- Programs operating in rural areas where long-distance transports are common should choose an aircraft with extended fuel range.
- Programs serving referral hospitals with small or limited-access helipads should choose an aircraft capable of landing in a relatively small area (small footprint).
- Programs that perform many critical-care transports should have an aircraft with a cabin large enough for the medical team and the necessary equipment.

Generally, the more of these criteria the aircraft meets, the more expensive it becomes. Since cost is nearly always a factor, the end product often represents a compromise between the ideal and the affordable. For example, a large aircraft is desirable if critical-care interhospital transports will comprise most of the program's activity. However, as aircraft get larger, they also become dramatically more expensive to purchase and to operate. Whereas the ideal aircraft in this case may be an S-76 or a Bell 214, the program may settle for a BK-117 or a Bell 430 and realize significant cost savings.

Programs with a mixed-mission profile may be forced to select an aircraft that is not ideal for any single mission type but that performs adequately in all categories. A program that performs critical-care transports and also makes scene calls may want an aircraft that is smaller than ideal for critical-care transports and larger than ideal for scene flights, but capable of performing adequately in both roles. Many scene-landing areas are small, and a large aircraft may have a hard time finding an area large enough to land in.

Another factor that must be considered in many urban areas is noise. A hospital-based program located in a residential area will usually want a low-noise aircraft with plenty of power to allow it to attain altitude quickly and minimize the disturbance to residents.

Aircraft Commonly Used for Air Medical Transport

A number of helicopters have been adopted for air medical use (Table 8-1). Historically, the first modern aircraft modified for continuous medical use was the Bell 47, the bubble-windowed helicopter made popular by the M*A*S*H movie and television series. That aircraft was little more than a motorized frame with a small cockpit for the pilot. Stretchers were attached to the skids on the outside of the aircraft, and patients were strapped to the stretchers and transported without benefit of medical care. Fortunately, significant advances have been made in aircraft design and technology over the last 50 years, and even the cheapest modern medical helicopter is a vast improvement over the Bell 47. However, that venerable aircraft must be acknowledged for the important role it played at the time. There are still many Bell 47s flying today, primarily as crop dusters and recreational aircraft.

Table 8-1 Helicopters Most Commonly Used for Air Medicine in the United States

Aircraft Type	Number of U.S. Programs Using	Percent of U.S. Programs Using
American Eurocopter BK-117	63	25%
American Eurocopter AS 350	29	11%
American Eurocopter BO-105	27	11%
Bell 222	25	10%
American Eurocopter EC-135	23	9%
Bell 206	23	9%
Augusta 109	17	7%
Sikorsky S-76	13	5%
American Eurocopter AS 365	10	4%
Bell 412	9	4%
Bell 230	8	3%
American Eurocopter EC-130	3	1%
American Eurocopter AS 355	3	1%
McDonnell Douglas MD-900	2	1%
Bell 212	1	0%

Source: FlightWeb AMT Registry
http://www.flightweb.com/AMT-Registry/index.php

Modern air medical helicopters are a marvel of technology. They are powered by turbine engines that are compact, light, and very powerful. For example, the engine in the Augusta 119 (Koala) weighs less than 200 pounds, produces more than 1000 horsepower, and is remarkably reliable.

The **avionics,** or electronics, used in more expensive AM helicopters are similar in design and sophistication to those used in commercial airliners. Many twin-engine aircraft (and a few single-engine) are instrument-flight-rated (IFR) and fully capable of flying in limited-visibility conditions. They have all the necessary instruments to bypass bad weather, make instrument approaches to airports, and fly safely in otherwise unsafe conditions. For example, with the global positioning satellite (GPS) coupled autopilot, the pilot programs a course and the aircraft will fly multiple legs and change direction as necessary to maintain that course. Color weather radar helps the pilot identify and fly around areas of bad weather. A recent development allows helicopters to fly directly to their landing pads using specialized GPS devices.

It must be noted, however, that these avionics devices are very expensive and that not all programs have access to this technology. Some programs fly only under visual flight rule (VFR) conditions, when visibility meets certain minimum requirements. In parts of the country where fog and low ceilings are not generally a problem, these programs can have a very high mission-completion rate.

Some of the aircraft that are widely used in the United States are discussed in detail below.

avionics
The electronic devices a pilot utilizes to set and maintain altitude and direction during flight.

Augusta A-109

The A-109 is a sleek and fast midsized twin-engine aircraft. It is currently available in two models, the A-109 Power and the A-109 K-2. The A-109 Power is equipped with two Pratt & Whitney 206C or two Turbomeca Arrius 2K1 engines controlled by a full-authority digital-engine control system (FADEC). It features a main rotor head constructed of titanium, with elastomeric bearings and blade grips. The blades are made of composite material. Improved aerodynamics and digitally controlled engines have reduced fuel consumption and increased range and payload. The pilot workload has also been reduced by digital avionics.

Large available space, easy access to the cabin, and a functional layout all allow a rapid role change from passenger transport to air medical configuration. As an air ambulance, the aircraft may be configured with one or two litters, two medical attendants, and two pilots. The cabin width allows easy movement between two stretchers placed lengthwise and offers total body access to the patients. The copilot seat is reversible for an additional medical attendant.

Entry and exit are made convenient by the large flush sliding doors on either side of the fuselage and the low level of the floor. The interior layout allows for the installation of all the medical equipment required for in-flight primary care of the patient. Standard equipment rails are installed on the rear bulkhead and on the two upper side panels. Distribution outlets for oxygen, air, vacuum, and electrical supply are also routinely provided in the ambulance configuration.

In its standard configuration the aircraft seats eight people, including one pilot. In air medical configuration it can transport two patients and up to three medical attendants. When two stretchers are in use, two medical attendants is more reasonable. Tall personnel may have difficulty in the A-109 as the patient compartment has a relatively low ceiling.

The A-109 K2 differs from the A-109 Power only in its engines and avionics. It is powered by two Turbomeca Arriel-1K1 engines, each generating maximum takeoff 771 shp. This ship was engineered to provide improved performance at high altitudes and in hot temperatures. It also allows for an improved margin of safety during single-engine operation. Available options include a searchlight and an instrument panel compatible with third-generation **night-vision goggles (NVG)** to improve **night vision.** Augusta A-109 K2's are already operating in mountainous areas of the United States, Europe, and Japan, and in the hot climates of Latin America and the Persian Gulf.

Augusta A-119 (Koala)

Introduced in 2001, the Koala is billed as the largest single-engine helicopter intended for EMS operations (Figure 8-1). The aircraft was certified in 1998 and deliveries began in 2000. It was designed for a range of

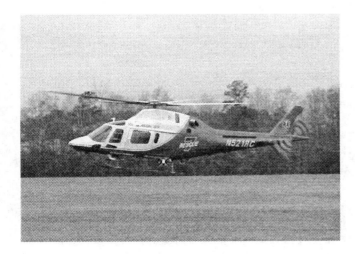

FIGURE 8-1
An A-119
Courtesy of Chuck Carter

Aircraft and Equipment   111

activities for which a single makes more economic sense than a twin. The Koala's big selling feature is its large "wide-body" fuselage. Augusta states that the cabin is 30 percent larger than that of any other single-engine helicopter in current production. The aircraft is large enough to accommodate two stretcher patients side by side and two medical personnel. Most other single-engine helicopters are equipped for a single stretcher because of limited space. The Koala has two large sliding doors, one on either side of the fuselage. As another bonus, the baggage compartment in the rear of the fuselage is accessible during flight.

The Koala features both an attractive price and a low cost of ownership. It takes advantage of many of the technologies developed for the A-109, including a main rotor head in titanium with composite blade grips and elastomeric bearings. This arrangement provides the benefits of a fully articulated rotor system while significantly reducing the weight of the rotor head and reducing maintenance requirements. The Koala is also equipped with a full complement of avionics designed to reduce the pilot's workload.

American Eurocopter AS-332 (Super Puma)

The Super Puma (Figure 8-2) is a twin-engine, medium-weight helicopter that makes extensive use of cutting-edge safety features. This is the only helicopter in the world that is certified without restriction for flight during icing conditions. It is one of the largest aircraft used for air medical purposes. However, because of its size and considerable cost, few of these aircraft are used in an exclusive air medical role. In its normal passenger configuration, it can transport up to 24 passengers. In air medical configuration, up to 6 patients and 3 or 4 medical attendants may be transported. The Super Puma is used in Australia and Europe more than in the United States.

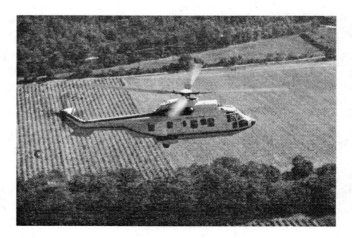

FIGURE 8-2
An AS-332
Courtesy of American Eurocopter

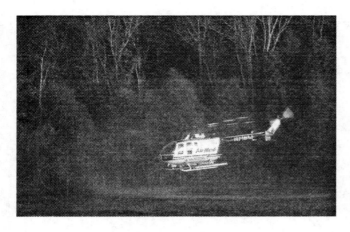

FIGURE 8-3
A BO-105
Courtesy of American Eurocopter

American Eurocopter BO-105

The BO-105 is a five-place, multipurpose, light-utility helicopter (Figure 8-3). Considered one of the most successful helicopter designs, it made its debut in 1964 and is widely used in both military and civilian settings. The most recent version is the CBS model, which has a fuselage 25 cm (10 inches) longer than its predecessor's and an extra window. It has a rigid rotor system that requires relatively little maintenance.

The BO-105 has a reputation for being a workhorse. It is reliable and takes abuse without complaint. However, the rigid rotor system produces a somewhat rougher ride than a similar aircraft with flexible rotor systems might. The aircraft also has a tendency to produce notable transitional shudder on final approach for landing. The shudder can be so pronounced as to cause anxiety in conscious patients. Some programs using this aircraft routinely warn patients ahead of time.

In standard passenger configuration this aircraft seats five, including two pilots or one pilot and a passenger in the front bucket seats and three passengers on a rear bench seat. In air medical configuration it transports two patients and one or two medical personnel. Access to the rear of the aircraft is limited during flight. The "tunnel" prevents accessing a patient's abdomen and lower extremities during flight. With its reasonable cost, low maintenance, and reliability, the BO-105 is a very popular air medical helicopter.

American Eurocopter AS-350 (A Star)

The A Star is a light-duty, general-purpose helicopter that is durable and reliable. The cabin is relatively wide and there is no midpost as in the Bell 206, with which it is often compared. The unobstructed cabin allows for easier movement and less restricted patient access. However,

Aircraft and Equipment   113

the cabin is somewhat shorter than in the 206, and the stretcher system extends from the front of the cabin nearly all the way to the rear, making it cramped for the attendant sitting at the head of the patient. The aircraft provides a relatively quiet and smooth ride.

The first commercially successful model was the AS-350. That model has since been replaced by the AS-350 B2, which has a more powerful Turbomeca Arriel 1D1 engine. The B2 has become popular because of its strong engine performance and excellent reliability. It has ample power for a patient and three medical attendants. Patient weight is almost never a factor; patient girth is more likely to halt a flight. A B3 model, recommended for hot and high environments, is also available.

The A Star cabin allows for one stretcher patient mounted lengthwise along the left side of the aircraft. One attendant can sit at the head of the stretcher. The aircraft is wide enough to hold two additional attendants. Several vendors offer an adjustable attendant seat, which is normally positioned at the side of the patient. Some vendors offer a second litter option, but it is stacked above the primary litter and access is limited. That arrangement also eliminates the attendant who would otherwise sit at the head of the primary patient.

American Eurocopter AS-355 (Twin Star)

The AS-355N is the latest twin-engine version of the A Star family. It is basically an A Star fitted with two Turbomeca Arriel 1A engines and a FADEC system. Its design makes use of composite materials. The cabin is similar to that of the AS-350 model in size and shape. The Twin Star is often an upgrade for programs that have used the A Star and like its design but want to add the redundancy and additional power of a second engine.

American Eurocopter AS-365N (Dauphin)

The AS-365N2 is a medium-weight multipurpose twin-engine helicopter (Figure 8-4). In addition to technological innovations (main and rear rotor blades made of composite materials, tail rotor built in the fin), the reliability and availability of this helicopter are highly valued worldwide. It is equipped with two Turbomeca Arriel 1C2 engines that offer excellent performance.

The AS-365N Dauphin 2, a twin-engine midsized utility helicopter, is one of Eurocopter's most successful designs and has found widespread use in corporate, police, media, EMS, and search-and-rescue roles worldwide. The AS-365N is a much-improved development of the original SA-365C

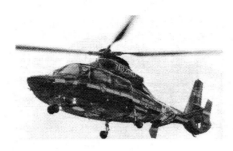

An AS-365N2
Courtesy of American Eurocopter

Dauphin 2. (Until January 1990 AS-365 models were designated SA-365. In 1992 Aerospatiale's helicopter division was incorporated into Eurocopter.) The AS-365N introduced more powerful Arriel 1C turboshafts, enlarged tail surfaces, revised transmission, main rotor, rotor mast fairing and engine cowling, and retractable tricycle undercarriage. The AS-365N first flew in March 1979, and deliveries began in early 1982. Deliveries of the improved AS-365N2 began in 1990. It features upgraded Arriel 1C2 engines, improved gearbox, increased maximum takeoff weight, redesigned cabin doors, revised interior, and optional EFIS instrumentation. The AS-365N3 was fitted with FADEC-equipped Arriel 2Cs engines designed to perform at high altitude and in hot environmental conditions. Deliveries began in December 1998.

The improved EC-155 (initially AS-365N4) features twin Arriel 2Cs equipped with FADEC, a five-blade Spheriflex main rotor, and bulged doors that help provide a 40 percent increase in main cabin size (Figure 8-5). Its first flight was in June 1997, and French and German certification was awarded in December 1998. Table 8-2 compares the AS-365N2 and the EC-155.

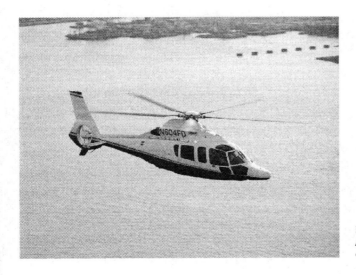

An EC-155
Courtesy of American Eurocopter

Aircraft and Equipment

Table 8-2 Comparison of AS-365N2 and EC-155

	AS-365N2	EC-155
Power plants	Two 550 kW (739 shp) Turbomeca Arriel 1C2 turboshafts driving a four-blade main rotor and Fenestron shrouded tail rotor.	Two 635 kW (851 shp) takeoff rated Arriel 2Cs driving a five-blade main rotor and Fenestron shrouded tail rotor.
Performance	Max cruising speed 154 kt, economical cruising speed 140 kt. Initial rate of climb 1380 ft./min. Hovering ceiling in ground effect 8365 ft., out of ground effect 5905 ft. Range with standard fuel 485 nm.	Max cruising speed at sea level 142 kt, economical cruising speed at sea level 136 kt.
Weights	Empty 2240 kg (4940 lb.), maximum takeoff 4250 kg (9370 lb.).	Empty 2353 kg (5187 lb), maximum takeoff 4800 kg (10,582 lb.).
Dimensions	Main rotor diameter 11.94 m (39 ft. 2 in.), length overall rotor turning 13.68 m (44 ft. 11 in.), height 3.98 m (13 ft. 1 in.). Main rotor disc area 111.9 sq. m (1205 sq. ft.).	Main rotor diameter 12.60 m (41 ft. 4 in.), length overall rotor turning 14.43 m (47 ft. 4 in.), fuselage length 12.70 m (41 ft. 8 in.), height 4.35 m (14 ft. 3 in.). Main rotor disc area 124.7 sq. m (1342.1 sq. ft.).
Capacity	One pilot (VFR) or two pilots (IFR), and maximum seating for 13 passengers (with one pilot). Standard passenger seating for eight or nine.	Standard seating for 14 including one or two pilots. Most recent model (EC-155) transports two patients and a medical crew of two or three.

American Eurocopter BK-117

The BK-117 is the most widely used EMS helicopter (Figure 8-6). It combines a relatively large patient compartment with good reliability and economy. It was developed as a collaborative effort between MBB of Germany (now part of Eurocopter) and Kawasaki of Japan, and the first production model (the BK-117 A1) was delivered in 1983. An updated model, the BK-117 A3, with higher maximum takeoff weight, was certified in March 1985. The BK-117 A4 was introduced in 1987. It features increased transmission performance, an improved tail rotor, and increased fuel capacity. The BK-117 B1, also certified in 1987, has more powerful engines and better performance. The BK-117 B2 is currently in production and has an increased maximum takeoff weight. The BK-117

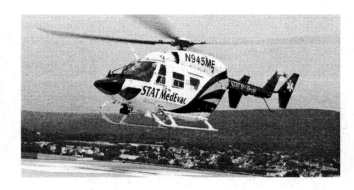

FIGURE 8-6
A BK-117
Courtesy of American Eurocopter

C1 is a German development with Turbomeca Arriel engines. The BK-117 C2 is currently under development and makes use of new avionics.

The BK-117 has a rear-loading configuration. Its rear "clamshell" doors open directly into the patient care compartment. The aircraft offers good size and patient access and can transport two stretcher patients and a medical crew of two. Table 8-3 compares the BK-117 A and B2.

Table 8-3	Statistics, American Eurocopter BK-117 A and BK-117 B2	
	BK-117 A	**BK-117 B2**
Maximum cruise speed	143 kt	134 kt
Initial rate of climb	1970 ft./min.	1900 ft./min.
Hovering ceiling out of ground effect	13,450 ft.	7500 ft.
Range with maximum payload	295 nm	With standard fuel tank 290 nm; with internal long-range fuel tank 381 nm
Maximum payload	3350 lb.	3846 lb.
Capacity	One pilot and seating for a maximum of 10 passengers.	In its EMS configuration the aircraft is capable of transporting two patients and a medical crew of two or three.

Aircraft and Equipment 117

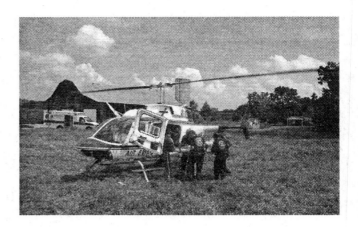

FIGURE 8-7
A Bell 206L4
Courtesy of Sheldon Cohen/Bell Helicopter

Bell 206L

The Bell 206L (LongRanger) is one of the most widely used helicopters in production (Figure 8-7). With its reasonable operating costs and low maintenance requirements, it is very popular in air medical configuration and with law enforcement agencies. The 206L is a descendant of the 206B, a shorter, five-place aircraft whose smaller space made patient access difficult and limited the medical crew to one.

The 206L offers a lengthened cabin and more powerful engine. In its normal configuration it has seating for seven. In air ambulance configuration it accommodates two stretchers and up to two medical attendants. The second patient is mounted on a rack above the primary patient. Access to both patients may be difficult, and the transport of two critical patients is not recommended.

Subsequent versions have been the 206L1 LongRanger II, introduced in 1978, the 206L3 LongRanger III, and the current 206L4 Long-Ranger IV, introduced in 1992. Each new version has featured a more powerful engine and other technical improvements.

The LongRanger was one of the most widely used single-engine air medical craft in the 1970s and 1980s. Older models (L1s and L2s) were very weight sensitive, and crew and patient weight were often limiting factors in transports. The L3 and L4 models have more power and are better suited for medical use.

Bell 212

The Model 212 is a medium-lift twin-engine helicopter. Bell announced its decision to develop the Model 212 in early May 1968 largely in response to a Canadian Armed Forces requirement for a twin-engine version of the CUH1H (Model 205), then entering military service in that country, and following successful negotiations with Pratt & Whitney Canada and the Canadian government. Development of the Model 212 was a joint venture between Bell, Pratt & Whitney Canada, and the Canadian government, the latter providing financial support. The resulting helicopter (designated CUH1N in Canadian and UH1N in U.S. military service) first flew in 1969 and was granted commercial certification in October 1970. The first commercial deliveries occurred in 1971.

The most significant feature of the 212 was the PT6T Twin-Pac engine installation. This consisted of two PT6 turboshafts mounted side by side and driving a single output shaft via a combining gearbox. The most obvious benefit of the new arrangement was better performance because of the unit's increased power output. However, the Twin-Pac engine system offered a major advantage in the event of engine failure: sensors in the gearbox would instruct the remaining operating engine to develop full power, thus providing a true engine out capability, even at maximum takeoff weight. These aircraft were widely used in the Vietnam War for troop transport, cargo movement, and air medical transport. Total seating capacity was 15, including 1 or 2 pilots.

Bell 214ST

The 214ST is Bell's largest helicopter. Although it shares a number with the 214 Huey Plus, the Bell 214ST is a much larger aircraft. It was developed to deliver better performance in hot and high environments. The 214ST features two General Electric CT7 turboshafts, a stretched fuselage seating up to 17 in the main cabin, glass-fiber main rotor blades, and lubrication-free elastomeric bearings in the main rotor hub. The ST suffix originally stood for Stretched Twin, reflecting the changes over the 214, but this was later changed to stand for Super Transporter. The 214ST first flew in February 1977. One hundred of the helicopters were built between 1980 and 1990. In passenger configuration this aircraft seats 2 pilots and up to 17 passengers. In air medical configuration 2 stretchers can be easily accommodated along with a medical crew of 3 or 4. In mass casualty configuration as many as 8 stretchers may be mounted.

Bell 222

The Bell 222 is a twin-engine light-utility helicopter widely used for corporate and air medical transport. Bell announced development of the 222 in 1974, following the positive response generated by a mock-up proposal displayed at that year's Helicopter Association of America convention. Taking note of potential customers' preferences and suggestions, Bell modified its design accordingly, and the subsequent development effort led to the Model 222's first flight in August 1976. A number of advanced features were designed into the 222, including the Noda Matic vibration reduction system developed for the 214ST, stub wings housing the retractable undercarriage, provision for IFR avionics, and dual hydraulic and electrical systems.

The 222 was awarded FAA certification in December 1979. Production deliveries began in 1980. Subsequent development led to the more powerful 222B, with a larger-diameter main rotor, and the 222UT (Utility Twin), which replaced the retractable wheels with fixed landing gear.

The 222 brought a new level of aerodynamics and flight stability to the helicopter market. Because of its inherently stable flight characteristics, the 222 was the first helicopter certified for single-pilot IFR without an autopilot. Bell produced 184 of these aircraft.

Bell 230

The Bell 230 was the successor to the 222, with Allison 250 turboshafts replacing the LTS 101 engines (Figure 8-8). The first flight of a 230 took place in August 1991. The aircraft was delivered with either skids or retractable wheels. The wheeled version yields greater speed but at the cost of the auxiliary fuel tanks normally mounted in the sponsons. The skidded version decreases cruise speed by 2 to 3 knots but adds approximately 84 nm of range. In the wheeled version the 230 has a cruise speed of 141 knots and a range of 301 nm. With skids, the range increases to 385 nm and the cruise speed decreases to 139 knots.

In passenger configuration the 230 accommodates one pilot and seven passengers. In air medical configuration it is capable of transport-

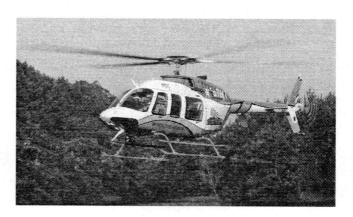

FIGURE 8-8
A Bell 230
Courtesy of Sheldon Cohen/Bell Helicopter

ing one patient and up to four medical personnel or two patients and two medical personnel. The Bell 230 is a desirable air medical platform because of its relatively low cost of purchase and maintenance and fairly roomy, quiet interior. For those operating in hot climates, the 230 has an exceptional air-conditioning system. A total of 38 230s were produced, the last delivered in 1995.

Bell 407

The Bell 407 is the successor to very successful 206B (Jet Ranger) and 206L (LongRanger) light singles (Figure 8-9). Development work on this aircraft dates back to 1993. The first production 407 flew in November 1995, and customer deliveries began the following February. As of early 2003 over 600 of these aircraft were in service, which makes the 407 the fastest-selling single-engine turbine helicopter ever. Extensive use of lightweight composite construction and on-condition maintenance give high payload and low operating costs.

In contrast to the 206, the 407 features a four-blade main rotor that uses composite construction, and the blades and hub have no life limits. Benefits of the four-blade main rotor include improved performance and better ride comfort. Another significant improvement over the Long-Ranger is the 18-cm (8-in.) wider cabin, which significantly increases cabin space. The 407 also has larger main cabin windows. Power comes from a more powerful Allison 250C47 turboshaft fitted with FADEC, allowing an increase in maximum takeoff weight and improved performance at hotter temperatures and/or higher altitudes. The tail boom is made from carbon fiber composites. Bell is considering fitting the 407 with a shrouded tail rotor. The aircraft is powered by a 700 shp Allison

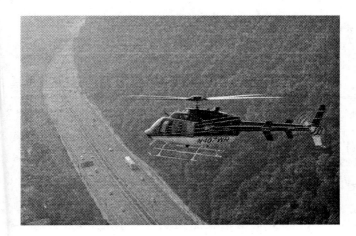

FIGURE 8-9
A Bell 407
Courtesy of Sheldon Cohen/Bell Helicopter

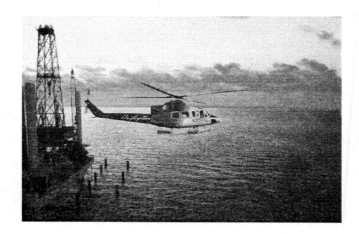

FIGURE 8-10
A Bell 412
Courtesy of Sheldon Cohen/Bell Helicopter

250C47 turboshaft driving a four-blade main rotor and two-blade tail rotor. In its passenger configuration the 407 seats one pilot and up to six passengers.

Bell 412

The 412 is a medium-lift twin-engine helicopter (Figure 8-10). It is an off-spring of the 212, the major change being a smaller-diameter, four-blade main rotor in place of the 212's two-blade unit. The upgrades from the 212 provide a 30 percent increase in airspeed. In its normal configuration the 412 seats 15 passengers. In air medical configuration it can carry up to six litters or, more commonly, two litters, two or three attendants, and an extensive line of equipment. With over 220 cubic feet of cabin space, the 412 is one of the largest helicopters used for air medicine. This aircraft is ideally suited for large medical teams or for the transport of patients who require specialized equipment (ECMO, balloon pumps, and so on).

Bell 427

The 427 is the latest addition to Bell's light twin lineup and serves as a replacement for the 206LT TwinRanger (Figure 8-11). The 427 was the first Bell helicopter designed entirely on computer. Compared to the 407, the 427's cabin is 33 cm (13 in.) longer and eliminates the roof beam that obstructs the cabin on the 206/206L/407. The fuselage makes extensive use of composite materials. The first flight of the 427 was in December 1997, and Canadian certification was awarded in November 1999. First customer deliveries followed U.S. certification in January 2000. U.S. FAA dual-pilot IFR certification was awarded in May 2000.

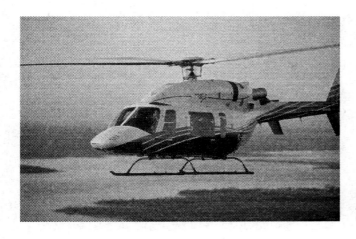

FIGURE 8-11
A Bell 427
Courtesy of Sheldon Cohen/Bell Helicopter

Power comes from two FADEC-equipped Pratt & Whitney 207D turboshafts with electronic control, driving the composite four-blade main rotor and two-blade tail rotor through a new gearbox. The aircraft is capable of full single-engine capability at maximum weight. The main rotor's soft-in-plane hub features a composite flexbeam yoke and elastomeric joints, eliminating the need for lubrication or maintenance. The 427's glass cockpit features an integrated instrument display system (IIDS). A hinged main cabin door is standard; a sliding door is optional. In passenger configuration the aircraft seats a pilot and up to seven passengers. When fitted with a medical interior, the aircraft is capable of transporting two litter patients and a medical team of two.

Bell 430

The Bell 430 is a twin-engine intermediate helicopter (Figure 8-12). It was introduced in 1995 as a stretched and updated version of the Bell 230. Its most notable upgrades include an 18-inch extension of the fuselage and a four-blade, bearingless, hingeless, composite main rotor. Other improvements over the 230 include a 10 percent increase in horsepower due to more powerful Allison 250 turboshafts (with FADEC). An optional EFIS flight-deck system is available. The 430 also features as standard a Rogerson Kratos IIDS. Engine and flight information are displayed on two large LCD panels. The 430 is offered with skids or retractable wheeled undercarriage. As with the Bell 230, the wheeled configuration decreases drag and makes the aircraft a few knots faster. However, addition of the retractable landing gear results in loss of fuel capacity. While the skidded version is slightly slower, it has greater fuel capacity and provides an additional 140 km (50 miles) of range. In 1996 this aircraft set the around-the-world helicopter speed record.

Aircraft and Equipment 123

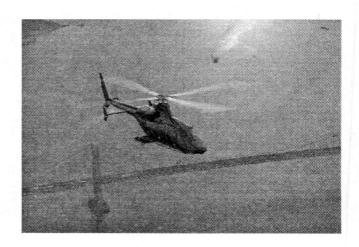

A Bell 430
Courtesy of Sheldon Cohen/Bell Helicopter

Standard passenger capacity is one pilot and nine passengers. The stretched fuselage provides a welcome addition of space to the patient compartment and makes the aircraft relatively roomy for air medical use. When fitted with a medical interior, it transports two litter patients and a medical team of two or three. It provides a very smooth and relatively quiet ride.

Boeing McDonnell Douglas Explorer MD-900

The MD-900 represents the first of a new breed of AM helicopter (Figure 8-13). Introduced in 1994, this was the first midsized twin to be equipped with the NOTAR system. The traditional tail rotor has been replaced with

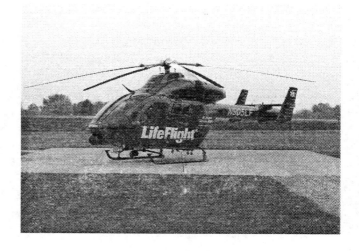

An MD-900
Photo copyright Terry Shepherd

an internal blower adapted from the smaller MD-520. A powerful fan located inside the tail boom forces air through a directional air outlet on the end of the tail. The pilot can vary the amount of air blowing through the outlet. As airflow is increased, lateral thrust increases, just as with a conventional tail rotor. The chief difference is that the "rotor" is totally contained within the fuselage, and the dangers associated with a traditional tail rotor are eliminated. The rotorless system also produces less noise than a traditional tail rotor. The unorthodox appearance of the aircraft, however, takes a little getting used to.

The Explorer is certified for single-pilot IFR operations and certified in the stringent Category A operation, which requires that the helicopter be able to continue takeoffs and landings with one engine inoperative.

The aircraft has a number of safety features incorporated into the fuselage and landing gear. The landing gear and airframe structures are designed to soften the impact of a hard landing. Seat supports absorb vertical impact energy, and two beams extending below the nose of the aircraft minimize the likelihood of rolling forward during a hard landing or crash.

The aircraft has small external dimensions—its overall length is only 38.3 feet—but the cabin is large enough for AM use. In its normal passenger configuration it seats one pilot and seven passengers. In air ambulance configuration it can accommodate one or two stretchers and two medical attendants.

MD-902

In September 1997 the improved Explorer 902 was introduced as an upgraded replacement for the MD-900. Features of the MD-902 include PW206E engines with higher single-engine performance ratings, revised engine air inlets, improved NOTAR inlet design, and a more powerful stabilizer control system. Benefits include improved range and endurance and increased maximum takeoff weight.

Sikorsky S-76

The S-76 is one of the larger helicopters commonly used for air medical service (Figure 8-14). This aircraft is considerably larger than the Bell 430, Dauphin, or BK-117. Sikorsky began design and engineering work on the S-76 in the mid-1970s and used technologies and experience gained from the military S70 Blackhawk program. The resulting S-76A was powered by two Allison 250C30S turboshafts. The first flight was in March 1977, and FAA certification was awarded in November 1978. The first improved model was the S-76 Mark II (introduced in March 1982) with more powerful Allison engines and avionics improvements. The S-76B is powered by two Pratt & Whitney

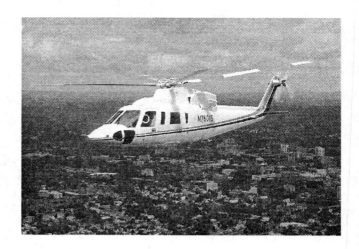

FIGURE 8-14
An S-76C+
Courtesy of Sikorsky Aircraft Corporation

Canada PT6B36s. The newer S-76C is powered by two Turbomeca Arriel 1S1 engines. The S-76A+ designation refers to S-76As that were retrofitted with Arriel engines.

The most current version of this aircraft is the S-76C+, which offers an 18 percent increase in horsepower and FADEC-equipped Arriel 2S1 engines. Certification of the C+ was awarded in 1996. Recent improvements include composite blades, a quiet tail rotor with curved blades, an active noise and vibration control system, and an advanced health and usage monitoring system. A three-LCD-screen integrated instrument display system for engine and rotor information is now standard, supplementing the four-screen Honeywell EFIS suite.

The S-76, with its relatively large interior space and fast cruise speed, is desirable as a critical-care air ambulance. In passenger configuration it seats a pilot and 12 or 13 passengers. In the air medical version two patients and a medical crew of three or four can be easily accommodated. Although the S-76 can be flown by one pilot, that option is rarely used because of the size of the aircraft. This aircraft may be too large for some smaller hospital landing pads.

Bell/Augusta 609

The Bell/Augusta 609 "tilt-rotor" represents a major turning point in the development of rotor-wing aircraft (Figure 8-15). Although the BA-609 is still in the testing stage, many customers have already placed orders. The aircraft has tremendous potential for air medical use and warrants some discussion. This will be the first commercial application of tilt-rotor engineering. The six-to-nine-passenger aircraft will combine the speed and range of a turboprop with the vertical takeoff and landing

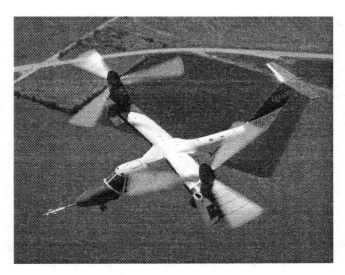

FIGURE 8-15
A Bell 609
Courtesy of Sheldon Cohen/Bell Helicopter

capability of a standard helicopter. According to promotional materials, the aircraft will have a cruise speed of 275 knots and an operating range of 750 nm. At 17.5 ft. the cabin is long enough to allow two patients to be positioned head to toe along one side. Three or four attendants can be seated along the opposite wall. The height and width of the cabin are similar to those of a Bell 430 helicopter.

The fuselage of the aircraft resembles that of a typical 8-to-10-passenger turboprop airplane. However, the one striking difference is the presence of tilting wing-mounted "nacelles." Each nacelle has three large blades and resembles a small rotor. The nacelles may be rotated so that they are vertical or horizontal in relation to the ground, thus allowing for vertical takeoff and landing. Following takeoff, they are slowly rotated forward into a more traditional fixed-wing propeller position, and the aircraft flies in a manner similar to that of a typical turboprop aircraft. According to promotional materials, the transition process will require roughly 20 seconds to complete.

The maiden flight of the BA609 took place in March 2003. Bell has received almost 70 advance orders for this craft, virtually assuring its commercial success.

While the technology is not yet proven, the appeal of a vertical takeoff and landing aircraft with this speed and range is obvious. The same aircraft could be used to make short interfacility transports and to move patients over long distances. The time saved by not having to move patients to and from an airport by ground ambulance will likely be enough to offset the airspeed, which is slightly slower than that of a conventional jet aircraft.

Table 8-4 shows the specifications of aircraft commonly used in air medicine.

Table 8-4 Specifications for Aircraft Commonly Used in Air Medicine

Aircraft	Max. Wt. (Gross)	Rotor Diam.	Engine(s) (HP Each) Max. Cont.	Cabin Size Pilot/Pass & Pat/Attend Cab. Cu. Ft.	Range (To Empty)	Fast Cruise
BK-117 A	6,173	36'1"	2 (600)	1-9 2-2 177	295	143
BK-117 B2	7,385	36'1"	2 (550)	1-9 2-2 177	290	134
BK-117 C1	7,385	36'1"	2 (692)	1-9 2-2 177	292	133
AS-332 L2	20,503	53'1"	2 (1657)	2-24 4-4 430	447	150
AS-350B	4,300	35'1"	1 (590)	1-6 1-3 106	395	125
AS-350B2	4,960	35'1"	1 (625)	1-6 1-3 106	360	133
AS-350B3	4,960	35'1"	1 (848)	1-6 1-3 106	360	134
BO-105 CBS-4	5,511	324"	2 (420)	1-4 1-2	300	110
BO-105 Super 5		324"	2 (420)	1-4 1-2	300	110
EC-135	6,250	33'5"	2 (571)	1-7 2-2 170	332	138
Bell 407	5,000	35'	1 (700)	1-6 2-2 125	312	115
Bell 427	6,000	37'	2 (543)	1-7 2-2 142	353	126
S-76C+	11,700	44'	2 (856)	2-12 2-4 244	439	155
S-76 Mk II	10,300	44'	2 (650)	2-12 2-4	404	125
Bell 206L2	4,150	37'	1 (500)	1-6 2-2 120	360	124
Bell 206L3	4,150	37'	1 (650)	1-6 2-2 120	360	110
Bell 206L4	4,450	37'	1 (630)	1-6 2-2 120	324	110

Model	Weight	Rotor	Engines	Config		
Bell 222	8,250	42'	2 (680)	1-7 2-2	390	130
Bell 230	8,400	42'	2 (700)	1-7 2-2	301 (wh) 380 (sk)	141 (wh) 138 (sk)
Bell 430	9,000	42'	2 (699)	1-9 2-3 224	272 (wh) 348 (sk)	138 (wh) 128 (sk)
Augusta 109E	5,730		2 (573)	2-6 2-2		
Augusta 109 MAX	5,997		2 (380)	2-6 2-2		
Augusta A-109 Power	6,283	36'	2 (567)	2-6 2-2	521	154
Augusta A-109 K-2	6,283	36'	2 (632)	2-6 2-2	435	143
Augusta 119	5,997	36'	1 (872)	1-7 2-2	535	140
Bell 412	11,900	46'	1 (1308)	1-14 2-4 240	356	127
Bell 412EP	11,900	46'	1 (1800)	1-14 2-4	402	124
Bell 214ST	17,500	52'	2 (1625)	2-17 2-4	418	130
AS-365N2	9,370	39'2"	2 (632)	1-12 2-3 177	485	148
AS-365N3	9,480	39'2"	2 (800)	1-12 2-3 177	427	148
EC-155	10,582	41'4"	2 (800)	2-12 2-4 235	424	144
MD Explorer-900	6,250	33'10"	2 (629)	1-7 2-2	302	136
MD Explorer-902	6,250	33'10"	2 (641)	1-7 2-2	302	136

Table 8-5 Air Medical Equipment List

Airway management equipment including

- oxygen
- mechanical suction
- intubation equipment
- ventilatory support equipment

Cardiac monitor/defibrillator

Advanced Cardiac Life Support drugs and therapeutic modalities (or equivalent specific to type of mission.)

Other electronic devices that may be essential in delivering specific patient care (i.e., pulse oximeter, N pumps, ETCo2 detector/monitor, external pacemaker)

Air Medical Equipment

As with ground ambulances, the equipment available on air ambulances may vary. Because of the complexity of patient types, most are equipped for both emergency and critical-care transports (Table 8-5). A typical inventory includes the basic equipment found in all ground ambulances such as oxygen, bag-valve-masks, oral and nasopharyngeal airways, blood pressure cuffs, cardiac monitor, and intubation kits. Most air ambulances are also equipped with a complement of invasive/noninvasive vital signs monitors, 12-lead cardiac monitor/defibrillator/pacemakers, full-service ventilators, neonatal isolettes, and a full range of medications. The various devices are often more compact (and expensive) than those used in the hospital setting and may operate differently (Figure 8-16).

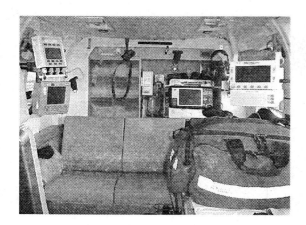

FIGURE 8-16
Aircraft interior showing medical equipment and configuration

Ventilator

Most air medical services have at least one full-service ventilator. It should have both pressure- and flow-controlled modes and should allow for operator-controlled adjustments to tidal volume, inspiration time, ventilation rate, positive end expiratory pressure (PEEP), and oxygen concentration. FIO_2 should be adjustable from 21 percent to 100 percent. The device should contain user-defined alarms loud enough to be heard in an operating aircraft. Alternatively, a blinking warning light may be used if the light is bright enough to be seen under any operating conditions.

Some programs keep a second, usually smaller and less sophisticated ventilator available for a second patient or in case of primary unit failure. The secondary unit is often an oxygen-powered transport ventilator. Transport ventilators are acceptable for backup use but should not be considered a replacement for a full-service model.

IV Pumps

IV pumps should be compact and user-friendly. Because of size and weight constraints, most flight programs use triple-channel pumps capable of regulating three flow rates simultaneously (Figure 8-17). While these devices are very reliable, a major component failure may result in

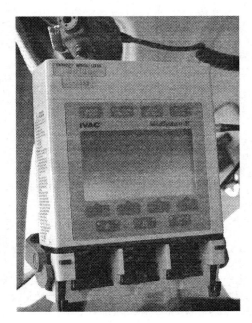

FIGURE 8-17
Triple channel infusion pump

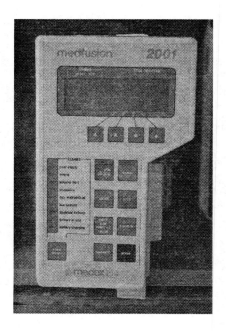

FIGURE 8-18
Enclosed syringe pump
Courtesy of MedEx Inc.

the loss of all three channels, leaving the flight crew with multiple IVs to calibrate manually. A backup IV pump should be carried as well.

Syringe pumps can be an effective way to administer certain medications (Figure 8-18). A syringe pump cancels the need to hang another bag of IV fluid and can save valuable space. It can be programmed to deliver very specific quantities of medication over a designated period of time. Some models have an enclosed syringe chamber to prevent damage to operating parts and to minimize the risk of tampering with medication administration rates.

Monitoring Equipment

A variety of invasive and noninvasive vital signs monitors are available. These devices may be set to record vital signs and other parameters at preset time intervals. The Protocol Propaq is one of the most widely used of these devices. It offers multiple functions in a relatively compact and reliable unit. Physio Control, Zoll, and others also offer high-quality devices suitable for air medical application.

Historically there have been cardiac monitor/defibrillator/pacing units and there have been vital signs monitoring units. Over the past several years these devices have become more similar, each adding features of the other. Within the next few years there will likely be one device that performs ECG monitoring, defibrillation, external pacing, and invasive and noninvasive monitoring.

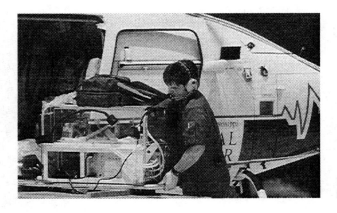

FIGURE 8-19
Neonatal isolette

Neonatal Transport Isolettes

Many AM programs offer neonatal transport services. These tiny patients require equipment often very different from that typically used for adult patients. Neonates are very susceptible to environmental changes and should be transported under tightly controlled conditions, generally in a neonatal isolette. The isolette is a self-contained device with an enclosed chamber that maintains temperature within a narrow range (Figure 8-19). It also contains a ventilator, pulse oximeter, and ECG monitor. It is generally designed to mount on a stretcher base that is compatible with the aircraft stretcher loading system. The setup also includes a battery, oxygen, and compressed air, so that it can operate independently during moves in and out of hospitals.

Neonatal isolettes are typically large and very heavy and cannot be stored aboard the aircraft when not in use. They are typically stored at the base of operation and loaded into the aircraft only when needed. The reconfiguration process usually requires the unloading of most of the adult equipment and replacement with the isolette and carry-on bags used by the neonatal transport team. This process can take 15 to 30 minutes, depending on the aircraft size and type.

Medications

Most AM programs staff with personnel capable of providing a full range of emergency and critical-care procedures, and a full complement of emergency and critical-care medications is essential (Figure 8-20). The choice of medications carried by a flight program is influenced by the philosophy of the medical director, the role of the flight program, and the capabilities of referring and receiving hospitals. The medical crew should have the capability to continue using medications that have been

Aircraft and Equipment   133

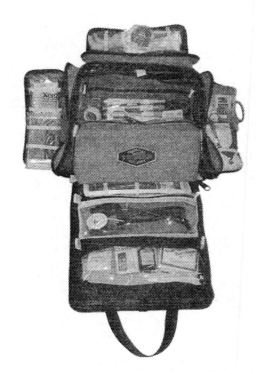

FIGURE 8-20
Aircraft medication kit
Courtesy of Thomas Transport Packs

started at the referring facility and to start indicated medications that may not have been available at smaller referring facilities.

Fibrinolytic Agents

Fibrinolytic agents should be carried by all programs that provide critical-care service. These drugs may be indicated for certain medical conditions, such as acute myocardial infarction, confirmed nonhemorrhagic stroke, or pulmonary embolus. Fibrinolytic agents have serious potential side effects, and the degree of risk increases as the elapsed time since onset of symptoms increases. The AM team must be capable of performing a thorough screening prior to administration. In some cases the availability of Computerized Axial Tourography (CT) at the referring facility is a prerequisite for administration of these drugs.

Nitric Oxide

Nitric oxide may be indicated for a select subgroup of neonatal patients. It is sometimes used in the management of hypoxic respiratory failure in full-term and nearly full-term infants. It decreases pulmonary hypertension and may be used as an alternative to ECMO in some patients. Although studies are inconclusive, there appears to be a significant amount of anecdotal evidence to support the use of nitric oxide.

Neuromuscular Blocking Agents

Neuromuscular blocking agents have become the standard of care for the management of patients with difficult-to-manage airways and when elective intubation is indicated. These medications have been used by both ground and air medical programs for years, and their safety and efficacy in the AM environment is well proved. Since airway management is such an important role for the AM team, it is essential that all medical team members have substantial experience in performing rapid-sequence intubation before being allowed to function as independent AM team members.

Antidotes and Antivenins

For programs that support smaller hospitals, the provision of antidotes and antivenins may be an important role. Smaller hospitals are often unable to maintain a complete supply of these expensive agents and refer patients to larger facilities. However, since many overdoses, poisonings, and bites or stings respond best to prompt treatment with reversing or inhibiting agents, the AM program may play a significant role in the management of these patients.

AM programs should maintain an adequate supply of antidotes for all poisonings and overdoses that may reasonably be anticipated in their service area. Although some of these agents may be used infrequently, the program may be relied upon to provide them when needed by referral sites. It is not practical for a program to stockpile all agents, such as snake and spider antivenins, but they should be acquired on an as-needed basis from a reliable source.

Providing this service may be easier and more cost-effective for AM programs that are based at a larger referral center. The AM program can establish a relationship with the hospital pharmacy and obtain medications as needed.

Sedatives and Analgesics

The relief of pain and suffering is one of the most basic tenets of the medical profession. Analgesics should be administered to patients experiencing moderate to severe pain where there are no contraindications.

Sedatives are indicated for patients who are intubated, undergoing certain medical procedures, or experiencing excessive preflight anxiety. Patients with closed head injury may require sedation to prevent struggling, prevent increases in intracranial pressure, and ensure their safety. Benzodiazepines such as midazolam, lorazepam, and diazepam are commonly used by AM programs for this purpose. Midazolam has gained popularity over the past several years and is the drug of choice. It has the added benefit of inducing anterograde amnesia, allowing patients to forget painful or disturbing procedures.

Some of the more commonly used narcotic analgesics are morphine, meperidine, and fentanyl. Each of these has its pros and cons, and the AM team should select an analgesic based on the needs and risks of the patient at hand. While morphine continues to be the standard by which all narcotic analgesics are measured, it does cause peripheral vasodilation and may cause hypotension in susceptible patients. Meperidine is an effective analgesic, but one of its metabolites (apomeperidine) may induce tachycardia. Fentanyl is a newer-generation drug and has the lowest incidence of side effects when administered appropriately.

Dissociating agents such as propofol may also be valuable tools in the management of select patients. Propofol has a very short half-life, and when the infusion is discontinued, the patient generally returns to a normal level of consciousness within a few minutes. The patient can be completely sedated during transport but recovers rapidly, so assessment by receiving physicians is not impeded by the medication.

Blood and Blood Products

Some AM programs may have a frequent need for blood or blood products. For programs using larger aircraft, the addition of a small refrigerator may be an option, and blood may be issued on a daily basis. More commonly, programs obtain blood from hematology labs as needed.

Summary

The aircraft is the main focus of the medical flight program. The capabilities and characteristics of the aircraft chosen will strongly influence program activities and performance. Cabin size, weight capacity, avionics, and range are all important features that must be evaluated. Most air medical programs perform both scene and interfacility transports and should utilize aircraft that perform well in each of those roles. In the United States, over 30 different helicopter models are used as air ambulances. The BK-117 is the helicopter most widely used by air medical programs. That aircraft has many desirable characteristics, notably a roomy patient compartment, instrument flight capability, and economical performance. However, other aircraft are available that also perform well in those categories.

As important as the aircraft is the medical equipment integrated into it. The flight team should have available medical equipment and supplies for all potential patient types. This equipment should be compact, lightweight, durable, and capable of performing at all altitudes. It should also be configured to be compatible with the medical interior of the aircraft. Larger items such as neonatal isolettes may require modification according to the aircraft type used. Program personnel should invest adequate time evaluating potential aircraft and medical equipment configurations prior to purchase.

REVIEW QUESTIONS

1. List five characteristics of the ideal medical helicopter.

2. Programs operating in areas where low visibility is a problem should choose a(n) _____ equipped aircraft.
   a. Air conditioner
   b. Emergency float
   c. Satellite tracking system
   d. IFR

3. A hospital-based program located in a residential area will usually want to consider a _____ aircraft with plenty of _____ to allow it to attain altitude quickly and to minimize the disturbance to residents.
   a. large, power
   b. quiet, power
   c. fast, rotor surface area
   d. large, rotor surface area

4. The rotor-wing aircraft that is most frequently used for air medical transport in the United States is the:
   a. Bell 430
   b. Sikorsky S-76
   c. American Eurocopter AS-350
   d. American Eurocopter BK-117

5. List one aircraft from each of the following manufacturers that is commonly utilized for air ambulance operations and describe the positive characteristics of each aircraft.
   Augusta
   American Eurocopter
   Bell
   Sikorsky

Flight
Physiology

Objectives

Upon completing this chapter, the reader should have a better understanding of the following topics:

* The effects of altitude on the eustachian tubes and inner ear

* The effects of altitude on the respiratory, cardiovascular, and gastrointestinal systems

* Methods of compensating for increases in altitude

* Airsickness and its potential impact on patients and crew members

* The impact of aircraft noise on patients and crew members

KEY TERMS

airsickness, p. 144

altitude, p. 140

barodontalgia, p. 142

barosinusitis, p. 141

barotitis media (ear block), p. 140

Boyle's Law, p. 143

decibel (dB), p. 145

eustachian tube, p. 141

motion sickness, p. 144

Introduction

Changes in altitude may result in a number of problems for those who fly. Even on pressure-controlled commercial airlines earache, headache, and sinus-related problems are relatively common during and after flight.

Fortunately, most of the discomforts associated with altitude changes are relatively minor. However, the implications for patients transported by air medical programs may be more significant. These persons may present with disease states that can be easily worsened by even slight changes in pressure or avilable oxygen. This chapter addresses the physiologic implications of air medical transport and those conditions most likely to be affected by changes in altitude.

The Effects of Altitude

altitude
Distance above sea level (ASL) or above ground level (AGL). Generally measured in feet or meters.

One of the unique characteristics of air medical programs is the fact that they operate at high altitudes. **Altitude** changes have potential implications for patients and crew members alike. Increases in altitude are associated with a decrease in both atmospheric pressure and oxygen concentration. These progressive changes have a number of predictable effects on humans. The clinical significance of these effects varies depending on the altitude and the underlying health of the air traveler. While most air medical helicopters operate at relatively low altitudes, there is still some potential for altitude-induced pathophysiology. Some of the more common conditions are described below.

Barotitis Media

barotitis media (ear block)
Trapping of air in the middle ear.

During ascent, barometric pressure decreases, leaving pressure in the middle ear greater than that of the environment. This can cause **barotitis media** (also called **ear block**). The higher-pressure air forces its way out through the **eustachian tubes,** which are located in the back of the nasopharynx (Figure 9-1). These tubes are approximately 1.5 inches long, soft, and easily collapsible, and they act as a sort of one-way valve to allow air to escape but not to reenter. However, airflow resistance (patency) is highly variable. Some individuals almost never have problems with middle-ear equalization, while others may experience discomfort in elevators.

As the aircraft begins to descend and environmental pressure increases, the tympanic membranes in the middle ear are forced inward. If patency in the eustachian tubes is poor and the pressure difference across the tympanic membrane becomes too great, pain results, and in extreme cases the membrane may rupture. Any condition that results in edema in the nasopharynx, such as allergy or infection, may obstruct airflow through the eustachian tubes and worsen barotitis media.

Certain maneuvers may be performed to equalize pressure in the middle ear. The simplest method is to press the tongue against the roof

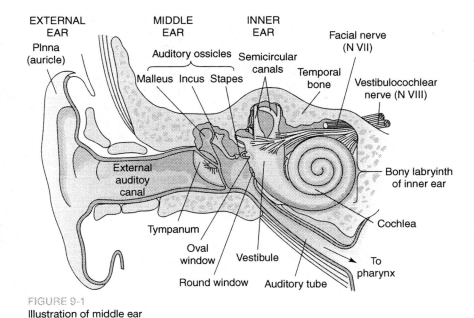

EXTERNAL EAR
Pinna (auricle)

MIDDLE EAR
Auditory ossicles
Malleus Incus Stapes

INNER EAR
Semicircular canals
Temporal bone

Facial nerve (N VII)

Vestibulocochlear nerve (N VIII)

External auditoy canal

Bony labryinth of inner ear

Tympanum

Cochlea

Oval window
Vestibule
Round window
Auditory tube

To pharynx

FIGURE 9-1
Illustration of middle ear

eustachian tubes
A tube lined with mucous membrane that connects the nasopharynx to the middle ear cavity.

of the mouth while simultaneously swallowing. That action forces the eustachian tubes to open, allowing air back into the middle ear. If that fails, the Frenzel maneuver may be attempted. Herman Frenzel was a Luftwaffe commander who developed this technique for dive-bomber pilots during World War II. The technique involves closing off the vocal cords, as though you are about to lift a heavy weight, pinching the nostrils closed, and making a "K" or guttural "guh" sound. This maneuver compresses air in the nasopharynx and forces air into the eustachian tubes. This technique can be performed repeatedly and in quick sequence.

If these techniques fail and pain continues, the pilot should be asked to level off or increase altitude and descend more slowly. Many flight programs discourage crew members from flying when they have upper-respiratory conditions likely to result in nasal congestion or infection. When transporting patients with decreased level of consciousness, the pilot should be asked to control the rate of descent as much as possible to avoid the possibility of ear damage.

Barosinusitis

barosinusitis
Sinus discomfort secondary to air trapping and air expansion within one or more sinuses.

The mechanism of **barosinusitis** (also called sinus block) is very similar to that of barotitis. The problem may occur either on ascent or descent,

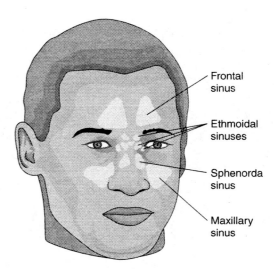

FIGURE 9-2
Illustration of sinuses

Frontal sinus

Ethmoidal sinuses

Sphenorda sinus

Maxillary sinus

but more commonly on descent. Sinuses are rigid, bony cavities lined with mucous membranes and connected to the sinus cavity by means of one or more small openings (Figure 9-2). If these openings become obstructed by edema of the mucous membrane lining, equalization of pressure becomes difficult. Inflammation and edema may be so complete as to prevent air from entering or exiting the sinus cavity.

The sinuses most often affected by pressure change are the frontal and maxillary. The most common symptom with the frontal sinuses is pain above the eyes. If the maxillary sinuses are affected, pain is generally felt on either side of the nose and under the cheekbones. Maxillary sinus pain may also be referred to the teeth and upper jaw and sometimes mistaken for a toothache (**barodontalgia**). The onset of sinus pain is usually sudden. Techniques for alleviating sinus pain are the same as those for barotitis media.

barodontalgia
Toothache that results from increased or decreased pressure due to a change in altitude.

The GI Tract

The GI tract is the area most often associated with complaints during ascent. As altitude increases and environmental pressure decreases, gas within the GI tract expands and consumes more space within the abdominal cavity. This may cause a feeling of fullness or abdominal discomfort. Belching or passing flatus generally relieves this sensation. Patients with underlying gastrointestinal disorders or trauma may experience increased discomfort. AM team members who frequently experience abdominal bloating or discomfort may obtain some relief by taking simethicone (Gas-X) with meals or before beginning a shift.

The Respiratory System

As altitude increases, atmospheric oxygen concentration decreases, diminishing the amount of oxygen inhaled with each breath. In a healthy traveler this effect becomes clinically significant only above altitudes of 10,000 to 12,000 feet. Patients who are already compromised by trauma or illness may begin to experience problems before reaching that level. Above 10,000 to 12,000 feet, decreasing oxygen concentration and the expansion of intestinal gases may decrease respiratory excursion and lead to impaired respiration. Patients with pressure-sensitive conditions such as pneumothorax, increased intracranial pressure, or barotrauma may need to be flown at lower altitudes when transported in nonpressurized aircraft. Patients who are already hypoxic may require incremental increases in oxygen flow rate to maintain acceptable oxygen saturation levels.

Patients who are intubated should be observed carefully for changes in respiratory status as altitude is increased. Also, the volume of air contained within the cuff of the endotracheal tube may increase or decrease with altitude. **Boyle's Law** states that the volume of a gas is inversely proportional to its pressure, temperature remaining constant. Practically speaking, this means that at 18,000 feet, where the pressure is approximately half that at sea level, a given volume of gas will expand to twice its initial volume (Figure 9-3). For example, the 10 cc of air typically injected into the cuff of an endrotracheal tube at sea level will expand to 20 cc at 18,000 feet, leading to increased intratracheal pressure and possibly to damage to the tracheal wall and/or larynx. Similarly, a small pneumothorax at ground level may expand and become clinically significant at altitude. Even at 10,000 feet, gases expand by 30 percent. For most air medical services these concerns are rarely serious. Programs operating in or around mountainous areas are more likely to see rapid increases and decreases in flight altitude.

Boyle's Law
The volume of a gas is directly proportional to the pressure exerted on that gas (e.g., as pressure decreases, volume increases, and vice versa).

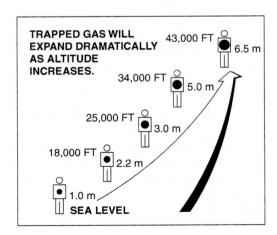

TRAPPED GAS WILL EXPAND DRAMATICALLY AS ALTITUDE INCREASES.

43,000 FT — 6.5 m

34,000 FT — 5.0 m

25,000 FT — 3.0 m

18,000 FT — 2.2 m

1.0 m
SEA LEVEL

FIGURE 9-3
The effects of gas expansion

Flight Physiology   143

The Circulatory System

The direct impact of altitude on the cardiovascular system is minimal. Indirect effects, however, may be substantial. For example, altitude-induced hypoxia may lead to tachycardia, worsen myocardial ischemia, or precipitate myocardial infarction in a patient being transported for partial coronary artery occlusion. Hypoxia-induced dysrhythmias may appear or worsen. Similarly, altitude changes may lead to decompensation in an otherwise stable congestive heart failure or COPD patient. Expansion of intestinal gases may increase intrathoracic pressure, increase myocardial afterload, and subsequently alter circulatory efficiency.

Airsickness

airsickness
Motion sickness that occurs as a result of the movements associated with flight.

motion sickness
A condition that results from prolonged exposure to erratic or rhythmic movement in any combination of directions. Nausea, vomiting, headache, and vertigo characterize severe cases.

Airsickness refers to the vertigo, abdominal discomfort, nausea, and sometimes vomiting that may result from the repetitive and often unpredictable movements of an aircraft in flight. The pathophysiology and manifestations are similar to those of **motion sickness** associated with boat or car travel. This is one of the most common maladies that affect air travelers, including team personnel and patients. When severe, airsickness can be debilitating. Fortunately, steps can be taken to decrease the incidence and minimize symptoms.

* Fly facing forward when possible.
* When not occupied with other responsibilities, look out a window at a fixed point on the ground or horizon.
* Do not read or continually gaze at a fixed object inside the aircraft.
* Eat a small meal or snack before flying. Airsickness is more likely to occur on an empty stomach.
* Oral antiemetic drugs such as promethazine (Phenergan), dimenhydrinate (Dramamine), hydroxyzine (Visteril), and meclizine (Antivert, Bonine) may be helpful, especially if taken prophylactically. To be most effective, these agents should be taken well in advance of the flight. This may be difficult for AM personnel, since most flights are unscheduled. The use of antiemetics should be taken very seriously, as these drugs may have sedative and hypnotic effects on some people. A crew member who repeatedly develops airsickness should discuss the problem with the program medical director before deciding on an antiemetic. Obviously pilots should never ingest any medication with the potential to alter mental status or alertness.

The problem is somewhat more complicated for patients being transported by air. Nausea and vomiting may have clinically significant implications. Fluid loss and development of electrolyte imbalances may have a negative impact on the clinical condition of a patient who is already unstable from other causes. The gag response can increase blood pressure, intrathoracic pressure, and intracranial pressure. Fortunately, patients can be managed more aggressively without concern for altered mental status. Parenterally administered antiemetics will relieve airsickness in most patients. In addition to the medications listed above, ondansetron (Zofran) is a particularly effective antiemetic when administered intravenously. Critical or potentially unstable patients should also have a nasogastric tube inserted prior to transport. Prompt administration of antiemetics may prevent the development of vomiting in high-risk patients.

Noise

Hearing is defined as the sense that enables us to perceive sound. Hearing is second only to vision in its importance to our overall well-being. We process thousands of sounds each day that help us make decisions, avoid danger, and experience pleasure. Without this ability, we would be severely handicapped in today's high-technology world. We would be unable to use a telephone, hear a radio or television, detect the alarm clock, or know when it is time to remove food from the oven. The importance of maintaining healthy hearing cannot be overstated. But most of us take hearing for granted and rarely think about protecting it.

decibel (dB)
The standard unit of measure of sound intensity.

Hearing involves the perception and differentiation of sound waves that impact our tympanic membranes. Different frequencies of sound waves are perceived differently by the listener. **The decibel (dB)** is the unit used to measure sound intensity. The bottom threshold of normal human hearing sensitivity is between −10 and +25 decibels. A person who cannot hear sound at 25 dB has abnormal hearing (hearing loss). The sound level of speech at typical conversational distances is between 65 and 70 dB. An increase of 3 dB from any starting level is equivalent to doubling the sound intensity (Table 9-1).

The ear is a very sensitive organ, and exposure to loud noises may result in permanent hearing loss. The degree of risk is determined by two factors: the loudness of the noise and the duration of exposure to the noise. The number of decibels required to cause permanent hearing damage depends on the period of exposure. As noise level increases, the time required decreases. For example, the OSHA limit for exposure to 90 dB is 8 hours per day. The limit for exposure to 115 dB is 15 minutes. Exposure beyond those time limits may result in permanent hearing loss. About 10 million people in the United States have noise-induced hearing loss, nearly all of which was caused by occupational exposure.

Table 9-1 Decibel Level of Various Activities/ Conditions

Activity/Condition	Decibel Level
Rustle of leaves	10
Whisper	20
Quiet business office	50
Conversational speech	60–70
Vacuum cleaner	65
Automobile interior at cruise	65–80
Lawn mower	95–100
Rock concert	100–110
Snowmobile/JetSki	120
Jet engine	130–150
Pain threshold	140–150
12-gauge shotgun blast	165

Noise is a factor in all phases of aircraft operation. A turbine engine may produce a noise level of 130 to 160 decibels. Exposure for even a few minutes may result in permanent hearing loss. Aircraft technicians should be required without exception to wear effective hearing protection when working on or near a turning helicopter. Unfortunately, with experience often comes complacency. Why walk back to the storage cabinet for the headset when the aircraft will only be running for a few minutes? Hearing protection must *always* be worn to avoid cumulative hearing loss.

While the cabin of a helicopter is generally quieter than the exterior, the noise level may still be above 100 dB. Crew members should continue to wear hearing protection inside the aircraft. If it becomes necessary to exit the aircraft while it is turning, the headset or helmet should be unplugged and kept in place until the wearer is safely away from the aircraft or until the aircraft is shut down. Some crew members wear foam earplugs under the helmet or headset for additional protection. Earplugs are much smaller yet more effective at noise suppression than headsets. When the two are combined, ambient noise is reduced even more. Many aircraft headsets have adjustable volume control, allowing the wearer to compensate for the additional sound dampening of earplugs.

Patients should have hearing protection applied before they are moved to the aircraft. This applies to all patients, regardless of level of consciousness or mentation. Although unconscious patients may not be aware of noise, they may still suffer hearing damage. If spinal immobilization or the presence of bandages makes the use of a headset difficult, towels or large ear pads may be used instead.

Noise may interfere with communication between the patient and crew. The auscultation of breath sounds, blood pressure, and heart tones may be particularly challenging inside a turning helicopter. For that reason some medical helicopters are equipped with built-in Doppler devices that are wired into the intracabin communications system.

Summary

The most obvious unique characteristic of flight programs is the fact that they operate at a variety of altitudes. The altitude changes associated with air travel may have physiological implications for patients and crew members alike. Two of the most common adverse reactions to air travel are barotitis media and airsickness. Barotitis media involves a pressure imbalance across the tympanic membrane and manifests as transient ear or facial discomfort. In susceptible persons, usually those with allergies or sinusitis, nasal congestion may result in more serious symptoms, including severe pain and potential rupture of the tympanic membrane. Airsickness results from the irregular movements of the aircraft as it encounters gusts of wind and air pockets during the course of flight. It is manifest as a feeling of queasiness or, in severe cases, nausea and vomiting. The impact of altitude change may be more significant for patients who are seriously ill or injured. Patients should be evaluated for potential problems before the flight begins. Patients who are compromised by cardiovascular or respiratory conditions may be at increased risk for decompensation during high-altitude flight. In particular, patients with pneumothorax may experience acute respiratory compromise due to gas expansion as altitude increases. These patients may require an increase in supplemental oxygen. Those at very high risk, for example those with large pneumothoraces, should be transported at lower altitudes or by ground ambulance.

Noise is also a factor for air medical programs. The noise level in a helicopter may be great enough to result in hearing loss in those not wearing hearing protection. Headsets should be required for patients and crew members alike. In addition to blocking aircraft noise, headsets also allow for easier communication among crew members and between patients and crew members.

While there are a number of hazards associated with changes in altitude, proper planning can account for these and allow for modifications necessary to offset negative effects. Medical team members should factor in the potential impacts of altitude changes when performing patient assessment and establishing a treatment plan.

REVIEW QUESTIONS

1. A condition associated with ascension and altitude, characterized by in increase in pressure in the middle ear, is:

   a. Barotitis media   c. Otitis media

   b. Barosinusitis   d. a and b

2. A technique that may be effective in relieving the symptoms of the condition referred to in question 1 is:

   a. Massaging the ear lobe on the affected side

   b. Drinking water while simultaneously gurgling

   c. Swallowing large gulps of air

   d. The Frenzel maneuver

3. Gas volume will become twice what it was at sea level at an altitude of approximately _____ ft.

   a. 6000   c. 18,000

   b. 12,000   d. 24,000

4. Discuss three techniques that may be utilized to decrease the probability and severity of airsickness.

5. Permanent hearing loss may occur after as little as _____ minutes of close exposure to a running turbine engine.

   a. 5   c. 15

   b. 10   d. 60

Common
Patient Types
and Principles
of Management

Upon completing this chapter, the reader should have a better understanding of the following topics:

* General principles of management of patients being transported by air

* The importance of history taking and the physical examination

* Basic and expanded scope-of-practice patient management skills

* The potential benefits of air medical transport by patient type

Introduction

This chapter presents an overview of the conditions commonly encountered by air medical teams. It is not intended to be an exhaustive source of medical information; numerous texts cover pathophysiology and disease processes in greater detail. This chapter will present aspects of medical care that are common to air medicine or that require special consideration because of the out-of-hospital and flight aspects of air medicine.

General Principles of Management

Air medical teams are called on to manage a variety of patient types. Most patients are of high acuity. Team members must be capable clinicians, adept at assessing and treating virtually all patient types. They must ensure that indications for treatment are acted upon in a timely manner. They typically have no backup, no one to catch omissions in assessment or shortcomings in diagnosis. Each program should have in place a comprehensive quality management and continuing education program to ensure that the medical team remains proficient.

Gathering Patient Information

The goal of patient assessment is to gather enough information so that the pathophysiology underlying the patient's medical or traumatic condition can be fully appreciated. The process is similar to assembling a jigsaw puzzle. Each piece of medical information fills in a piece of the puzzle. As additional information is gathered, the picture becomes more complete and easier to comprehend. The history, vital signs, physical examination, ECG, laboratory results, and so on are each equal to one puzzle piece. The puzzle pieces may not be the same size. For a patient with overlapping and complex medical conditions, the history may provide information that is very valuable (equivalent to a large puzzle piece). Other information, such as allergies, may provide little useful information (smaller puzzle piece). In some cases it may be fairly simple to assemble the puzzle, and in others very challenging. The goal is always the same: to end up with a puzzle that is as complete as possible given the circumstances.

The History

The patient assessment process begins with the gathering of a medical history. When combined with the chief complaint, this information often serves as a starting point for the hands-on physical examination. Most patients picked up for an interfacility transport are evaluated prior to arrival of the flight team. The history is generally available from the referring health care team or from family members and should include:

chief complaint, associated complaints, history of present illness, past medical history, medications, and pertinent family medical history. The history should also note interventions provided by the referring health team and the patient's response.

Obtaining a history in the prehospital setting may be a bit more challenging. Patients may be unconscious or mentally compromised and unable to provide meaningful information. In such cases, relatives, friends, or witnesses may be consulted for information. Medical bracelets or necklaces occasionally provide a clue. If the history cannot be obtained during the early phases of patient management, the medical team is forced to rely more on assessment skills and intuitive thinking.

The Physical Examination

When combined with the history, a physical examination serves as the basis for all treatments that follow. While a complete head-to-toe examination may not be indicated for every patient, the exam should be comprehensive in regard to the chief complaint and medical history. The flight team must be adept at recognizing which body system(s) requires evaluation for each chief complaint and patient type.

The physical examination begins with a search for conditions that may pose an immediate threat to life or limb (Figure 10-1). The airway is opened and checked for patency. Breathing is evaluated for rate and depth. The chest is checked for open pneumothorax or other conditions that may impair the patient's ability to move air. The patient is rapidly assessed for exsanguinating hemorrhage. If at any point during this preliminary assessment any conditions are noted that may be a threat to survival, they are immediately corrected before the examiner moves on to the next step.

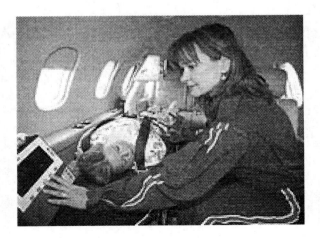

FIGURE 10-1
Medical team member performing physical examination
Courtesy of Air Ambulance Specialists, Inc.

Common Patient Types and Principles of Management

Next, a focused examination is performed. The focused exam involves a more thorough and detailed evaluation of body areas or systems that are most likely to be associated with the chief complaint and associated complaints. At this stage, the goal is to either confirm or rule out potential causes. For example, if a patient is complaining of chest pain, the goal is to first determine potential causes. Diseases involving the heart, lungs, musculoskeletal system, or alimentary system may cause chest pain. Since cardiac implications are most significant, the examiner begins with an assessment of the cardiopulmonary system. Other potential causes should also be assessed, such as environmental or emotional stress, gastroesophageal reflux disease (GERD), costochondritis, and gallbladder disease. Evaluation should include each area of the body that may provide relevant clues.

The final phase of the physical examination is the head-to-toe assessment. All body parts and all body systems are assessed for abnormalities. There are situations in which the head-to-toe exam either is not warranted or is precluded by the need for ongoing stabilization of a higher priority. In other cases this may be the only part of the physical exam that provides any meaningful information—for example, with a patient who is unresponsive, with unknown complaint and unknown history. Similarly, a patient with multisystem trauma should receive a head-to-toe examination to identify specific traumatic injuries.

All phases of the physical exam should be performed in a thorough, confident, and unrushed manner. This examination is very different from the nursing assessment typically performed in the emergency department. That assessment is grossly inadequate for the air medical setting. The exam should more closely resemble that performed by an experienced acute-care physician. It should involve much more than going through the motions. For example, palpation of the abdomen is of little value if the examiner is uncertain what she is palpating for. Similarly, heart tones can be easily auscultated by anyone with a stethoscope, but recognizing and assigning significance to the sounds produced by each phase of the cardiac cycle can be more challenging.

Analysis of Laboratory Values

A laboratory workup will have been completed on many of the patients transported from one facility to another. While the AM team may not always have the resources necessary to correct abnormalities identified by these tests, members should be adept at interpreting the more common test results.

When time permits, laboratory findings should be carefully reviewed prior to beginning transport. Clinically significant abnormalities should be questioned and if indicated, treated in a timely fashion. Blood glucose is one of the most commonly utilized tests. Glucose is the primary energy source within most cells and is oxidized in cell respiration to carbon dioxide and water to produce energy in the form of adenosine triphosphate (ATP). Nerve tissue is especially dependent on glucose as its source of energy and permanent damage may occur if the glucose level falls too low.

The complete blood count (CBC), basic metabolic panel (BMP), arterial blood gas (ABG), and cardiac enzymes (CE) are the most frequently available lab diagnostic studies for flight teams at the time of transport. ABGs provide valuable information regarding oxygenation and pH of the blood. Cardiac enzymes are indicators of myocardial damage generally resulting from myocardial infarction. Creatine phosphokinase (CPK) or creatine kinase (CK) and troponin are the most commonly utilized cardiac enzymes.

The CBC consists of several tests that quantitate the absolute and relative values of blood components. Included in the count are red blood cells (RBCs), hemoglobin (Hgb), hematocrit (Hct), platelet count (PLT), and white blood cell (WBC) count. The RBC count measures the number of RBCs per cubic millimeter. By measuring the number of grams of hemoglobin/100 ml of blood, the Hgb concentration of the red blood cells can be determined. Values that are below normal may indicate anemia or acute blood loss. Increased values may be indicative of polycythemia.

The hematocrit (Hct) is an indication of the percent volume of RBCs in whole blood. That value is roughly three times the hemoglobin concentration. Decreased Hct may indicate acute blood loss, overhydration, or anemia. An elevated Hct may indicate polycythemia or dehydration.

The platelet count is a part of the CBC that is sometimes overlooked. However, it can be an important step in evaluating the clotting process. The WBC count is a measurement of the number of WBCs in a cubic millimeter of blood. Increases in WBCs may result from infection, trauma, immune deficiencies, sepsis, or leukemia.

The basic metabolic panel (BMP) includes a group of tests that are bundled for reimbursement convenience purposes. The group includes calcium (Ca), chloride, CO_2, creatinine, glucose, potassium (K), sodium (Na), and urea nitrogen (BUN). Calcium (Ca) is an extracellular and intracellular cation that acts as a catalyst in the transmission and conduction of nerve impulses and stimulates the contraction of skeletal, smooth, and cardiac muscles.

Creatinine is the byproduct of phosphocreatine, a source of energy for muscle contraction. Elevated levels of creatinine can be seen in cases of advanced or end stage renal disease.

A pocket guide to laboratory tests and values should be kept in the aircraft for backup reference and may be helpful in evaluating less common results.

Test	Normal Values	Indications to Check
Glucose	70–110 mg/dl	Altered mental status, dehydration
CPK	5–35 U/ml	Chest pain, anginal equivalents
Troponin I	0–0.1 ng/ml	See Creatine phosphokinase (CPK)
Troponin T	0–0.2 ng/ml	See CPK
RBC—Male	4.2–5.6 M/ul	Hemorrhage, hydration changes, blood dyscrasia
RBC—Female	3.1–5.1 M/ul	As above
Hgb—Male	14–18 g/dl	Hemorrhage, anemia, blood dyscrasia
Hgb—Female	11–16 g/dl	As above
Hct—Male	39–54%	Hemorrhage, hydration changes, electrolyte disturbances, neoplasia
Hct—Female	34–47%	As above
WBC (lymphocytes)	15–44%	Infection
Calcium	8–11 mg/dl	Suspected electrolyte disturbance
Chloride	96–112 mEq/L	Acidosis, hydration derangements
CO_2	21–34 mEq/L	Acidosis, alkalinity
CO	>10% saturation	Exposure to smoke or noxious gases
K	3.5–5.5 mEq/L	Suspected electrolyte disturbance
Na	135–148 mEq/L	Suspected electrolyte disturbance
BUN	6–23 mg/dl	Suspected renal disease, CHF
Creatinine	.6–1.6 mg/dl	Suspected renal disease, kidney disease

Some flight programs use a portable laboratory evaluation system such as I-STAT. Portable clinical analyzers are freestanding test stations capable of determining a number of laboratory values. They perform tests relatively quickly and with minimal input from the operator, including blood glucose, electrolytes, hemoglobin, and hematocrit. Programs that perform a large number of critical-care or neonatal transports may benefit from the availability of a portable analyzer. Team members should be thoroughly trained in its use.

Interpretation of Diagnostic X Rays, CTs, and MRIs

Many patients will have had X rays, CT, or MRI tests performed as part of their prior evaluation. Members of the flight team should have some basic ability to interpret radiologic films and to recognize pneumothorax, hemothorax, simple cervical fractures, and long bone fractures. Since these skills may be used only infrequently, annual recurrent training is essential.

Establishing a Treatment Plan

Once all the available information has been collected, the medical team must develop a working diagnosis and a matching treatment plan. The treatment plan should be specific to the patient and should be based solidly on the results of the assessments listed above. The plan will generally coincide with previously implemented patient treatments—that is, patients with a pertinent medical history are likely to receive treatments that are similar to those received in the past. That is not to say that the treatment plan should be based solely on history. Conditions change, and the treatment plan should take current findings into account as well.

Patient Management Skills

Airway Management

Airway management is often the most important role of the air medical team. AM team members are expected to manage even the most challenging patient airway situations. Sometimes the flight team may be dispatched to retrieve a patient simply because others have been unable to establish a definitive airway. Multiple prior attempts at intubation may result in trauma and disruption of the patient's airway, making the procedure even more challenging. Each member of the medical team should be adept at orotracheal and nasotracheal intubation and should be comfortable in the role of managing difficult airways. Laboratory and surgery rotations addressing difficult airway management should be a routine part of new employee orientation.

Rapid-sequence intubation facilitated by the use of neuromuscular blocking agents and sedatives has become a routine procedure for air medical teams. It is often used electively by the flight team to facilitate various treatments and to enhance safety during the transport of potentially disruptive patients. Sedatives and paralytic agents relax the muscles and decrease passive resistance.

Team members should also be well versed in the use of alternative airway management techniques. While the intubation success rate for AM team members should approach 100 percent, there is always the chance of failure with a particularly difficult patient. Use of a secondary device, such as a laryngeal mask airway (LMA) or a Combitube, may be indicated. Since these devices are used only rarely, they should be covered in detail during new employee orientation and recurrent training.

For interfacility patients, the airway should almost always be secured prior to moving the patient to the aircraft. The hospital environment is more amenable to the performance of intubation and other airway management techniques. The lighting is better, there is more room, and there is more help. Once in the aircraft, noise, vibration, and limited space can make airway management a greater challenge, especially in smaller aircraft.

Scene flights present a somewhat different situation. The patient is often in an uncontrolled environment, perhaps trapped in an automobile or entangled in farm machinery, and may need to be intubated while suspended in an awkward position or with limited access. A patient with anaphylaxis and laryngeal edema may be hypoxic and fighting violently. AM team members should be capable of performing intubation even in these atypical presentations.

Digital intubation may be the only practical method for some patients. For example, a near-apneic patient trapped in a badly damaged car may be in such a position that a laryngoscope cannot be introduced or the patient's mouth cannot be visualized. However, an experienced flight nurse or paramedic may still be able to intubate the patient digitally. An atypical presentation may require an atypical management technique.

While it is generally desirable to establish a definitive airway at the earliest opportunity, there may be times when it is best to wait until the patient is in the aircraft—in weather extremes, for example, or when the safety of the crew is threatened. However, in most cases the patient with respiratory compromise should be ventilated and intubated where found.

Transtracheal Jet Insufflation

If a patient cannot be intubated and the airway cannot be acceptably managed by conventional or alternative means, a surgical airway is indicated. In many flight programs the AM team is not allowed to perform that technique, in which case transtracheal jet insufflation may be a viable option (Figure 10-2). This technique involves the insertion of a

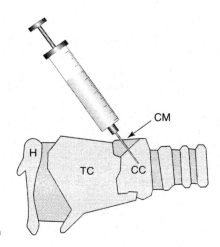

FIGURE 10-2
Transtracheal jet insufflation

large-gauge needle or over-the-needle catheter through the crycothyroid membrane and directly into the trachea. A tube connects the catheter to a high-pressure oxygen delivery device and the patient is ventilated by the systematic insufflation of oxygen followed by passive expiration.

An alternative technique involves the use of a dilator to enlarge the small opening created by the needle stick. The hole may be enlarged enough to allow insertion of a small endotracheal tube or a similar commercial device. Transtracheal jet insufflation by simple needle insertion is generally not considered a surgical procedure. The use of a dilator or scalpel to enlarge the needle stick site makes the scope of the procedure less clear, and some states may classify it as a surgical procedure. Classification and associated scope-of-practice issues should be resolved before nonphysician personnel are allowed to perform this procedure.

Surgical Airways

In some systems, AM teams are allowed to perform surgical airway procedures. Flight nurses and flight paramedics may perform them in some states. This technique should be performed only when an airway cannot be established through more conventional means. Formal instruction from an experienced physician, followed by mannequin or cadaver lab practice, must be a prerequisite for performing this technique on live patients.

Other Expanded-Scope Procedures

Needle Thoracentesis

Blunt or penetrating thoracic trauma may result in tension pneumothorax. If not treated promptly, this condition can result in death. Needle thoracentesis is a relatively simple procedure that can relieve intrathoracic pressure and serve as a temporary stabilizing measure until a tube thoracostomy can be performed (Figure 10-3). All medical team members should be competent in this procedure.

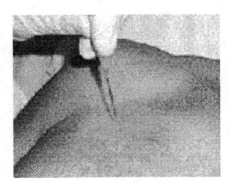

FIGURE 10-3
Needle thoracentesis

Common Patient Types and Principles of Management 157

Tube Thoracostomy

Some AM programs allow their medical personnel to perform tube thoracostomy. For programs staffing with physicians this is not an issue, as tube thoracostomy is a standard skill for physicians who are residency-trained in emergency medicine or trauma. It is also taught in the ATLS course offered by the American College of Surgeons. In some states flight nurses and/or flight paramedics are allowed to perform the procedure; in other states they must receive special approval from the appropriate governing body. For programs that transport large numbers of trauma patients, this option should be considered when possible. In lower-volume programs, skill maintenance may be an issue.

Escharotomy

Programs operating in areas where one or more burn units or burn centers are located may transport relatively high numbers of burned patients, who have special care needs. Patients with circumferential burns may experience compromised circulation and possible tissue death. Loss of hands or feet may occur. In extreme cases involving the thorax, respiratory excursion may be impaired to the point where adequate ventilation is not possible. In both cases, prompt treatment is necessary to prevent permanent damage. Escharatomy consists of making one or more incisions through the fascia to relieve the constriction (Figure 10-4). This procedure is generally not included in the scope of practice of nurses or paramedics, although some states allow these personnel to perform it with special justification and training.

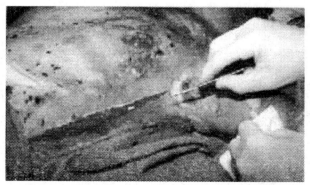

FIGURE 10-4
Escharotomy being performed

Categorizing Patients by Potential for Benefit

AM teams are generally capable of providing a level of care that exceeds the care available from a typical ground ambulance service. They have a more thorough knowledge of emergency medicine and critical care and greater access to technology, and the AM drug kit is more comprehensive. The flight team also generally sees more high-acuity patients and therefore has more experience managing that type of patient. However, there has been little research demonstrating significant improvement in outcome for patients transported by air ambulance rather than ground ambulance. Studies show significant variation in benefit by patient type. Some patients have much to gain from involvement of the AM team, while others have little.

Medical patients generally have the most to gain. The flight team should be able to provide most of the treatments available in a hospital setting for medical patients. Management of cardiac arrest, airway difficulties, angina, acute myocardial infarction, electrolyte disturbances, and other conditions is clearly within the capabilities of the AM team. With these expanded capabilities, extended scene time or time in a referring hospital may be indicated prior to transport.

On the other hand, a flight team may have little to offer badly injured trauma patients. While the establishment of a definitive airway, the relief of a tension pneumothorax, and the administration of blood products are certainly prerequisites for a good outcome, the most important treatment the flight team can give these patients is rapid delivery to a trauma center. AM team members should not be lulled into thinking otherwise.

Trauma

Trauma is defined as a physical injury or wound caused by external force or violence. In the United States, trauma is the leading cause of death for those between 1 and 44 years of age. Trauma is significant not only as a cause of death but also as a cause of temporary and permanent disability. For each person who dies as a result of trauma, two are left disabled. Some of the more common causes of trauma are motor vehicle crashes, gunshot wounds, knife wounds, blunt force injuries, falls, and burns. Trauma may account for 50 percent or more of total flights in some programs, notably those based at regional trauma centers.

Damage due to trauma may be classified as primary or secondary. Primary trauma is delivered and completed at the time of the traumatic event. Little can be done to undo the damage. Secondary injury occurs or develops after and as a result of the primary event. It evolves as a result of anatomic and/or physiologic changes precipitated by the primary event. Examples include increased intracranial pressure or development of compartment syndrome. Secondary injury may be prevented or minimized if proper medical treatment is performed in a timely manner. Air medical teams may play a vital role in limiting the development or progression of secondary injury by reaching patients quickly, providing stabilization, and facilitating quick delivery to a medical facility with trauma management capabilities.

One of the secondary complications of trauma is hypothermia. This condition can develop in patients who are exposed to cold temperatures for an extended period. However, traumatic injuries may compromise the normal compensatory mechanisms and hypothermia may develop even in moderate temperatures. Even patients who are adequately shielded from the cold may suffer a decrease in body temperature and require active rewarming.

Significant traumatic injuries can be managed definitively only in the operating room. While trauma patients may be managed supportively, the importance of prompt delivery to a facility where trauma surgeons are available cannot be overemphasized. The Golden Hour concept remains one of the most important components of prehospital and in-hospital trauma management. Patients who are discovered quickly, stabilized on scene, and delivered to definitive care generally have better outcomes than those not receiving that degree of care.

Types of Trauma

Multisystem Trauma

Multisystem trauma refers to traumatic injuries involving multiple anatomic systems within the body. This type of injury often produces a higher-acuity patient than does a traumatic injury involving a single system. Multisystem injuries are generally more complex and require a team approach for adequate management. The treatment of choice is rapid extrication, prompt immobilization/stabilization, and delivery to a trauma center. For primary responses, scene time should be minimized, and, beyond establishment of ABCs, treatments should be initiated during transport.

Single-System Trauma

This involves injuries to a single body system. An example is multiple fractures occurring without head, thoracic, or abdominal involvement. Although single-system injuries may be life-threatening, they are less likely to be so than multisystem injuries. They may be an indication for air transport if potentially life- or limb-threatening.

Penetrating Trauma

Penetrating trauma is endemic in the United States. Projectile injuries and stab wounds are relatively common sights for flight team members. Firearm-related injuries are commonly seen in inner city and rural areas alike. These injuries are particularly challenging, as the extent of damage is often difficult to assess outside the operating room, particularly in the early stages of injury. For example, it may be difficult to determine whether tachycardia is caused by pain and anxiety or by developing hypovolemia. It may be difficult to tell whether mild dyspnea is secondary to guarding or due to developing hemothorax or pneumothorax. This is one injury type for which overtriage can often be justified. If the pathway of the projectile indicates potential damage to a vital organ, aircraft use may be warranted even in the absence of early clinical compromise. In the presence of a mechanism of injury that may be life-threatening, it is better to overmobilize than to undermobilize.

Blunt Trauma

Although the impact of AM programs on the outcomes of trauma patients is the subject of some controversy, several studies have indicated a positive impact on the outcomes of victims of blunt trauma. This type of injury is typically associated with deceleration and falling. Automobile crashes may result in the transfer of tremendous physical energy to passengers. Although three-point seat belts and air bags may significantly reduce the incidence of blunt trauma, not all drivers use them. In high-speed crashes, significant trauma may occur even when restraint devices are in use.

Falls are often associated with blunt trauma. Life-threatening injuries may develop secondary to falls of relatively short distances, especially in the elderly. Significant internal injury can occur with little or no external manifestation. During scene responses it is extremely important that medical team members conduct a thorough hands-on assessment before accepting a refusal from a patient presenting with blunt trauma, especially when the mechanism of injury is indicative of potential internal injury. While it is possible that symptoms may not manifest until long after the incident has occurred, a thorough physical will elicit findings in most cases.

Blunt trauma associated with failing vital signs indicates catastrophic internal injury and has a very high mortality rate. If these patients are transported by air, rapid delivery to the operating room is the most valuable service the AM team can provide. Only the most essential stabilizing techniques should be performed on scene. All other interventions should be carried out during transport.

Patients with cardiac arrest occurring secondary to blunt trauma have a survival rate of less than 1 percent. Using an aircraft to transport these patients is almost always a futile effort. It is an inefficient use of resources and should be discouraged. Conversely, victims of blunt trauma

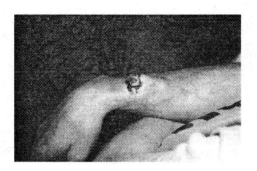

FIGURE 10-5
Patient with fracture

with potentially serious injuries but relatively stable vital signs may benefit from helicopter transport.

Orthopedic Injuries

The enhanced safety devices that are now routinely integrated into passenger cars have led to a significant increase in survival rates in crashes. Passengers frequently survive crashes now that would have been considered fatal only a few years ago. However, the restraint and airbag systems in most passenger cars are directed at protecting the patient's head and torso. They are less effective at preventing extremity injuries and in some cases may even cause or contribute to such injuries. The result is that more passengers are surviving, but often with significant orthopedic injuries (Figure 10-5).

Orthopedic injuries alone, while painful and potentially debilitating, are rarely life-threatening. In most cases management involves immobilization and splinting. If perfusion is compromised, prompt realignment may be required to salvage the distal extremity. The flight team should be adept at assessing and managing orthopedic injuries and performing realignment and reduction procedures when indicated.

Fractures, especially those that are grossly displaced, are often unnerving and may distract less experienced medical personnel from more serious injuries. When responding as a secondary unit to scene requests, the flight team should always double-check to make sure that more serious injuries have not been overlooked. In many cases the first responders have already packaged the patient and access may be difficult. It is generally not appropriate to unpackage the patient just to reassess. However, if there is any suspicion that injuries have been missed and that additional treatment may be indicated, the flight team should not hesitate to reassess. This can generally be done in the aircraft so as to avoid transport delays (and also to avoid offending prehospital personnel).

When there are no contraindications, pain management should be a priority. Prompt pain management is not only humane, it also decreases physical and mental stress and may lead to a reduction in recovery time. In the absence of contraindications there is rarely a valid reason to withhold narcotic analgesia from patients with moderate to severe pain. Contraindications may include traumatic brain injury, undiagnosed abdominal pain, hypovolemia, multisystem trauma, hypotension, and the ingestion of other CNS depressants. A thorough history and physical examination should always precede the administration of narcotic analgesics.

Head Injury

Patients presenting with traumatic brain injury require specialized medical care available only at select tertiary care centers. The early involvement of a neurosurgeon is essential to maximize outcome potential. This type of injury is so specialized that other members of the health care team are essentially helpless to provide any degree of definitive care. However, the flight team is qualified to start treatments to prevent the development of secondary injury, including establishment of a definitive airway, monitoring and regulation of oxygen saturation levels, and administration of sedatives and neuromuscular blocking agents to prevent nonpurposeful movements that may increase intracranial pressure. When appropriate and when authorized to do so, the flight team may administer steroids and/or osmotic diuretics to help limit cerebral edema.

Spinal Injuries

Patients with unstable spinal injuries are often transported by air medical services. While many have complete injuries and prehospital stabilization is of little significance, others may benefit substantially. For example, patients with incomplete spinal disruptions (i.e., subluxation), which have the potential for worsening, may benefit from the relatively smooth ride offered by a helicopter. In areas where roads are less than ideal, the difference in ride quality may have a significant impact on outcome. These patients may also benefit from the availability of medications such as methylprednisolone that the flight team has access to but many ground ambulances do not.

Patients with actual or potential spinal injuries should be thoroughly assessed and either cleared or completely immobilized prior to transport. (Figure 10-6) Air medical personnel should be trained to implement a prehospital c-spine clearance protocol. For scene responses, any patient for whom the flight team cannot easily rule out injury should be immobilized prior to movement.

Interfacility transports are generally less challenging. Patients have typically been assessed and spinal injuries have either been ruled out or confirmed. The flight team must use caution, however, in relying on the assessment of physicians who are not trained in emergency medicine. Some AM programs have protocols specifying that all patients who are being transported to a referral center and who have not been assessed

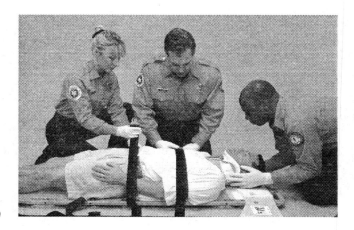

Patient in complete spinal immobilization

and cleared by a physician trained in emergency medicine, trauma management, or neurosurgery be transported in an immobilized state regardless of perceived radiology findings.

Patients who have been immobilized for long periods may be subject to secondary injuries from prolonged lack of movement and contact with a hard surface. Unpadded spine boards may cause soft-tissue injury to the occipital region of the scalp and the sacral and coccygeal regions of the back. Padded boards or vacuum devices are much less likely to cause this type of injury. The patient's normal anatomic position must also be taken into consideration when using spinal immobilization equipment. Some patients, notably the elderly, may have kyphosis or other abnormalities in spinal contour and require extensive padding prior to attachment to an immobilization device.

Prehospital Management of Trauma

Many cases of prehospital trauma are secondary to motor vehicle crashes or entanglement in machinery (Figure 10-7). Prehospital treatment should involve appropriate medical extrication. Standing passively by while rescue personnel disentangle a patient from a vehicle is an inadequate approach. It is essential that the medical team gain control of the patient immediately upon arrival, that a reasonable assessment be done, and that stabilization procedures be initiated as soon as the patient becomes accessible. Spinal immobilization, airway control (including intubation), and IV insertion can all be accomplished during the extrication process. Effective medical extrication may require the periodic interruption of the physical extrication process for reassessment of the patient and/or to provide necessary stabilization. The medical team should ensure the safety and ongoing treatment of the patient during all phases of the process.

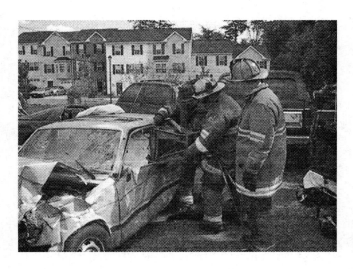

FIGURE 10-7
Wrecked vehicle with patient trapped inside
Photo courtesy of www.Seatpleasantfire.com

Upon removal of the patient from the vehicle, immediate life threats should be corrected (if possible), and the patient immobilized and promptly moved to the aircraft. Establishing an airway and performing pleural decompression or tube thoracotomy may be valid reasons for briefly delaying transport. All other procedures, including the establishment of IVs, should be performed in the aircraft during transport. The AM team's most valuable contributions when dealing with high-acuity trauma patients are immobilization to prevent secondary injury, preservation of vital signs, and rapid delivery to a trauma center.

The use of blood and blood products during the initial stabilization process may be beneficial. However, due to logistics this is an uncommon practice. Hospital-based programs have an advantage in this area. They can sign out a limited quantity of O negative blood from their emergency departments when blood is likely to be needed for prehospital or interfacility transports. Larger aircraft may even have small refrigerators in the patient compartment for this purpose.

Interfacility Management of Trauma

There are two basic scenarios for trauma patients being moved from one facility to another—those who have been stabilized and those who haven't. In many rural areas, hospitals do not have the personnel or equipment to stabilize trauma patients. The air medical crew may be called on to provide initial stabilization at the referring facility prior to transport and to continue the stabilization process during transport. Patient care should be very similar to that provided in the prehospital setting. An airway and adequate ventilation should be established immediately where the patient is found. Other procedures that have been shown to have less impact on outcome (IV, urinary catheter, etc.) should be performed during transport.

Patients who have been stabilized by referring personnel may be treated slightly differently. They generally will have a secure airway, will be ventilating adequately, and will have received fluid or blood products. Some may have received preliminary surgical stabilization. The flight team should avoid unnecessary delay but may take a slightly less rushed approach. An adequate physical examination should be performed and all pertinent medical information should be obtained prior to transport. A special effort should be made to maintain normal body temperature.

Medical Conditions

Cardiovascular Conditions

Patients presenting with myocardial disease processes are often of high acuity and may be candidates for air medical transport. Acute myocardial infarction, unstable angina, cardiogenic shock, aortic dissection, and refractory dysrhythmias may all be justification for aircraft use. The medical team should be adept at managing these patient types. Rotor-wing air ambulances should be equipped with 12-lead ECGs and have a full complement of cardiac medications including fibrinolytic agents, anticoagulants, beta-blockers, and glycoprotein inhibitors.

anxiety

An emotional state precipitated by a stressful situation. Many patients become anxious when they learn they are about to fly in a helicopter.

There has been concern about subjecting cardiac patients to the stresses of flight. Evidence suggests that the **anxiety** induced by flight may elevate catacholamine levels and increase myocardial oxygen demand, thereby increasing the risk of complications. Indeed, the mere thought of flying in a helicopter creates anxiety in some patients, and steps should be taken to relieve the anxiety before beginning the move to the aircraft. Interacting with the patient and family members in a caring and informative way may be all that is needed to relieve minor anxiety. In more refractory cases, anxiolytic medications may be indicated. Morphine sulfate, the drug of choice for pain of cardiac origin, also has anxiolytic properties and will relieve anxiety in most patients. If analgesia is not indicated, a benzodiazepine such as lorazepam or midazolam may be effective. In rare cases where the patient's fear of flying does not diminish and sedation is refused, ground transport should be arranged.

Cardiac Networks

Over the past several years it has become clear that a significant percentage of acute myocardial infarction patients do not respond to fibrinolytic therapy. These patients require prompt invasive treatment in order to maximize their outcome potential. In some areas of the country, cardiac networks have been established to ensure that these patients are promptly moved to hospitals capable of providing definitive care, namely cardiac catheterization and cardiovascular surgical capabilities. AM programs have proved useful in this process, especially when tertiary-level facilities are a long distance away.

The specifics of these systems vary according to the capabilities of pre-hospital personnel operating in the area. Under ideal circumstances, ground and air ambulances have 12-lead ECG capability and cardiac patients can be screened prior to transport. Patients presenting with indications of unstable angina, myocardial injury, or myocardial infarction can be routed directly to a definitive care facility. If the nearest facility is far away or requires much longer transport time, the patient may be taken to a nearer facility for initial stabilization. If the patient requires critical care capabilities or if the nearest appropriate definitive care facility is a long distance away the patient may benefit from involvement of the AM team program at that point.

Left Ventricular Assist Devices

Air medical programs may be called on to transport patients with frank left ventricular failure. These patients may be dependent on left ventricular assist devices (balloon pumps or IABCs, intraaortic balloon counterpulsation devices) to maintain effective cardiac output (Figure 10-8).

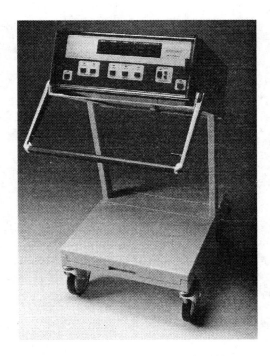

FIGURE 10-8
Left ventricular assist device
Courtesy of Thoratec Corporation

Common Patient Types and Principles of Management 167

The availability of these devices may have a significant impact on patient outcome. The IABC device is very effective at buying time until a patient's own left ventricle can recover or until more definitive therapy becomes available. The device is typically large and cumbersome, so it is difficult to secure in most helicopters. Ideally, the use of these devices should be factored in during the design of the medical interior of the helicopter. Aircraft can also be retrofitted, or the device can be strapped to the tracks that secure movable seats.

Extracorporeal Membranous Oxygenation

Extracorporeal membranous oxygenation (ECMO) is similar to the heart-lung bypass machine often used during cardiac bypass surgery. The patient is attached to the machine by way of two tubes. One tube circulates deoxygenated blood from the patient to the machine. As the blood moves through the machine, it is brought into contact with a series of semipermeable membranes that are in close proximity to a high-concentration oxygen source. As the blood moves past the membrane, oxygen diffuses into the blood and carbon dioxide diffuses from the blood into the machine. The newly oxygenated blood is then pumped back into the patient.

ECMO is a subspecialized service available only at tertiary-care facilities. Hospitals offering this service may accept high-risk, high-acuity referrals from surrounding hospitals. In some cases an ECMO device may be mounted aboard a helicopter and used during transport. Larger helicopters are needed to accommodate the machine, which is larger and heavier than a balloon pump, and personnel are required to operate it. A specialty care team should always be in attendance during these transports, along with at least one member of the core medical team.

Aortic Aneurysm

Patients presenting with dissecting aortic aneurysm are at risk for rapid deterioration during transport. In many cases they require prompt cardiovascular surgery to survive. The goal of the medical team should be to stabilize and deliver the patient to the cardiovascular surgeon as quickly as possible. Anxiety and hypertension must be controlled. Anxiety results in sympathetic stimulation, which precipitates vasoconstriction, increases stroke volume, and ultimately increases blood pressure. As stroke volume and blood pressure increase, the aorta is further stressed, increasing the probability of further dissection and aortic rupture.

It is extremely important that these patients be calmed and sedated if necessary before they are moved to the aircraft. Blood pressure should be closely monitored and kept in the low normal range. Beta-blockers may be effective in decreasing sympathetic tone and controlling blood pressure. The goal is to reduce intraaortic pressure so as to reduce the amount of pressure being placed on the damaged aortic wall. However, blood pressure should not be lowered so much that adequate tissue perfusion is threatened.

In case of sudden decrease in perfusion status, ruptured aneurysm must be suspected. The administration of fluids and blood products to reestablish adequate perfusion and the rapid delivery of the patient to a cardiovascular surgeon should be the primary concerns. In these cases rapid deterioration and death are common.

CNS Disorders

Stroke

Since the advent of fibrinolytic use for embolic/thrombotic strokes, the role of the air medical program has become more important in the management of those patient types, especially in rural areas. There are still many rural hospitals that do not have CT machines or physicians willing to administer fibrinolytics to stroke patients. In such cases the use of an aircraft may significantly reduce the amount of time between onset of symptoms and administration of fibrinolytic therapy. Ischemic stroke patients may benefit substantially from air transport. In contrast to most other medical patients, the greater benefit is from prompt delivery to a facility with CT and fibrinolytic capabilities than from the medical care available from the flight team.

In rural areas where community hospitals are long distances from referral centers, the use of a helicopter may save valuable time and enable the patient to be seen within the window of opportunity for fibrinolytic administration. A cooperative effort in which prehospital personnel notify the flight team as soon as the patient is encountered can speed this process, sometimes dramatically. The aircraft can acquire the patient directly from the scene or, if a hospital is located nearby, can rapidly retrieve and transfer the patient from that hospital to a referral facility.

As the management of stroke patients continues to evolve, more patients are being taken to an interventional laboratory, where a catheter is threaded directly into the cerebral vessels holding the clot. Fibrinolytic agents can then be administered directly into the blocked vessel in higher concentrations than would be possible otherwise. This procedure can be done beyond the time frame allowed for systemic administration of fibrinolytics. Unfortunately, it requires equipment and personnel available only at a small number of U.S. hospitals. An air medical service operating in an area where this treatment is available may be justified in transporting patients directly to the center even if it means a longer transport time.

A number of studies are evaluating a variety of potential neuroprotectants. It is the goal of researchers to design a substance that will preserve cerebral tissues in the presence of prolonged hypoxia. Such a medication would extend the window of opportunity for administering fibrinolytic agents or other definitive therapies that may be developed.

Seizures

Patients presenting with refractory tonic-clonic seizures (status epilepticus) may be candidates for air medical transport. Often they have seized for some time prior to involvement of the flight team. They have likely received large quantities of anticonvulsants, including benzodiazepines and other CNS depressants. The flight team may have to deal not only with ongoing seizure activity but also with the cumulative effects of those medications.

Patients who seize for extended periods (longer than 20 or 30 minutes) may develop hypoxic and/or toxic brain damage and should be managed aggressively. The goal is to stop not only the physical manifestations of the seizure but also the underlying electrical activity. High-dose benzodiazepines, barbiturates, phenobarbital, and other antiepileptic medications should be used as directed by protocol.

Some of these patients also have underlying medical conditions that put them at additional risk. Sustained tonic-clonic seizures subject the patient to a tremendous amount of physical stress. The energy expenditure associated with a seizure is equivalent to that of a strenuous athletic event. Patients who are already in poor physical health are at risk for developing secondary complications. In particular, patients with arteriosclerosis may be at increased risk for developing myocardial infarction or hypoxic stroke and should be frequently reassessed for vital signs, ECG, and oxygen saturation. Benzodiazepines such as lorazepam and diazepam remain the mainstay of seizure management for adult patients. These drugs eventually halt seizure activity in over 90 percent of patients. When administered as directed, they have a high success rate and a relatively low incidence of side effects. Respiratory depression and hypotension can be significantly reduced if these drugs are administered in small increments over several minutes. Fear of causing respiratory compromise should never delay the administration of these medications. If the patient does develop respiratory compromise, the airway should be controlled and maintained as with any other patient type.

The use of neuromuscular blocking agents for patients presenting in refractory status epilepticus is rarely indicated. While these drugs control the outward manifestation of seizures, they have little effect on electrical activity within the brain. By masking the signs of seizures, they may delay more aggressive treatment aimed at stopping the actual seizure. If seizure activity continues despite adequate doses of standard medications, general anesthesia may be the only option for stopping the seizure activity.

Patients who develop seizure activity as a result of head trauma are at additional risk for secondary injury. Tonic-clonic seizure activity increases intracranial pressure and may have a negative impact on outcome for those patients. Here again aggressive treatment must be provided to prevent secondary brain damage.

Pulmonary Diseases

Patients with chronic pulmonary disease may experience acute compensation of a critical nature. They may be ventilator-dependent, require close monitoring, and are often transported by helicopter. These patients may be particularly sensitive to environmental changes. They are often precariously balanced between compensation and decompensation, and any change in oxygen availability may lead to deterioration in clinical status. Altitude changes that are clinically insignificant for other patient types may have a notable effect on these patients. Efforts should be made to fly at low altitudes when transporting patients with pulmonary disease. When that is not possible, altitude changes should be made as slowly as possible and oxygen delivery should be carefully titrated to compensate.

Chronic lung disease patients who have not been intubated should be monitored carefully. They may normally maintain oxygen saturation and blood gas values that are outside the normal range. For these patients, relative readings and trends are of more value than snapshot values. Patients with advanced disease often benefit most from a conservative approach regarding airway management. For a patient who is maintaining oxygenation status within a reasonable range of normal, it is often best not to intubate as the patient may become ventilator-dependent and weaning can be difficult. As with any other patient type, if acute decompensation occurs, the airway should be managed by any means necessary to restore adequate oxygenation.

Burns

Air medical programs are frequently called on to transport critical burn patients. In many areas of the country, there are few burn centers and patients may have to be transported long distances. During the acute phase of burn management, medical personnel should focus on stopping the burn process, establishing an appropriate airway, preventing infection,

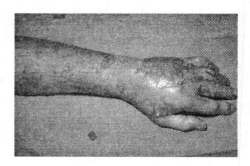

FIGURE 10-9
Patient with second- and
third-degree burns
Shout Pictures

controlling pain, and maintaining hydration. Patients with respiratory involvement may be at high risk for glottic and laryngeal edema with subsequent airway closure and must be managed promptly and aggressively to maintain airway patency. AM teams are well suited to perform the procedures necessary to maintain the airway in the high-risk burn patient.

Infection is almost always a concern for patients with significant burns (Figure 10-9). AM personnel should minimize the risk of introducing bacteria to the burned area. Loose debris should be brushed away and sterile saline used to irrigate contaminated surface areas. In most cases it is appropriate to cover the burned area with dry, sterile linens. If there are extensive second-degree burns with much pain, the application of cool sterile saline to the linen may ease pain. However, it may also increase the risk of contamination. For moderate to severe pain, narcotic analgesics should be administered. In addition to being in pain, burn patients are often anxious and confused. Narcotic analgesia also puts patients at ease and helps them to be more cooperative.

Fluid management is another important issue with burn patients, who lose fluid rapidly and in proportion to the burn surface area. The AM team should be capable of rapidly assessing the patient's fluid deficit and longer-term infusion requirements. The two most commonly employed formulas for determining fluid replacement needs for the adult patient are the Parkland Formula and the Modified Brooke Formula. Children have greater body surface area in relation to body weight, and determining adequate fluid replacement may be somewhat more difficult than with adults. The Shrine Burn Formula is commonly used when dealing with children.

Burn patients may have circumferential burns of the thorax and/or extremities. Badly burned tissue may become hard and inflexible. If that occurs around the thorax, respiratory excursion may be compromised. Prompt intervention is necessary to maintain respiratory status. Circumferential burns of the extremities may lead to loss of distal perfusion and, if not managed promptly, threaten the survival of distal tissues.

Either of these circumstances requires the performance of escharotomy. This should be a standard skill for programs that transport significant numbers of burn patients. In some states only a physician may perform escharotomy; others allow flight nurses or flight paramedics to perform the skill if a need can be documented and if adequate training is provided.

A recent study suggests that most burn patients transported by air medical programs had injuries that did not require critical-care management and that air transport simply added to the patient's medical bill. That may be because burn centers are sparsely located in many areas of the country and transport to a burn center can be a complicated process. In any case AM programs should have a protocol for determining if a burn patient has injuries significant enough to warrant use of an aircraft.

Other Roles

To some extent the role of an AM program may vary by location. For example, programs operating in urban areas may do more interfacility transports and relatively few scene responses. Those based in rural areas may see more scene responses, but also be called on to transport patients between hospitals. The availability and education level of prehospital providers may influence air medical activity. In areas where paramedics are readily available aboard ground ambulances, the number of air medical scene responses is generally lower than in areas where paramedics are not available.

The geography and placement of hospitals is another factor that affects response patterns and volume. In regions where there are many community hospitals and ground ambulances have shorter transport times, the incidence of scene flights may be lower. In mountainous or difficult-to-access areas, there may be more scene flights.

Business agreements may also influence the types of transports done. Financial incentives may result in new or modified response patterns, patient types being transported, modifications to crew composition, and protocol usage.

Some less traditional roles for AM programs are discussed below.

Organ Procurement

Some AM programs allow their aircraft to be used to deliver an organ harvest team and/or transport donor organs. While this may not always be the most economical way to provide this service, it is certainly an appropriate use for a medical helicopter. In some areas AM programs transport a large percent of organ donors. Programs interested in becoming involved in such activities should contact their state or regional organ recovery agency for information.

Delivery of Blood and Pharmaceuticals

In rural areas smaller hospitals may not have the volume of patients necessary to stock infrequently used pharmaceutical agents, antivenins, or large volumes of blood and blood products. If a facility runs out of a vital blood product or drug while managing an emergency patient, an AM team may be used to deliver the products. In most cases the patient will also be secured by the flight program and transported to a larger referral facility.

Search and Rescue (SAR)

Search and rescue (SAR) involves the use of the aircraft and flight crew to locate a missing person or persons. AM programs are generally used only in cases with potential medical implications. Law enforcement agencies generally have their own aircraft for performing SAR in criminal activities. In some areas there may be overlap. Air medical programs should use extreme caution before allowing their aircraft to be used to search for a felon who does not want to be found. There have been cases where medical aircraft have been fired on. (See Appendix E for additional information on SAR.)

Summary

The flight team manages a variety of patient types. Many patients are critical, and the actions taken by the flight team may have a significant impact on outcome. The medical team should be adequately prepared to manage virtually all emergency and critical care situations. To do so, each member of the team must be knowledgeable and experienced at history gathering and patient assessment. A systematic approach helps to minimize the risk of overlooking clues.

Air medical teams may respond to two very different types of requests. Scene flights are less controlled and have more potential dangers. Patient information may be sketchy or completely lacking. These patients benefit most from a flight team that is competent in prehospital and emergency medicine. In contrast, interfacility transports usually involve patients who have been evaluated by a physician, and more information is available. Those patients benefit more from critical-care knowledge and skills.

The flight program may also function in nonstandard roles that go beyond typical patient transport. These roles vary by location and according to the needs of the medical community. Examples include organ procurement and the delivery of blood products and/or pharmaceuticals. The flight program should be prepared for all contingencies.

REVIEW QUESTIONS

1. This skill may be utilized as a temporary fix when a surgical airway is indicated but when air medical personnel are not permitted to perform that skill.
   a. Auricular decompression
   b. Transtracheal jet insufflation
   c. Crichopectoralis decompression
   d. Pericardiocentesis

2. This procedure may restore blood flow to an extremity in a patient with a circumferential burn.
   a. Escharotomy
   b. Tracheostomy
   c. Pneumonectomy
   d. Pleural decompression

3. Patients presenting with this type of traumatic injury may benefit from the relatively smooth ride offered by the rotor-wing air ambulance.
   a. Muscle strain
   b. Fracture of the radius
   c. Pneumothorax
   d. Spinal injury

4. Patients presenting with this condition and who remain anxious about air medical transport may require ground transport.
   a. Acute myocardial infarction
   b. Femur fracture
   c. Septic shock
   d. Snakebite

5. A specialty care team should always be used when patients receiving this treatment are transported.
   a. Dopamine infusion
   b. Ventilator with PEEP setting
   c. Continuous administration of analgesics for gall stones
   d. Extracorporeal membranous oxygenation

6. Discuss the implications of air medical transport of patients with pulmonary disease.

CHAPTER 11

Preparing the Patient for Air Medical Transport

Objectives

Upon completing this chapter, the reader should have a better understanding of the following topics:

* The general approach to preparing the patient for transport

* Patient assessment and management

* The importance of communication with the patient, family, and referring medical personnel

* The approach to interfacility transports and scene responses

* Management of violent patients

* The pros and cons of allowing family members to accompany a patient

Introduction

In order to transport patients safely and efficiently, an air medical program must use a systematic approach to patient assessment and management. While this approach may vary somewhat depending on the type of transport and the specific patient pathophysiology, the basic approach should remain the same.

The patient should be adequately assessed from physical and psychological perspectives. Medical needs must be anticipated and prepared for. The patient's mental status and activity level must be evaluated as a possible safety threat before the patient is moved to the aircraft. Conscious patients may require calming or sedation if there is significant anxiety about flying or any potential for violence. Safety concerns dictate that this process be more thorough than it would be with a ground ambulance operation.

General Approach

The role played by each crew member depends on the number of crew members available, the patient type, and whether the patient is being acquired from a prehospital site or from a referring hospital. Each member's role should be determined well in advance of encountering the patient. While team members should confer with one another over assessment and treatment-related decisions, each should have separate, specific responsibilities. A suggested approach is for one team member to proceed immediately to the patient and begin the assessment process. The other team member makes contact with referring medical personnel or, if a scene flight, witnesses and bystanders. The two then combine their information, form a preliminary diagnosis, and develop a treatment plan.

Patient Assessment

Each member of the medical team must be capable of performing a thorough physical examination, including assessment of all body systems, breath sounds, heart tones, cranial nerves, and so on. That is not to say that every body system of every patient should be assessed. Each patient should be assessed to the extent warranted by circumstances. For some patients that may mean a head-to-toe assessment of all body systems. For others, such as a patient with an isolated extremity fracture, the assessment may be more focused. In any case the exam should be complete enough to explore all reasonably likely pathologies.

For interfacility transports a thorough exam should be a routine part of the patient acceptance process. Accepting and moving a patient to the aircraft without assessment should be done only under extenuating circumstances. The well-being of the patient and the credibility of the flight team may hinge on this assessment.

Pain status should also be evaluated for each patient. In the era of modern health care there is rarely a valid reason for allowing pain to go untreated. For scene responses there may be relative or absolute contraindications to the administration of narcotic analgesics. For isolated extremity injuries and burns, pain management should be considered a priority and should be initiated at the earliest opportunity, often before the patient is moved from the scene.

Airway Management

For all patient types, the assessment and stabilization of immediate life threats is the first priority. The medical team should be certain that every patient transported has a patent airway. For critical or unstable patients an endotracheal tube should be placed prior to transport. Even patients who are stable but have significant potential for deterioration may benefit from elective intubation. That may be particularly true for patients with head injury where movement may increase ICP.

If the patient has an existing ET tube, placement should be assessed. Obvious displacement may be recognized by visual or tactile assessment. Breath sounds should be auscultated bilaterally in at least two locations. The epigastrum should be auscultated for sounds of gastric insufflation. If breath sounds are normal, there should be secondary confirmation using a reliable technique. The simplest way to do this is with a bag-valve-mask that incorporates a carbon dioxide detector. Portable commercial devices that measure expired CO_2 and oxygen saturation are effective. The use of an endotracheal aspiration bulb may also be adequate.

If findings indicate a misplaced tube, prompt corrective action should be taken. A tube that is totally dislodged should be removed and the patient ventilated via bag-valve-mask until a new tube can be inserted. If a tube is still in the trachea but has been displaced distally, the cuff should be deflated, the tube retracted until breath sounds normalize, and the cuff reinflated.

The use of neuromuscular blocking agents (NMBAs) is a must for all critical-care transport teams. Used in conjunction with benzodiazepines and/or fentanyl, NMBAs facilitate intubation. Benzodiazepines are effective agents for maintaining sedation during transport. Propofol is also effective, especially for patients with potential neurologic compromise. The drug has a very short half-life and neurologic status returns to baseline within minutes after the infusion is discontinued. Receiving physicians can then perform a neurologic assessment shortly after the AM team delivers the patient.

The intubated patient should be carefully monitored before and during transport. Breath sounds should be assessed and reassessed frequently. Ancillary devices should be used for confirmation. Pulse oximetry is useful for monitoring trends in oxygen saturation. CO_2 detectors are better suited for the detection of acute changes as may occur with tube displacement or compromises in airway patency.

Ventilator-dependent patients should be checked for airway patency. If secretions or mucous plugs are noted in the airway or the endotracheal tube, they should promptly be removed with a suction device. Patients with chest trauma and decreased oxygen saturation levels may have pneumothorax, hemothorax, airway disruption, or foreign material in the airway. Surgical airways are options for flight programs that either staff with physicians or allow expanded scope of practice for nurses or paramedics. This should be considered only in cases where an airway cannot be established by more conventional means. All AM programs should have a viable contingency plan for difficult airway management.

For interfacility transports the task is somewhat simpler. One crew member should approach and assess the patient while the other communicates with referring medical personnel and obtains patient information that may already have been gathered. In no case should this information be accepted as fact without reassessment. There is always a possibility that something has been missed or that the patient's condition has changed since the last set of information was acquired.

All necessary monitoring equipment should be taken to the bedside and attached before patient movement. Most flight programs use a lightweight multifunctional monitor such as the Propaq. That device monitors ECG, invasive and noninvasive blood pressure, arterial pressure, oxygen saturation, central venous pressure, and intracranial pressure. Other monitoring devices commonly used by flight programs include the Lifepak 12 and Matrix CCT.

IV lines should be changed out, infusions reestablished at the correct rate/dose, and all other ongoing treatment modalities evaluated and reestablished at the appropriate level. Spinal immobilization should generally be maintained at this point. The majority of trauma patients transported by an AM program have been exposed to significant forces, and any existing spinal precautions should be maintained. While it may be appropriate for AM personnel to assess spinal status and determine whether immobilization is needed in the prehospital setting, that should generally not be done for interfacility transports where a physician assessment has already been completed.

The Bispectral Index Monitor

The Bispectral Index Monitor (BIS), which has traditionally been used in the operating room, has begun to make its way into critical-care units and some AM programs. This device may be of value when transporting patients who have received neuromuscular blocking agents and are sedated. The BIS quantifies sedation and pain levels by performing two measurements of electrical activity: frontal lobe electroencephalogram (EEG) and electromyography (EMG). These data are obtained through a probe that attaches to the patient's forehead. The BIS uses an algorithm to correlate the two data streams and produces a single number, or BIS value, that represents the patient's level of consciousness. This number is displayed on a large screen on the front of the device. The scale ranges from zero, no activity (dead), to 100, fully alert.

As a patient's level of consciousness decreases, so does the BIS score. In an operating room, surgery is generally performed when the BIS score is in the 40–50 range. A score of 70 generally indicates that sedation is adequate to ensure that recall doesn't occur. The BIS device can also be used to determine whether a patient is experiencing pain and whether the amount of analgesia administered is adequate. Use of the BIS allows medical personnel to more accurately maintain sedation and pain relief while minimizing the incidence of both over- and undermedication.

Communication

Communication is key to getting the patient prepared in an efficient manner. The medical flight team must communicate with first responders, nurses, physicians, or anyone else who may have pertinent information regarding patients and their prior medical care. While the general approach to patient preparation is similar, specific actions may vary depending on whether the patient is being acquired from a medical facility or from an out-of-hospital site.

Communication with the Patient

The thought of a helicopter flight can be very traumatic for some patients, especially when the flight is necessitated by a medical emergency. Conscious patients should be psychologically prepared for transport before they are moved to the aircraft. They should be informed of their medical condition, of the need for transport by air, and of the name and location of the destination hospital. After they have been moved to the aircraft, they should be informed of the upcoming sequence of events, including noises and movements, and continually updated as new stressors occur. Crew members should establish rapport with every conscious patient. Too often AM personnel get caught up in the medical side of patient care and forget the personal side. They must remember that they are caring for people and not just nameless faces.

Emotional stress can have a negative impact on immune function and may result in prolonged recovery time. It is important to relieve as much anxiety as is reasonably possible. Some patients may become calmer in response to a reassuring voice or touch. If a patient becomes exceedingly anxious about flying, and if no contraindications exist, sedation should be considered. If tachycardia and/or hypertension are a concern (AMI, increased ICP), sedation and the use of beta-blockers or other appropriate agents should be considered (according to local protocol) prior to moving the patient to the aircraft. If a patient's level of anxiety may complicate the existing medical condition and sedation is not an option, ground transport should be considered.

Communication with the Family

Communication with family members should be considered an integral role of the flight team. While this applies primarily to interfacility transports, there are also times when family members are present at scene responses. Family members should be considered part of the air medical transport equation. They are typically emotionally distraught, and for many this is their first encounter with an emergency department or an air medical program. They may not have been told anything about the patient's condition before the flight team arrives. All the activity and unfamiliarity of the medical environment may lead to confusion, frustration, and impatience.

It is important that family members be oriented as soon as possible. They should be given an explanation of the patient's condition and the need for air transport. They should be told where the patient is being taken and given directions to the facility if necessary. Some programs hand out brochures that include the name of the receiving facility, directions to the facility, and a list of pertinent telephone numbers. Taking the time to do this not only helps relieve their anxiety but ensures a more tolerable experience for everyone.

Communication with Referring Medical Personnel

During interfacility transports, the primary source of information is referring medical personnel. In most cases the patient has been under their care for some time. They will likely have conducted a physical examination, gathered a history, and performed some degree of diagnostic testing. While the flight team may need to perform additional assessments, the information from referring personnel should be used as a starting point (Figure 11-1).

It is essential that all members of the flight team, including pilots, understand the importance of good interpersonal skills. Often referring personnel do not have the capability to provide definitive care and have called the AM team to move the patient to another facility where definitive care is available. The fact that they do not have the necessary equipment and expertise may result in frustration and impatience. Whether or not this behavior is appropriate, team members must maintain their composure and project a positive attitude.

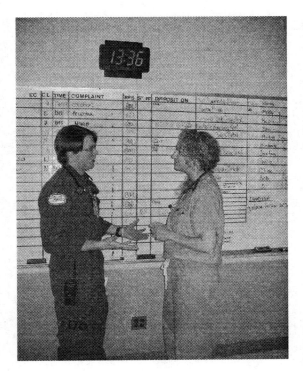

FIGURE 11-1
Flight team member speaking with referring medical personnel

Flight personnel are received differently at different facilities. In some places they may be treated as dignitaries; in others their presence may be all but ignored. Some referring physicians leave all decision making and treatments to the flight team; others want to direct every detail of treatment. The team must be capable of adjusting to different situations while maintaining professionalism and treating others with dignity and respect.

Intracabin Communication with the Patient

Hearing protection is a must for all patients, regardless of level of consciousness (Figure 11-2). Disposable earmuffs or earplugs generally work well for unconscious patients. If bandaging is in the way, padded gauze should be secured over the patient's ears. All conscious or semiconscious patients should have a headset. Some programs have a dedicated headset that plugs into the intracabin communications system for patient use. The design allows the patient to hear the flight team and to respond via a voice-activated microphone. The flight crew has the

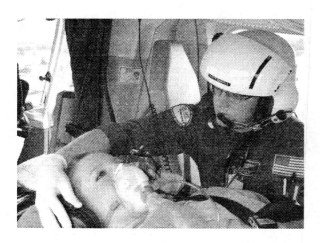

FIGURE 11-2
Crew member applying hearing protection
Photo by Mark Galtelli

option of switching the patient's headset receiver on and off as necessary. Crew members must remember that the patient can hear what is being said and should mute the patient's headset before discussing medical information that may be troubling to the patient, such as the pros and cons of a particular treatment.

Interfacility Transports

Generally, there is some degree of medical information available when the flight team responds to a medical facility. Depending on the capabilities of the referring facility and the area of the hospital from which the patient is being acquired, that information may range from a preliminary assessment to a thorough workup that includes radiographs and lab tests. At the very least the patient's admission form and a summary of assessment and treatments should be obtained prior to transport. Ideally, there should be copies of all medical records and radiographs. However, for patients presenting with time-sensitive conditions, the need for prompt transport may outweigh the need to wait for complete medical records. For example, a patient presenting with multisystem trauma should be transported immediately, with or without complete records.

The aircraft stretcher should be taken to the patient's bedside. If the stretcher does not have wheels, it should be placed on a rolling gurney supplied by the hospital. The patient should be secured to the stretcher and the stretcher secured to the rolling gurney before leaving the hospital. That precaution makes the move from the hospital cot to the aircraft more predictable and safer for all.

In an aircraft cabin, any loose item has the potential to become a projectile in the event of turbulence or a hard landing or crash. All equipment

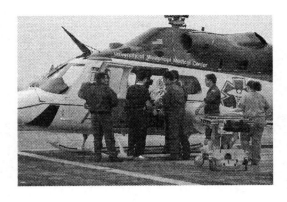

FIGURE 11-3
Patient being loaded into aircraft

must therefore be mounted or securely attached. The FAA provides strict guidelines regarding the amount of force that mounting brackets must be able to withstand. Bringing extra equipment aboard without an acceptable means for securing it may not only violate FAA regulations but subject crew members and patients to unnecessary danger. The pilot should screen all items loaded into the aircraft.

For patients the most vulnerable phase of AM transport is loading and unloading. IV lines are often dislodged, patients may be inadvertently extubated, and equipment may be dropped. Those errors can be easily prevented if assistants are closely supervised and the move is made carefully (Figure 11-3). Some steps that should routinely be performed when securing a patient from a referring hospital are as follows.

1. Questionable IV lines should be discontinued and restarted. A critical patient should have a minimum of two functional IVs prior to transport. A noncritical patient should have at least one patent line.

2. All collection bags should be emptied. A patient who is conscious, stable, and does not have a urinary catheter should be offered the opportunity to void before leaving the referral facility.

3. The patient's airway should be secured in a definitive manner. If there is any doubt as to the patient's ability to self-maintain the airway during transport, the patient should be sedated, paralyzed, and electively intubated.

4. Any noncritical patient who is anxious about flying, is nauseated, or has a history of motion sickness should be medicated accordingly. Insertion of a nasogastric tube should be considered in patients with abdominal or gastrointestinal injuries or diseases. Nausea and vomiting may have clinically significant implications for patients with certain disease processes. The simultaneous, violent muscle contractions and glottic closure associated with vomiting may result in increased intraabdominal, intrathoracic, and intracranial pressures (Figure 11-4).

Preparing the Patient for Air Medical Transport   185

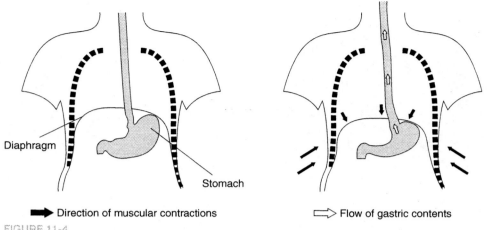

Diaphragm

Stomach

→ Direction of muscular contractions   ⇨ Flow of gastric contents

FIGURE 11-4
Illustration of effects of vomiting

Patients with any condition that may be negatively impacted by increases in any of these pressures may deteriorate if vomiting occurs. Such patients should be treated aggressively to prevent vomiting. The administration of an antiemetic as early as possible prior to flight and the insertion of a nasogastric tube may be effective. The nasogastric tube may also serve as a conduit for the administration of antacids and gastric coating agents. These are actions that can be taken by the referring facility prior to arrival of the aircraft.

5. IV lines should be shortened or looped and secured to the patient or to the stretcher to minimize the risk of entanglement.

6. Oxygen supply tubing should be looped and secured to the patient or to the stretcher.

7. If the patient is intubated, one person should be assigned to keep the tube secured and ensure that patient ventilation is uninterrupted.

8. All equipment (cardiac monitor, Propaq, CO_2 detector, and so on) should be secured to the stretcher. Often the best place to position equipment during movement is at the foot of the stretcher between the patient's feet or knees.

9. The patient and all equipment and other paraphernalia should be moved to the aircraft in a slow and controlled manner. The aircraft crew must monitor this process carefully. Overeager assistants may copy what they have seen on television, try to rush the process, and cause unnecessary problems. Running is almost never appropriate in the vicinity of an aircraft.

10. A reliable assistant should carry items that cannot be secured to the stretcher.

11. Anyone who is not essential to the move should be kindly thanked for their offer to help but should be kept away from the stretcher, the patient, and the aircraft.

12. Only members of the flight team should open aircraft doors. Over-stressing a hinge may disable the aircraft and require repairs and inspection to make it airworthy again.

13. The patient should be loaded into the aircraft only by the flight crew. If extra help is needed, assistants should be directed and monitored very carefully by a member of the flight team.

14. Only flight team members should close aircraft doors, making sure there is no IV or oxygen tubing protruding.

15. Crew members should make certain that all bystanders are at a safe distance from the aircraft during start-up and preparation for departure. Ideally, the helipad should be secured by law enforcement or security personnel prior to approach and departure. When that is not possible, the flight crew has to assume that responsibility.

Pediatric Patients

Pediatric patients may require extra effort on the part of the flight team. When conscious, they are often anxious and emotionally labile. Their anxiety tends to rise when they are confronted by strangers who want to take them away from their families to an unfamiliar vehicle that is crammed full of medical equipment and makes lots of strange, loud noises.

Pediatric patients must be approached in a calm and nonthreatening manner. When time permits, the flight team should build rapport with a child before attempting to move him to the aircraft. If that is not possible, the patient will either have to be moved in an anxious state or be sedated. A sedated child is preferable to one who is anxious and difficult to control. A disruptive child who is large enough or strong enough to threaten the safety of the transport should be managed as an adult and should never be transported in an agitated state.

A pediatric patient must be handled in a calm and compassionate manner. The patient may be critically ill or injured and family members may not see her alive again. The family must drive to a hospital that may be far away. They may not be familiar with the hospital or the medical care system and feel like outsiders. In some cases they may feel additional anxiety concerning the safety of flying.

Pediatric patients over the age of eight or ten may be easier to deal with. Parent separation may be less of an issue, and they can often be distracted from their medical or traumatic conditions by the flight experience. But sedation should be considered for any pediatric patient who continues to have significant anxiety, especially if the anxiety may compromise the patient's medical condition.

Neonatal Transports

Neonates are a group with unique needs. These patients are very small and fragile and require a specialized transport environment with strict environmental control. A neonatal isolette is a self-contained device that encloses the patient and provides all the tools necessary for monitoring and treatment. Most modern isolettes have integrated ventilators, infusion pumps, cardiac monitor, and other necessary monitoring devices. They also have their own source of compressed oxygen and compressed air for air mixing and operation of the ventilator. The isolette generally replaces the adult stretcher when mounted into the aircraft. Use of an isolette may also require reconfiguration of the aircraft to allow for the equipment and supplies needed by the neonatal team. Isolettes are typically heavy (over 200 pounds) and may require adjustments in the number of crew members and in weight and balance.

One or more neonatal nurses or physicians generally accompany neonatal patients. The specialty care needs of these patients typically require specialized drugs and equipment. However, as for all other patient types, at least one member of the core medical team should be aboard the aircraft to ensure safety and consistency.

Neonatal transports do not proceed at the same pace as most other transports. Extra time is required prior to liftoff to assemble the transport team and to reconfigure the aircraft for the isolette and necessary supplies. Once at the referring hospital, on-scene stabilization time may be considerably longer than for typical adult or pediatric patients. An hour or more is common; two to three hours is not unheard of in complicated cases. Neonatal transports are often scheduled in advance. Once the aircraft has been reserved for a neonatal flight, it is no longer available for other responses. To avoid conflicts and misunderstandings, AM programs should establish limits on how far in advance the aircraft may be reserved by the neonatal team.

Scene Responses

Scene responses can be more challenging than interfacility transports. A number of safety-related variables may come into play. AM teams are entering a less controlled environment and frequently do not have the backup support that is commonly available at a referring hospital. Scene

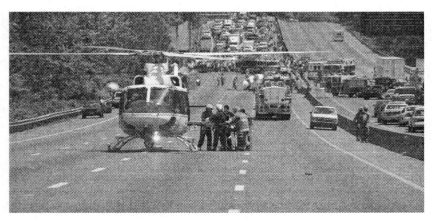

FIGURE 11-6
Helicopter landing at the scene of an accident
Courtesy of Sheldon Cohen/Bell Helicopter

responses more closely resemble a typical paramedic ground ambulance response, and the approach should be similar (Figure 11-5).

One advantage that AM personnel have over ground ambulance personnel is the aerial perspective. The entire scene can be viewed from above before landing. Potentially hazardous conditions may be spotted before the team even sets foot on the ground. For example, if an armed perpetrator is spotted in the area, the AM team should ensure that law enforcement has the scene under control before proceeding with the landing. Ideally the flight team is alerted beforehand by ground personnel, but that doesn't always occur. Once safety issues have been resolved, the team's attention should turn to patient care.

For scene flights the role of medical team members may vary according to the number of patients and the specific circumstances. For a typical one-patient scenario, both team members approach the patient. One begins the patient assessment while the other provides initial stabilization and begins supportive care. One member should question EMS personnel regarding their findings, impressions, and treatments. In a well-developed EMS system the patient has already been stabilized and most of the treatment has been started and sometimes completed. The actions of the flight team from that point depend on the type of patient and whether or not the patient has been adequately stabilized.

The gathering of medical information during a scene flight may be more difficult and time-consuming than for an interfacility transport. The environment is less controlled, and the patient may be unconscious or mentally compromised and incapable of providing information. A good working relationship with EMS personnel can speed and enhance the gathering of information. They have often had more time to interact with the patient and with law enforcement and other people on scene who may have information regarding what happened and about the specific patient. In rural areas it is not uncommon for EMS personnel to know a patient personally.

Patients who have been packaged prior to arrival of the AM team should remain packaged. Splints and bandages should generally not be removed for additional assessment. If information concerning covered injuries proves to be inaccurate, that information should be conveyed to the appropriate medical director or quality officer so that corrective action may be taken.

Some aircraft are designed in such a way that patient access may be limited once the patient is loaded into the aircraft. For example, the American Eurocopter BO-105 has a "tunnel" into which a patient's lower body is inserted during flight. Once the patient is in place, the medical team cannot access the lower abdomen or lower extremities. All necessary stabilization involving that part of the body must be provided before the patient is loaded into the aircraft. This is generally not an issue with medical patients, with whom scene time is less of an issue.

Conversely, multisystem trauma patients have little to gain from extended scene times. They should receive prompt initial stabilization, be immobilized and packaged appropriately, and be moved to the aircraft and transported as soon as possible. Patients should not be moved off EMS spine boards without good reason. Doing so subjects them to an unnecessary move, possibly complicating existing injuries.

Cardiac Arrest

An air medical program should rarely transport a patient who is in cardiac arrest. Medical patients should be worked where they are found and either stabilized or pronounced dead. For a routine cardiac arrest there is nothing to be done by the flight team at the bedside that cannot be done in the hospital. Interruptions in chest compressions and shifting the focus from patient care to patient movement often dilutes the resuscitation effort, and the patient's chance of being successfully resuscitated is generally decreased. The only common exception to this rule is the patient who is hypothermic.

Trauma patients presenting with cardiac arrest also have dismal outcomes. The patient who develops cardiac arrest secondary to trauma generally has a significant anatomical disruption and, outside the surgical suite, has a very poor prognosis.

Refusals

Occasionally a scene patient will adamantly refuse to be transported by helicopter. Nothing the medical team does will persuade the patient otherwise. The appropriate course of action will depend on other resources available and the patient's acuity level. For a patient with a high-acuity condition, abandonment should not be considered an option. Arrangements should be made to have the patient transported by ground ambulance. In rare cases where a patient is likely to deteriorate without continuing medical care, it may be appropriate for medical personnel to consider accompanying the patient during transport by private vehicle. While that is certainly unorthodox, it may be the only way to prevent patient deterioration.

Violent or Potentially Violent Patients

Any patient who has the potential to disrupt aircraft operation or become a danger to crew members during flight should *not* be loaded into the aircraft. This applies to both scene flights and interfacility transports. These patients should either be restrained chemically or transported by ground. Physical restraint alone should generally not be relied on, as there is always the possibility of escape. A patient capable of escaping a medical restraint device is capable of wreaking havoc in an aircraft. Physical restraint may provide extra peace of mind if used in conjunction with chemical restraint.

Each flight program should have in place a protocol for the management of patients who become agitated or violent during flight. That protocol should not involve having to contact a medical director first. These patients should be immediately and aggressively controlled. Drugs with proven track records include benzodiazepines, buterophenones, neuromuscular blocking agents, and narcotic analgesics. If a neuromuscular blocker is used for emergency restraint, the patient's airway must be rapidly secured. Any patient who receives an NMBA should be sedated as soon as possible afterward. Paralysis without sedation is inhumane.

Passengers

Whether or not to allow family members or friends to accompany a patient during helicopter transport is a controversial issue. Some programs allow passengers; others either discourage or prohibit the practice. In any case safety should be the overriding concern. If a family member appears to be anything other than absolutely cooperative and under control, the option should not be considered. When smaller aircraft are involved, this may not be an issue at all, since either there is no room for a passenger or the added weight may exceed maximum gross weight limits.

Even when larger aircraft are involved and weight or space is not an issue, there are pros and cons to this practice. Passengers may become excitable and distract the flight team or interfere with patient care. They may even endanger the safety of the medical team and the aircraft. However, if strict guidelines are followed, these possibilities are all but eliminated. In some cases the practice may be beneficial, as in the transport of a conscious pediatric patient, often a child with respiratory distress. The child may become very anxious when taken from the parent, so much so that her medical condition deteriorates. The options are to transport the child in the anxious and decompensated state, sedate the child, or allow the parent to accompany the child during the transport. Sedation may decrease anxiety, although it may also complicate the patient's medical condition.

Another case where the presence of a passenger may be of benefit is when a prisoner is being transported. In fact, some law enforcement agencies do not allow a prisoner to be transported without an officer escort. The prisoner is generally unconscious or chemically restrained, and the officer is there not to ensure that the patient is subdued but because the law requires an escort. AM programs should use caution in allowing the presence of loaded firearms aboard an aircraft. An inadvertent discharge could prove disastrous. While this rarely occurs, each program should have a policy addressing this issue.

Summary

The responsibilities of the flight team go well beyond the transport process. Patient stabilization and preparation for transport may have an impact on patient outcome that equals or exceeds that of the transport process. The specific approach taken will vary according to whether the patient is in the prehospital or in-hospital setting and based on the patient's specific medical condition and needs.

The flight team should obtain a medical history and perform a physical examination appropriate for the situation. The focused examination may vary considerably depending on the patient type and location. A prehospital assessment will generally be more comprehensive and an in-hospital assessment more focused. When indicated, pain and sedation status should be assessed. Airway patency and adequate breathing should be confirmed. If either is compromised a definitive airway should be established.

Unstable medical patients should be stabilized to the extent possible before being moved to the aircraft. In many cases the flight team is capable of delivering the same treatment available at a referral hospital, and there is no reason to delay that treatment. Trauma patients with extensive injuries require a different approach. Definitive stabilization is often impossible outside the operating room. These patients benefit most from rapid transport to a trauma center. The flight team should focus on minimizing delays providing temporary stabilizing measures.

For all patient types, the safety of the flight team and of the aircraft is always the highest priority. Any patient who presents an obvious or potential danger should not be moved to the aircraft until the flight team is satisfied that the danger has been alleviated. A violent patient may wreak havoc in a moving aircraft. Chemical restraint is the preferred method for controlling these patients. Physical restraint should be used as a failsafe. Physical restraint alone should never be relied on for an air medical transport. Each program should also have a policy regarding nonpatient passengers. It may sometimes be appropriate for a calm and responsible family member or friend to accompany a patient during transport.

REVIEW QUESTIONS

1. Discuss the importance of a thorough patient assessment prior to an interfacility transport.

2. Which of the following techniques are acceptable for confirming endotracheal tube placement?
   a. Pulse oximetry
   b. Assessment of breath sounds
   c. CO_2 detection devices
   d. All of the above

3. Discuss the importance of keeping family members informed regarding a patient's condition.

4. For patients the most vulnerable phase of air medical transport is:
   a. Takeoff
   b. Loading and unloading
   c. Landing
   d. Cruising at altitude

5. When transporting a neonatal patient:
   a. A specialty team is required
   b. The core medical team should remain behind during these transports
   c. Stabilization at the referring hospital may require hours
   d. a and c

6. Any noncritical patient who is anxious about flying, is nauseated, or has a history of motion sickness should be medicated accordingly.
   a. True
   b. False

7. Discuss precautionary measures that should be taken when moving a patient to and from the aircraft.

8. Regarding patients who become violent while aboard the aircraft:
   a. These patients should be immediately and aggressively controlled. Chemical restraint should be available without need for a verbal order.
   b. These patients should be left alone as much as possible so as to avoid provoking them further.
   c. These patients are often just frustrated and should not be seen as a threat.
   d. The medical team should defer to the pilot regarding a method for controlling these patients.

CHAPTER 12

Medical Direction

Objectives

Upon completing this chapter, the reader should have a better understanding of the following topics:

* The role of medical direction in the flight program

* Types of medical directors and specific roles of each

* The qualifications of a medical director

* Selecting a hospital destination (scene responses)

Introduction

EMTs, paramedics, registered nurses, respiratory therapists, and others who are employed by ambulance services (including flight programs) provide medical care under the guidance of a physician medical director. This oversight is typically required for ambulance licensure. It is also necessary in order for nonphysicians to legally perform certain medical skills, whether or not members of the flight team are licensed or certified as nonphysician practitioners. The input and oversight provided by the medical director is referred to as **medical direction** (or **medical control**). Medical direction is an essential component of all flight programs.

The involvement of physicians knowledgeable in emergency medicine and other appropriate specialty care areas is essential for the success of a program. Emergency medical services, including air medical programs, have evolved as an extension of emergency medicine, and most medical directors are emergency medicine specialists. It is important that emergency medicine residents develop a strong basic understanding of air medicine, as they may be called on to help establish or participate in these programs. In the latest position statement of the Air Medical

medical direction (medical control)
A process whereby knowledgeable physicians provide guidelines and oversee the practice of paramedics, nurses, and other nonphysician members of a health care team.

Physicians Association, there are three levels of priorities for prehospital and out-of-hospital medical care:

1. Safety of the crew, patient, and vehicle
2. Provision of appropriate patient care
3. Appropriate utilization of medical transport resources and cost-effective patient transport

Medical Directors

Medical direction occurs at two basic levels: off-line and on-line.

Off-Line Medical Director

The *off-line medical director* is administratively responsible for all medical aspects of the program, including training and development of protocols and standing orders. This person has ultimate authority in regard to all medical matters and should also have a well-defined role with respect to nonmedical components of the flight program. The off-line medical director is typically an experienced and well-respected physician in the medical community. This person may be called on to help resolve disputes between the flight program and other physicians or hospitals and must be knowledgeable, well spoken, and diplomatic.

The off-line medical director may be active in day-to-day activities or may serve more in the background. Both approaches are acceptable so long as she is kept current regarding program activities and actual or potential problem areas. A typical arrangement is for the off-line medical director to be available for consultation and problem solving, to have input into hiring of new personnel, and to ensure that protocols and medical procedures are kept current.

On-Line Medical Director

The *on-line medical director* is responsible for day-to-day and concurrent medical activities and is the person with whom the medical flight team consults regarding patient care. The flight team generally interacts more with the on-line than with the off-line director. This is the go-to person for medical problems. The on-line director may designate others as acting on-line medical directors (*designated on-line medical directors*) in his absence. As with the off-line medical director, contact between the medical flight team and the on-line medical director may vary from program to program depending on organizational structure.

Medical Direction

Medical direction takes three forms: prospective, on-line, and retrospective.

Prospective Medical Direction

Prospective medical direction involves all activities that occur prior to patient contact. This may include education and orientation, assessment of personnel competence, and the establishment of practice guidelines (protocols). This is the single most important component of medical direction. Protocols generally include *standing orders,* or advance directives that may be implemented without (or prior to) physician contact. Standing orders are intended to allow the flight team to function autonomously when there is a need to minimize treatment delays. Most air medical programs make extensive use of standing orders.

The responsibilities of an air medical director may vary from state to state and region to region. Statute and/or administrative policy, as promulgated by a state board of health or similar agency, generally specifies the medical director's authority and scope of practice and influence. Generally, the off-line medical director is the ultimate authority concerning the medical care rendered within a system.

On-Line Medical Direction

On-line or *concurrent medical direction* involves real-time communication between the flight crew and the medical director by radio or telephone. On-line consultation may be required before performing invasive, high-risk, or elective procedures. For example, the flight team may have standing orders to administer nitroglycerin, aspirin, morphine, and beta-blockers to a patient with chest pain but have to consult with the on-line medical director before administering a glycoprotein inhibiting or fibrinolytic agent.

On-line medical direction is most effective when it is offered as a two-way discussion of patient condition and options for patient management. The prehospital or air medical provider should be actively involved in the decision-making process. Each member of the air medical team should be viewed as an independent thinker with knowledge and experience that may be of value in the management of the patient at hand. While the medical director should have the authority to make the final decision, that decision should incorporate the impressions and suggestions offered by the AM team.

Visual Medical Direction

visual medical
direction

A specific type of on-line medical control whereby the medical director accompanies the flight team and provides on-scene medical direction. Also referred to as medical director ride-along.

Visual medical direction is a specific type of on-line medical direction in which the medical director accompanies the flight team and provides medical direction directly to the team during patient care. This may be done as a component of the quality management process. Visual medical direction does not occur frequently.

Retrospective Medical Direction

Retrospective medical direction involves after-the-fact follow-up and includes chart audits, case reviews, and evaluation of individual performance. This is an important component of the quality assurance and improvement process. Information gained retrospectively should be used to plan continuing education sessions and should strongly influence planning and prospective aspects of medical direction.

Flight programs generally employ a small number of highly qualified medical personnel and opt for strong prospective and retrospective medical direction, allowing medical personnel some degree of discretion in real-time decision making. In many cases patients are stabilized and transported without any direct communication between the flight team and the on-line medical director. Consultation with the medical director is reserved for cases in which the flight team is unsure how to proceed or where there may be conflict regarding the specifics of patient care. The on-line medical director should be available to resolve disagreement between the flight crew and medical personnel at a referral site.

Responsibility for Medical Direction

The off-line and on-line medical directors are generally responsible for providing medical direction for the air medical team. However, there may be situations in which the responsibility for medical direction is less than crystal clear. During scene flights there may be a physician on scene who gives orders to the flight team. During interfacility transports a referring physician may order care that does not coincide with the policies or protocols of the flight program. These conflicts should be promptly resolved so that the patient does not suffer as a result of the inconsistency. Any disagreement that cannot be worked out between the flight team and the referring physician should be referred to the on-line medical director for resolution.

On-Scene (Intervenor) Physicians

Air medical programs that make scene flights should have a policy for dealing with on-scene volunteer physicians. In most cases these physicians are trying to help, but most do not have a strong background in emergency care and their orders may not be in line with mainstream emergency medicine. Most programs have adopted policies requiring the medical team to tactfully explain to the volunteer physician that policy prohibits them from deviating from protocol.

Referring Physicians

Medical control for patients being transported from one hospital to another can be a touchy issue. Historically, the referring physician retained responsibility for the patient being transferred until arrival at the receiving hospital. As emergency medical services systems began to develop in the 1970s, that began to change. These systems incorporated their own medical control plans and their own off- and on-line medical directors. Responsibility for patient care began to move away from the referring physician toward the EMS system medical director. More recently the accepted practice has been for EMS systems to define the responsible physician in a formal policy, generally a medical control plan. In most states a department of health has to approve the plan before it becomes functional. At that point the medical director role is formalized.

Qualifications of the Air Medical Director

The medical director has a tremendous amount of influence on the flight program. This person should be carefully selected based not only on medical knowledge and experience but also on personal interest in the program and interpersonal skills.

The minimum requirements of a medical director of an air medical service should be:

- Licensure in the jurisdiction(s) that serves as a base for the air medical service
- Familiarity with EMS system design and operation

- Familiarity with the various medical care providers operating within the air medical program and their respective scopes of practice
- Active involvement in the care of critically ill and/or injured patients
- Education, experience, and expertise in those areas of medicine commensurate with the scope of care of the air medical service
- Familiarity with aircraft operation and safety issues
- Familiarity with medical and legal issues specific to EMS and air medicine

Desirable (ideal) qualifications for an air medical director include:

- A significant amount (2 years or greater) of EMS/air medicine experience
- Experience or training in out-of-hospital medicine (e.g., Base Station Course)
- Knowledge and understanding of flight physiology
- Board certification in Emergency Medicine or a closely related area
- Active and ongoing practice of emergency or critical care medicine
- Knowledge of EMS laws, rules, and regulations
- Completion of an air medical (or EMS) fellowship or preceptorship
- Knowledge of air medical dispatch and communications

Selecting a Hospital Destination

The selection of a hospital destination can be a complicated process. Is the nearest hospital most appropriate? Should the nearest hospital be bypassed and the patient delivered to a facility with specific medical capabilities matching the patient's needs? Who makes the decision? The underlying goal when selecting a hospital destination should always be to maximize the patient's potential for a good outcome.

Scene Flights

Scene flights involve patients with a variety of medical needs, physician preferences, and hospital preferences. At times these needs and preferences may be in conflict, and the AM team and on-line medical director have to determine the most appropriate receiving hospital. That may be done in real time or resolved by way of protocols. In most cases the air medical team has some freedom to select a destination based on the situation at hand. While this is rarely a black-and-white process, there are several criteria that may simplify the process.

1. *Medical needs of the patient:* These should always be the dominant factor. It is all too easy to get caught up in politics and administrative policies to the extent that the patient is forgotten. A conscious effort is required to prevent that from happening. The patient must be the first priority. All hospital policies regarding the selection of patient destinations should be written around that premise.

2. *Patient preference:* If an air medical program operates in an area served by two or more hospitals, patient preference may play a role in determining the destination. If a patient's medical needs can be met by the preferred hospital and there is no valid reason to do otherwise, the patient should be transported to the facility of her choice.

3. *Distance to potential hospital destinations:* When dealing with a patient who presents with a time-sensitive medical or traumatic condition, time until definitive treatment must be taken into consideration. That is not to say that the nearest hospital is always the best choice; this is only one of several variables to consider.

4. *Capabilities of potential hospital destinations:* It does no good to take a patient with multisystem trauma to a hospital that lacks surgical capabilities, or a patient with a closed head injury to a hospital with no neurological capabilities. Taking every patient requiring specialty care directly to a facility offering that care will not always be possible, but program policies should facilitate matching as much as possible.

5. *Volume status of potential hospital destinations:* In many areas of the country, emergency and critical care units are periodically overtaxed. Under those conditions hospitals may occasionally go on full or specialty care diversion. The air medical team must determine an appropriate destination for each patient, and in some cases may ignore the diversionary status of a particular hospital.

EMTALA
The Emergency Medical Treatment and Active Labor Act. Passed in 1986, this law defines requirements for participating hospitals to treat emergency patients.

If the air ambulance is owned or operated by one specific hospital, **EMTALA** requirements may require that the patient be transported to that hospital. Transporting directly to another hospital without first completing the necessary transfer papers may result in a significant fine. However, formal agreements among area hospitals or an approved state or regional trauma plan can preempt that requirement.

In some cases a patient or family member may insist on a hospital that the medical crew knows does not have the capability to manage the patient's condition. The team should educate the party to the benefits and risks of not going to the recommended facility. It may be necessary to transport a patient to a facility other than the one preferred even without the patient's consent, such as in an organized trauma system.

Interfacility Transports

EMTALA requires that, during an interfacility transport, each patient be attended by personnel qualified and capable of managing any reasonably foreseeable complication that may develop during the transport. The referring physician is responsible for ensuring that transporting personnel meet those requirements. However, where an organized EMS authority exists, the on-line medical director is typically responsible for the patient's care during transport.

Summary

Medical control is an integral component of air medicine. A majority of medical team members are nonphysicians and the involvement of a physician medical director is required. There are two basic types of medical directors, on-line and off-line. The off-line director is administratively responsible for the entire medical program. The on-line medical director reports to the off-line director and is responsible for day to day medical operations. A medical director should be knowledgeable in emergency and critical-care medicine and, ideally, will have formal education and experience in EMS and/or air medicine. He will play a key role in representing the AM program in the medical community and in handling complaints or concerns that come from the medical community.

Medical control is delivered in three basic formats, prospective, on-line, and retrospective. Prospective medical direction involves the development of protocols and standing orders. On-line medical control occurs when there is real time communication between a member of the flight team and the on-line medical director during the course of patient assessment and/or treatment. Retrospective medical control involves program performance assessment and follow up.

Medical control may also come into play when determining a hospital destination following a scene response. The development of hospital destination guidelines should be strongly influenced by the medical director. Specialty care patients may be transported directly to specialty care centers even if other hospitals are bypassed. Medical control may become slightly more complicated when dealing with interfacility transports. Referring physicians may become involved in the process and there may be some blurring of responsibility for oversight of patient care. However, in well-developed systems the off-line and on-line medical directors will generally always have final say regarding patient care provided by the flight program.

REVIEW QUESTIONS

1. The physician who is administratively responsible for all medical aspects of an air medical program is known as the:
   a. On-line medical director
   b. Off-line medical director
   c. Administrative medical director
   d. Physician advisor

2. This type of medical direction involves all activities that occur prior to patient contact.
   a. Prospective
   b. Retrospective
   c. Concurrent
   d. Visual

3. The type of medical direction in which the medical director accompanies the fight team and provides direction directly to the flight team during patient care is:
   a. Prospective
   b. Retrospective
   c. Concurrent
   d. Visual

4. Which of the following criteria should be considered when selecting a hospital destination for a patient acquired on scene?
   a. The patient's ability to pay for services rendered
   b. The location of the patient's family physician
   c. The patient's medical condition
   d. The pilot's preference

5. Which of the following situations involves a potential EMTALA violation?
   a. Administering a medication to a patient without approval of the patient's family physician
   b. Discussing a patient's medical information with a friend after work
   c. Making copies of a patient's ECG strip for use in a cardiology course
   d. A hospital-owned air ambulance that transports a scene patient directly to a hospital other than the owner without an existing agreement

CHAPTER 13

Quality Management

Upon completing this chapter, the reader should have a better understanding of the following topics:

* The role of quality management in an air medical program
* The components of the quality management process
* The steps in the design of the quality management program
* Patient confidentiality
* The CAMTS accreditation process and its potential benefits

Introduction

One of the underlying principles of an air medical program must be that the program will provide its patients with medical care of the highest possible quality. However, quality can be difficult to define. While there are a number of widely accepted definitions, each program should establish the specific principles on which to base its quality program. Goals, objectives, or benchmarks, and a reasonable time line should all be part of that process. Program personnel should all know exactly what the standard is and should be provided with the tools to meet it.

quality assurance/ quality improvement/ quality management Ongoing programs designed to monitor and improve the performance level of employees and systems.

Quality management (QM) involves the oversight of medical performance and the steps taken to maintain and improve the quality of patient care. There seems to be a different catch phrase for this process

205

every year or so: total quality management (TQM), continuous quality improvement (CQI), performance improvement (PI), and others. But the underlying objective has remained constant since the advent of total quality management, over 40 years ago: to minimize the incidence of errors and improve customer satisfaction. That goal may be accomplished through ongoing assessment and improvement of human performance and systematic processes.

There are three broad components of a quality management (QM) program: people, processes, and commitment. These three elements must be addressed individually and as a combined unit. In order to have a QM program that functions efficiently and produces the desired outcomes, all components must be regularly assessed.

KEY TERMS

quality assurance (QA)/quality improvement (QI)/
quality management (QM), p. 205

Personnel

The importance of people cannot be understated. They are the single most valuable resource in any organization. In order for personnel to produce the best possible outcomes, they must have the requisite mental capability, knowledge, skills, and experience. Most AM programs have the luxury of being able to select their employees from a large pool of highly qualified applicants.

In the unlikely event that a qualified applicant is not available to fill a position, the program director should consider temporary staffing options until a qualified applicant appears. It is far better to suffer hardship in the short term and wait for the right person than to hire hastily and be forced to live with the consequences. It is very difficult to transform a poor employee into an exemplary one.

The Quality Management Officer

Each flight program should have a quality management officer. That person should be charged with overseeing day-to-day medical performance and advising the medical director and the program director of actual or potential problem areas. The QM officer has a great deal of influence on the program and on practice habits of the flight team. In programs with a full-time medical director, the director may also function as the QM officer. When the medical director is not readily available, it may be more appropriate to have a senior-level nurse or paramedic in this position. In any case the person filling this role must respect the importance of the QM process and be willing to invest the necessary time and energy to see that the program is of the highest quality.

The role played by the QM officer may vary somewhat according to the organizational structure under which the AM program falls. If the program is part of a hospital system, the sponsor facility and its accrediting body dictate much of the quality assurance/performance improvement plan. The QM officer may have considerably more control and influence in shaping the plan in a program that is not hospital based or affiliated.

Quality Management Advisory Committee

Some programs have a quality management advisory committee that periodically assesses the performance level of the QM program and makes recommendations for modifications. The committee should be multidisciplinary, composed of the QM officer and members of the flight team as well as physician specialists, critical-care practitioners, prehospital representatives, and others who have a vested interest in the program or possess expertise that may benefit the program. The program medical director often chairs this committee. For hospital-based programs this function may fall to a hospital-wide committee that considers quality issues throughout the institution. The purpose of these committees is to provide an outside perspective and to advise the medical director, quality officer, and program director.

Processes (Systems)

The second component of the QM program is process. Even the best employees may not be able to provide high-quality results if they are operating within a poorly designed or maintained system. For employees to function at maximum capacity, the system must be designed to eliminate obstacles to the delivery of high-quality patient care. Obstacles may include a lack of knowledge or skill, inadequate equipment or supplies, personal or professional distractions, and complacency. Lack of personal motivation to perform at a given level may also be considered an obstacle.

Eliminating obstacles requires providing employees with adequate orientation, continuing education, and the tools to perform their jobs safely and efficiently. It also means establishing a supportive administrative structure whereby the program director, medical director, chief flight nurse, and quality officer stand firmly behind their employees.

Each component of the QM system must be clearly defined. The quality management advisory committee should discuss performance expectations and make recommendations to the medical director and program director regarding benchmarks and measurement criteria. One of the most important steps in establishing a quality program is setting the bar high and making it clear that each team member is expected to reach that bar. When everyone understands that anything less will be considered unacceptable, it becomes easier to perform at the higher level.

The QM process must incorporate regulations and guidelines set forth by regulatory and accrediting bodies. At the national level these agencies include the National Highway and Safety Administration, Department of Transportation, and Occupational Safety and Health Administration. At the state level the various Departments of Health and offices of emergency medical services also have policies and procedures that affect the QM program. Some states even have a statewide performance improvement process that all ambulance providers must participate in.

While the required policies, procedures, and guidelines of these national and state entities should be incorporated into the QM plan, they should not be seen as a complete product that may be used to replace a program-specific plan. One of the dangers of standardized QM is that the minimum standard will be accepted as the de facto practice standard. The likely result is a program that fails to perform as well as it has the potential to.

The QM process should include prospective, real-time, and retrospective elements to be maximally effective. However, given the high caliber of employees of most air medical programs, prospective and retrospective components should assume the most significance.

Commitment

It is possible for a QM program to have good people and good processes and still fail. The third variable and the one that maintains the focus of the QM program is commitment. Commitment is the drive to keep the QM program active and productive. It is difficult, but not impossible, to teach commitment; it must come from within.

Too often QM is adopted by an organization without any real commitment to the concept. It is adopted because it has worked for other organizations. There is often a financial motivation behind the move toward quality. Administrators may believe that a QM program will reduce the incidence of costly mistakes or improve morale and reduce turnover. This is not genuine commitment. In fact, administrators often have little understanding of the concept of QM. They are looking for a quick fix for a problem or series of problems. This lack of commitment often dooms these programs to failure or, at best, mediocrity. Occasionally, an exceptionally competent person is hired to develop and lead the program, and that person's commitment may produce the desired benefits. However, without the comprehension and true commitment of upper-level managers, the process is much more difficult.

Designing the Quality Management Program

The National Highway Transportation and Safety Administration has proposed the Malcolm Baldridge Quality Program as a model for designing a quality management program for emergency medical services agencies. The Baldridge program identifies seven key action areas. The following version is slightly modified to meet the specific needs of air medicine.

1. *Leadership:* Those at the top must have vision and an understanding of the direction the program is to take. They must lead by example and provide support and motivation. They must believe in the program.

2. *Information and analysis:* The key is to gather relevant data and to analyze it in a pragmatic manner. In regard to quality management, data decreases in value as time passes. Data that is gathered, processed, and analyzed in a timely manner will have more impact than data that is allowed to age before being applied.

3. *Strategic quality planning:* Both long- and short-term organizational objectives should be developed. Outcomes quality standards should be determined and benchmarks identified to determine if objectives are being achieved.

4. *Human resource development and management:* This involves the efforts undertaken to develop the full potential of the EMS workforce. This category includes recruiting, screening, training, orientation, evaluation, and disciplinary actions. Employee motivation is a prerequisite for effective outcomes in this category. Employees support a quality management plan when they are asked for input into the shaping of the plan.

5. *Process management:* This refers to the improvement of work activities and work flow across functional or departmental boundaries by the creation of systems and systems management. The purpose of process management is to ensure that obstacles to quality are eliminated or managed as efficiently as possible, and that processes are put into place to identify potential obstacles and deal with them proactively when possible. The ultimate goal is to predict so well that problems are eliminated before they occur.

6. *System outcomes*: This involves the evaluation of intermediate and terminal outcome measurements. For this process to be effective, appropriate measurement tools must be used. Those involved must know the appropriate data to measure and the appropriate process for performing those measurements.

7. *Customer satisfaction*: The program's primary customers are patients. But there are other customers as well. Family members are "near patients"—that is, they may not need medical care, but they often need information and compassion. Family members should never be ignored and, when time permits, should be given as much information about the patient as is reasonably possible. Other secondary customers are the prehospital providers who stabilize and refer patients, the referring medical personnel who call for assistance, and physicians and other health care professionals with whom the AM team interacts.

The QM officer should review and critique all patient transports in a timely manner. Ideally, all run reports should be reviewed within 48 hours of transport. Feedback has a greater impact if provided early, when the details of the transport are fresh in the mind of the caregiver. However, that is sometimes impractical, and a period of one week is considered acceptable. Beyond that period, memories begin to fade and the desired effect of the process may be compromised.

There must be a formal written plan prescribing the management of problem areas and personnel. This should include loop closure and follow-up. The quality assurance officer must have the authority to discipline personnel when indicated.

The quality officer may be a senior-level flight nurse, flight paramedic, or physician. This person must be well educated as to the importance of the quality improvement process, must be knowledgeable concerning all aspects of AM transport, and must have the respect of other team members.

The quality assurance process may be divided into two categories, one for scene responses and one for interhospital transports. The standard of care may differ significantly between these two settings. In the prehospital setting, patient assessment and treatment may be less precise and less definitive and the approach more subjective. There has been less time for data gathering and for considering all possibilities. In contrast, the interfacility patient has already been seen in a hospital and has had the benefit of the expertise and technology available there. The diagnosis and treatment plans should be more accurate and detailed.

This process begins with an assessment of existing quality (quality assessment). This baseline may be determined by reviewing patient charts and determining if protocols are followed and by examining skills success rates. However, the most valuable information is the correlation of diagnoses between the flight team and the admitting physician. While diagnostic refinement is to be expected following arrival at a referral center, there should be a reasonable amount of overlap between the air medical diagnosis and that of the admitting physician. If benchmarks have been previously set, compliance rates may also be a reasonable indicator of quality.

Cost-Effectiveness

Quality may be difficult to define and equally difficult to achieve. Building a good QM program requires extensive manpower and commitment at all levels. That generally translates into a significant financial commitment as well. However, as in virtually all other areas of medicine, cost-effectiveness has become an essential consideration. Fortunately, there is a growing body of knowledge regarding quality management, and some of that knowledge can be copied and applied at minimal cost.

A Note on Individualism

In recent years a disturbing trend has developed relating to quality management. The system is often held responsible for all mistakes. This has resulted in a hesitancy to hold individuals responsible for their actions. While systems design does have the potential to significantly improve the quality management process, it is only half of the equation. The other half is individual performance. Even the most detailed QM program cannot anticipate every patient care situation. Individual preparation, decision making, motivation, and achievement must be part of any medical care program.

Patient Confidentiality

In all areas of medicine, patient confidentiality is an absolute requirement. Recent changes in government regulations have reinforced the importance of confidentiality from a legal standpoint. The Health Insurance Portability and Accountability Act of 1996 (HIPPA), an amendment to the Internal Revenue Code of 1986, made significant changes in the federal requirements placed on health care organizations regarding patient confidentiality. HIPPA addresses the issue of exactly who has the right to access personally identifiable health information. Following the release of HIPPA, questions were raised concerning its interpretation and application. In an effort to clarify the intent of the act, the Standards for Privacy of Individually Identifiable Health Information (the Privacy Rule) took effect on April 14, 2001.The Privacy Rule creates national standards to protect individuals' personal health information and gives patients greater access to their medical records. The privacy standards:

1. Limit the nonconsensual use and release of private health information
2. Give patients new rights regarding access to their medical records, including the right to know who else has accessed them
3. Restrict the disclosure of individual health information to the minimum required
4. Establish criminal and civil penalties for improper disclosure
5. Establish new requirements for access to records by those requesting to do research

The implications for health care providers, including air medical programs, are obvious. Violations of HIPPA requirements may make a hospital or other health care organization the target of criminal or civil legal action. AM programs must be proactive in educating personnel and establishing policies that strictly control access to patient information to avoid intentional or inadvertent disclosure.

Air medical programs that are not associated with a hospital may be at particular risk, as HIPPA language may be difficult to decipher. Those programs should consult with attorneys or other experts in the field to establish policies and procedures.

Accreditation

Quality management is a complicated process requiring the input and oversight of a knowledgeable person or persons with the time and resources to build the program and keep it on track. While it is possible to create a quality program from within, it is difficult to maintain objectivity over the long term. A periodic evaluation by an outside person or group with no vested interest in the program provides a more objective view of the program's performance. That is the role of the accrediting body.

Accreditation is a voluntary process through which an air medical program progresses over a given period of time. The process requires that the program adopt certain performance standards relating to all aspects of the program and its operation. The intent is that these new standards will become a part of the program and not just a temporary goal to be met in order to attain accreditation. The program is then evaluated to determine how successfully the new standards have been met.

The organization offering accreditation for air medical programs is the Commission on Accreditation of Medical Transport Systems (CAMTS). CAMTS is a not-for-profit organization dedicated to improving the quality and safety of medical transport services. Its board of directors is composed of representatives from 16 member organizations: Aerospace Medical Association, Air Medical Physicians Association, Air and Surface Transport Nurses Association, American Academy of Pediatrics, American Association of Critical Care Nurses, American Association of Respiratory Care, American College of Emergency Physicians, Association of Air Medical Services, Emergency Nurses Association, National Air Transportation Association, National Association of Air Medical Communications Specialists, National Association of EMS Physicians, National Association of Neonatal Nurses, National Association of State EMS Directors, National EMS Pilots Association, and National Flight Paramedics Association.

The scope of the accreditation process is not limited to matters of quality management. The majority of standards address safety and patient care as well as issues such as minimum personnel qualifications, training, the role of the medical director, organizational structure, outreach, the role and influence of program personnel in the medical community, safety, and certification requirements.

The accreditation process consists of ten basic steps:

1. The AM program considers the pros and cons of seeking accreditation.

2. The AM program determines that there is a tangible benefit to gaining accreditation.

3. The AM program contacts the accrediting body and obtains the requirements for accreditation, including the accreditation standards.

4. The AM program familiarizes itself with the accreditation standards and does an informal self-assessment to determine the extent of its current compliance with the standards.

5. The AM program uses the results of the self-assessment to formulate a plan of action that will ultimately bring the program into compliance with the standards.

6. A formal self-study is done as prescribed by the accrediting body. It is signed by all the principals and submitted to the accrediting body.

7. The accrediting body evaluates the self-study and identifies areas that are unclear or require further discovery. The accrediting body and the AM program agree on a date for a site visit.

8. A site visit team is assembled. The team generally consists of two experts in the field, one of whom is a physician. The team is provided with all the information that has been gathered about the applicant program, including the self-study, and a list of questions and concerns that are to be addressed during the site visit.

9. The site visit is conducted. It generally consists of meetings and interviews with key members of the AM program, including the program director, medical director, chief flight nurse, hospital administrator (if applicable), communications supervisor, lead pilot, and members of the medical team. The team also reviews a sampling of program documents.

10. Following the site visit, the accrediting body issues a response to the application. The response may award full accreditation or probational accreditation with further action necessary to bring the program into full compliance, or it may withhold accreditation.

Cost

The CAMTS fee for completing the accreditation process ranges from $5,500 to more than $10,000. The exact cost is based on a formula that incorporates the number of transports made during the most recent year, the number of program sites, and the number of vehicles operated by the program. Higher numbers in each of these categories lead to a higher cost for entering the accreditation process. The process also requires a substantial investment of personnel time and effort. It generally takes four to six months to prepare for the site visit.

Benefits of Accreditation

Given the cost of seeking entry into the accreditation process, it seems only reasonable that there would be substantial benefit to completing the process and being awarded CAMTS accreditation. While the degree of benefit may vary by program, there is almost certainly something to be gained by achieving accreditation. Simply going through an accreditation process is a learning experience for program personnel. It forces personnel at all levels to reflect critically on their individual performance and on the structure and performance of the program as a whole. Anytime there is self-evaluation to that extent, weaknesses and more effective ways of accomplishing goals will be identified.

From a more tangible perspective, some insurance companies recognize the enhanced safety standards promoted by CAMTS, and accredited programs may be eligible for lower aviation insurance premiums. In some areas CAMTS-accredited programs may bid on exclusive contracts they would otherwise be ineligible for. The accreditation award is often a newsworthy event, providing the air medical program with positive media exposure. Accreditation may also enhance a program's credibility and give it a competitive edge over other area services.

Summary

Quality management and improvement should be an integral component of all air medical programs. There are two basic elements of quality management: personnel and process. The recruiting and hiring of well-educated and motivated flight team members is a prerequisite for success and should be a priority of program managers. There must also be a well-defined quality assessment and improvement process in place to provide the structure and support that personnel require to perform at maximum efficiency.

Accreditation is one means for strengthening a program's quality management program. The accreditation process forces a program to perform a thorough and critical self-assessment. It also offers a program access to the advice and solutions of others who have gone through the process. Completing the self-study and the site visit often leave program personnel with a new perspective and renewed enthusiasm and commitment.

REVIEW QUESTIONS

1. The general process that involves the oversight of medical performance and the steps taken to maintain and improve the quality of patient care is:
   a. Maintaining a balanced program budget
   b. Medical auditing
   c. Quality management
   d. Recertification

2. The three broad components of a quality management program are:
   a. People, processes, and commitment
   b. People, processes, and funding
   c. People, funding, and management
   d. People, resources, and medical direction

3. The single most valuable resource in the air medical organization is:
   a. People
   b. The aircraft
   c. Educational opportunities
   d. The state board of nursing

4. The National Highway Transportation and Safety Administration has proposed the _____ Quality Program as a model for designing a quality management program for emergency medical services agencies.
   a. John Barnes Noble
   b. Cashmere
   c. General Motors
   d. Malcolm Baldridge

5. The first step to building an effective quality management program is:
   a. Determining goals and objectives
   b. Setting benchmarks
   c. An assessment of existing quality
   d. Evaluating the recruiting and hiring process

6. A voluntary process through which an air medical program progresses over a given period of time and which is intended to improve safety and patent care is:
   a. Convocation
   b. Certification
   c. Registration
   d. Accreditation

7. The organization that specializes in accrediting air medical programs is known as:
   a. Joint Commission
   b. Committee on Accreditation of Medical Transport Systems
   c. Department of Transportation
   d. American Ambulance Association

Finance

Upon completing this chapter, the reader should have a better understanding of the following topics:

* Budgeting

* Aircraft acquisition options

* Income and expenses

* Subscription plans and service contracts

Introduction

A basic understanding of air medicine cannot be complete without a discussion of budgeting and finance. Many readers of this book will at some point take part in the operation of an air medical program. Emergency medicine residents in particular may, at some point in their careers, be called upon to help start a new program and will certainly have an influence on any existing programs with which they become associated. They should have a basic understanding of the financial aspects of these programs.

Budgeting

Establishing a budget is essential for the efficient operation of any business. A *budget* is a projection of all income and expenses over the upcoming year. Budgeting involves some degree of speculation. While projections are rarely totally accurate, they should be reasonably close. Projecting a budget should be a systematic process that evaluates all available data, including previous years' budgets, trends in call volume, population changes, changes in contract status, increases or decreases in

FIGURE 14-1
Sample budget

Income		
Patient revenues	$3,650,000	
Hospital subsidy	1,000,000	
Donations	15,000	
Contracts	$150,000	
Total Income		$4,815,000
Expenses		
Personnel	576,000	
Benefits	158,400	
Insurance	88,000	
Facilities maintenance	65,000	
Fuel	86,000	
Contracts with vendors	1,146,600	
Debt write-off	2,350,000	
Miscellaneous other	75,000	
Total Expenses	$4,545,000	
Capital Expenditures		
Medical equipment	185,000	
Fuel dispensing station	85,000	
Total Capital Expenditures	$270,000	
	Total Expenses	$4,815,000
Net Surplus/Deficit		0

insurance reimbursement rates, subsidies, and changes in the number of competitors.

The budget is generally divided three sections: income, expenses, and capital expenses (or equipment) (Figure 14-1). The income section should list all sources of income line by line. Those individual items are then combined into an income total. The second section of the budget includes all anticipated expenses, also listed line by line. For medium and larger operations, budget items are grouped by category. For example, many government and educational organizations use the categories Contractual, Commodities, Equipment, and Personnel. Each heading is followed by the line item expense in each category.

The budget concludes with the budget balance, which is the difference between income and expenses. The goal in budget planning is for those two numbers to be equal, that is, for the budget to be balanced. If there is more income than expenses, the excess income is known as a surplus. If there are more expenses than income, a negative balance, or deficit, results.

Once the budget has been completed and approved by the appropriate parties, it serves as the organization's financial map for the upcoming year. The manager is expected to stick to the budget unless unforeseen expenses arise, in which case the budget must be rebalanced. Since income is generally beyond the manager's control, expenses must be reduced to keep the budget in balance. In the unusual event that income exceeds projections, expenses may be increased.

Capital expenditures, or equipment, bear further discussion. The expenses associated with large acquisitions, such as aircraft or expensive medical equipment, may be spread over more than one year's budget. For example, few organizations have $4 million or more readily available to purchase a new aircraft. A more realistic scenario is for the organization to take out a loan to purchase the aircraft and pay the loan back over several years. The loan payments are included in capital expenses for each year in which payments are made.

Acquisition Options

Helicopters are expensive. A new medium twin-engine helicopter with a reasonable avionics package can cost $4 million or more. The annual operating budget for a single-aircraft program can easily exceed $1 million. Fortunately, hospitals have a number of options when starting a new program. If money is no object, the hospital can buy all the machinery, hire all the necessary personnel, and operate all aspects of the program. Few hospitals are that fortunate, and most choose other options.

At the other end of the spectrum is the *turnkey operation*, in which the hospital contracts with a vendor to provide major components of the program. In most cases the vendor provides the aircraft, pilots, mechanics, and all maintenance. The hospital typically provides medical personnel and equipment. This frees the hospital from having to start an entirely new operation from scratch. In order to minimize start-up costs, many hospitals lease or lease-purchase their helicopters. Leasing eliminates the large up-front purchase price and shifts the risk for repairs and upkeep to the vendor. Operating costs are typically included in the lease payment.

While vendors are willing to assume the risk for unanticipated repairs, they must budget for large, randomly occurring expenses. The result is a monthly and hourly charge that includes a significant markup above projected costs. Using this method, the vendor has a decent profit during bad times and a hefty profit when costs are low. In the long run it is significantly cheaper for a hospital to buy its own aircraft. The hospital still has the option of contracting with a vendor for pilots and maintenance. Under this arrangement the hospital retains ownership of the aircraft at the end of the contract, whereas with a lease the vendor keeps the aircraft. That fact alone can make a big difference in the cost of the program. Medical helicopters retain their value and in some cases may even appreciate in value.

Another option is to participate in a lease-purchase program. The hospital enters into a long-term lease agreement with a vendor but at the end of the lease has the option of purchasing the aircraft at a token price. The lease-purchase option offers the hospital a way to purchase an aircraft without having to go through the formal purchase process and produce a large amount of money at start-up.

Regardless of whether a hospital elects to lease or purchase, knowledgeable hospital personnel should be involved in the aircraft selection process. The needs of the program should be clearly defined and matched to aircraft capable of meeting those needs. Once a list of eligible aircraft has been prepared, a cost-effectiveness analysis should be conducted to narrow the list to those aircraft that perform most efficiently. Cost-effectiveness and cost efficiency may be determined by calculating anticipated operating costs. Those costs are compiled and published periodically in the *Aircraft Cost Evaluator* by Conklin and de Decker.

Operating Costs

The annual operating cost for a typical single-helicopter program may range from $1 million to well over $2 million per year, depending on aircraft type and flight volume (Table 14-1). Compared to other medical programs, personnel costs constitute a relatively small percentage of these expenses. Maintenance and upkeep are by far the most expensive areas. Aircraft mechanics typically perform preventive maintenance and replace parts on a daily basis. It is strongly recommended that each flight program have its own aircraft mechanic. A busy air medical program with two aircraft may require two mechanics working alternating shifts.

Helicopters consume large quantities of fuel. A typical midsize twin burns 70 to 100 gallons of fuel per hour of flight. Additional fuel is consumed during start-up and idling after landing. Fuel may be purchased in one of two basic ways, from an airport vendor or by the truckload from a wholesaler. Virtually all cities large enough to support a flight program have an airport nearby. Buying from an airport may be the simplest way to start out. However, airport fuel is very expensive, and significant savings may be realized by installing a tank

Table 14-1 Estimated Annual Operating Costs for a Twin-Engine Single-Aircraft Operation

Item	Amount
Amortization of aircraft	$450,000
Preventive maintenance	30,000
Major repairs/parts	100,000
Fuel	100,000
Personnel (including 20% benefits)	
Pilots (4.5)	300,000
Aviation technician (1.5)	100,000
RNs (4.5)	300,000
Paramedics (4.5)	230,000
Program director	80,000
Communications technicians (4.5)	150,000
Secretary/administrative assistant	32,000
Training/recurrent training	15,000
Weather radar/cable TV subscriptions	3,000
Medical equipment	22,000
Medical supplies	20,000
Communications equipment amort./rental	20,000
CE/educational materials	10,000
Outreach/PR	15,000
Space (offices, crew quarters, etc.)	24,000
Finance/accounting/billing	50,000
Total	$2,051,000

and fuel pumping system (Figure 14-2). When purchased in bulk, Jet A fuel generally costs 40 to 50 percent less than fuel purchased at an airport. A program that uses 6000 gallons of fuel per month could save $8,000 to $10,000 per month in fuel costs. Those savings can offset the cost of installing a fuel system in as little as one year. In the long run this is the most economical way to go. It also allows for re-fueling at the program's own heliport, saving wear and tear on the aircraft and eliminating the extra fuel cost associated with flying back and forth to an airport.

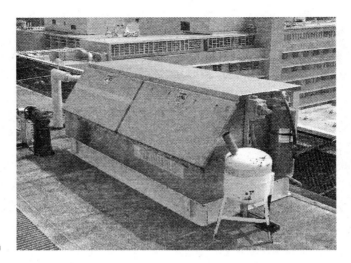

FIGURE 14-2
Heliport fuel system

Income

Most flight programs charge a liftoff fee and a loaded mileage fee. Some programs also charge a professional service fee. Changes in governmental reimbursement regulations now preclude billing for most "add-on" fees such as IVs and medications. In April 2002 the Centers for Medicare and Medicaid Services (CMS) implemented a new Medicare fee schedule, under which new rates began to be phased in over a four-year period and will be fully implemented in January 2006 (Table 14-2). During this period, reimbursement will be determined by blending a portion of the existing payment rate with a portion of the fee schedule payment rate.

Under this new system, air medical services will fare better than ground ambulances. When fully implemented, the base rate for helicopter

Table 14-2 Fee Schedule Implementation

Year	Existing Payment	Fee Payment
2002	80%	20%
2003	60%	40%
3004	40%	60%
2005	20%	80%
2006	0%	100%

transport will be $2,690.96 and that for fixed-wing ambulances will be $2,314.51.

Subscription Plans

Membership programs offer an air medical program a guaranteed and relatively predictable cash flow. For a set fee, an individual or family purchases an annual membership, and when they use the service under medically appropriate circumstances, they do not receive a bill. For patients with medical insurance a subscription program is basically an offer to have their deductible waived. The insurance carrier is still billed for the full amount of the transport.

Subscription programs are controversial. Some authorities believe these programs are nothing more than thinly disguised insurance plans and warn that there may be significant legal risk in offering them. However, a number of air medical programs have offered subscription plans quite successfully for many years and have seen no legal ramifications. Some states require the posting of a substantial bond before allowing the establishment of a subscription plan. Any program considering a subscription plan should look carefully not only at financial projections but at potential legal issues as well.

Payer Contracts

Payer contracts are agreements with hospitals, insurance companies, and other groups that may be in a position to pay or reimburse for air medical transport. To be effective, these agreements must offer an incentive to both parties. Generally, the incentive for the air medical program is guaranteed, prompt payment. The incentive for the hospital is a discount in the billing rate. Receiving hospitals also benefit by gaining rapid access to critical-care transport and the patients that may be secured through its use.

Guaranteed Payment

A few flight programs require a guarantee of payment prior to launch on interfacility transports. While this may be an acceptable policy in regard to elective and nonemergency transports, it should be avoided when emergency or potentially unstable patients are involved. Requiring prepayment or a guarantee of payment before agreeing to accept an emergency transport is unethical and suggests a loss of focus. This practice may also alienate referring physicians and result in a loss of future referrals. While flight programs must remain fiscally sound, financial arrangements should be established in advance in the form of contracts and mutual aid agreements.

Summary

Budgeting and finance are often viewed as necessary evils in the management of an air medical program. Although flight crew members would prefer to focus on more humanistic issues, air programs require a steady stream of money in order to survive. Maximizing income and controlling expenses are essential for long-term survival and growth. Program managers must be diligent in looking for opportunities to establish new contracts and finding ways to increase funding.

As health care reimbursement continues to be trimmed, program administrators must seek out new ways to make their programs more cost effective. That generally means finding ways to cut costs without compromising quality or safety and finding new sources of income. Cost sharing among several sponsoring hospitals is one effective method for generating new income and sharing program costs.

REVIEW QUESTIONS

1. A budget is defined as:
   a. A projection of income and expenses over the upcoming year
   b. The total of all expenses for a given period of time, generally one year
   c. The total of all sources of income for a given period of time, generally one year
   d. A businesses operating plan

2. The three sections of a budget are:
   a. Income, expenses, and personnel
   b. Income, expenses, and charitable contributions
   c. Income, capital expenses and charitable contributions
   d. Income, expenses, and capital expenses

3. The type of aircraft acquisition where a hospital contracts with a vendor to provide all major equipment and services is known as a _____ operation.
   a. Turnkey   c. Lease-purchase
   b. Minerver Cheevy   d. Package agreement

4. Advantages of a lease-purchase option include:
   a. It ensures that a vendor will provide an aircraft without a formal contract
   b. It ensures that the term of an agreement will be for at least 5 years
   c. There are no real advantages to the lease-purchase option
   d. It allows an organization to purchase an aircraft without having to go through the formal purchase process and without having to produce a large amount of start-up money

5. Discuss how it may be cheaper for an air medical program to purchase its own fuel storage and pumping system than to buy fuel at retail prices.

15

Benefits of an Air
Medical Program

Objectives

Upon completing this chapter, the reader should have a
better understanding of the following topics:

* The medical or humanistic benefits of the air medical
  program

* The financial benefits of the air medical program

* The educational and secondary benefits of the air
  medical program

Introduction

We must begin with the assumption that air medical programs have
something of value to contribute to patient care and improved
outcomes. Otherwise it becomes difficult to justify the high cost of these
programs. They are expensive, and that fact alone will continue to make
them potential targets as financial analysts look for ways to save money
in a very tight health care environment. An AM program must be able to
demonstrate that it is not only effective but also efficient.

At present a number of fairly conclusive statements can be made regarding the benefits of air medical programs. These benefits can be divided into two categories: medical (humanistic) and financial.

KEY TERMS

catchment area, p. 232

Medical Benefits

Most rotor-wing air medical programs are staffed and equipped to manage even the most challenging patients. The aircraft itself offers superior speed of transport and the ability to significantly reduce out-of-hospital time. These two attributes alone would seem to make air medical transport the superior mode of transportation for critical patients. While the literature is not always conclusive, some well-designed studies suggest that air medical programs have much to contribute to the management of certain categories of patients.

Patients presenting with multisystem trauma, stroke, and unstable cardiac conditions have been shown to benefit from treatment and transport by air medical programs. Patients with unstable fractures that may deteriorate with excessive movement may also benefit from the more stable ride provided by an aircraft. In particular, patients with unstable spinal injuries (subluxation) may have a lower incidence of transport-induced complications.

Referring physicians seem to take some comfort in knowing that a highly qualified flight team will manage their patients. The acuity level of patients transported by AM programs provides the medical team an opportunity to gain extensive experience in a relatively short time. The volume also provides the medical team with ongoing experience to keep their knowledge and skills well honed. The expertise and experience of the team often decrease the perceived medical/legal liability of referring physicians and make them more likely to use the service. They may also call on the flight team to help with difficult procedures prior to transport.

Literature Review of Air Medicine and Patient Outcomes

It may be hard for those directly involved with an air program to maintain objectivity when the effectiveness of their program is questioned. Crew members tend to form strong personal attachments to their flight programs and may find it difficult to accept outside criticism. However, patient outcomes data is what drives modern medical care (and reimbursement). Ultimately, every medical treatment is studied and proved to be effective or ineffective. Treatments with a positive impact on patient outcomes will generally be continued, while those with no impact or a negative impact will be discontinued.

There are two basic types of data relative to patient outcomes. The first, known as anecdotal evidence, involves personal experiences. A treatment provided by an individual or team under a given set of circumstances either works or fails to work. The individuals involved may form opinions about that particular treatment based on a few experiences.

The other type of data results from well-organized research that generally involves large groups of patients and compares outcomes of those receiving a particular treatment to those receiving an alternate treatment. In many cases this involves comparing patients receiving the standard of care to those receiving a new or experimental treatment. These studies are often double blind, meaning that neither the researchers nor the patients know which of the two (or more) treatments they are receiving. Conclusions can be formed regarding the effectiveness of the new treatment as compared to the old. Relatively little research has been done comparing patients treated and transported by air medical teams to those treated and transported by ground.

Of the studies that *have* been done, some have demonstrated benefit, especially in the area of trauma management. However, because so little meaningful research has been done, this mode of patient treatment and transport has yet to be fully legitimized by the scientific medical community. Some of the more significant studies are highlighted below.

Trauma Patients

As with any costly treatment modality, the use of helicopters in the management of trauma patients has been controversial. In a study by Urdaneta et al., 40 percent of patients benefited from helicopter transport.[1] Moylan et al. studied the impact of air medical transport on trauma patients with trauma scores of 5–10.[2] The results indicated a significant improvement in survival rates among the group transported by air.

Thomas et al. conducted a retrospective study that combined trauma registry data from five urban Level I trauma centers.[3] After correcting for age, sex, receiving hospital, and prehospital level of care, the study concluded that helicopter transport provided a significant reduction in mortality for patients presenting with blunt trauma.

On the other side of the issue, a number of studies show the involvement of helicopters in the management of trauma patients to be less beneficial. Braithwaite et al. examined the records of 162,730 patients treated at 28 accredited trauma centers in Pennsylvania[4] and found that while patients transported by helicopter were younger, were more seriously injured, and had lower blood pressure than comparable patients transported by ground, helicopter transport did not affect the estimated odds of survival. Koury et al. studied a group of trauma patients requiring urgent surgical intervention secondary to traumatic injury.[5] The study failed to identify any outcome benefit for the patients studied.

A few studies directly compared outcomes for patients transported by ground ambulance and air medical team. Oppe and De Charro conducted a retrospective analysis of patients who had been victims of accidents between May 1995 and December 1996.[6] They compared the death rate for patients treated by ground ambulance and air medical teams. The authors corrected for the fact that patients transported by air presented with more life-threatening injuries than those transported by ground. They concluded that use of the air medical program had little effect on patients with devastating injuries and those with relatively minor injuries. However, they found a significant benefit for patients with an intermediate probability of survival.

Kerr et al. conducted a comparative study involving the entire state of Maryland.[7] Data were obtained from the Maryland Institute of Emergency Medical Services System (MIEMSS). Among patients with a high index of injury severity, the mortality rate was lower among those transported by helicopter. This study is of particular interest because the air medical programs in Maryland are all staffed identically to ground ambulances. This finding removes medical capabilities and isolates the mode of transportation alone.

A recent multicenter study examined trauma registry data from five urban Level I adult and pediatric trauma centers. The study, which comprised 16,669 blunt trauma patients, found that the group transported by helicopter showed a significant mortality reduction of 24 percent over those transported by ground.[8] Other studies show less favorable results.

Given the limited data currently available, it appears that air medical transport is associated with a significant benefit for some injured patients, particularly those presenting with blunt trauma, and may offer little if any benefit to other trauma patient types.

Another study examined the effects of closure of an air medical program. The researchers found no increase in trauma mortality or morbidity. However, it did show a significant decrease in the number of patients seen at the sponsoring hospital. That study may be of greater interest to administrators than to medical personnel.

Medical Patients

Few studies have evaluated the outcome benefits of air medical transport for medical patients. Many of the studies that have been done involved the analysis of relatively small numbers and resulted in conclusions that are less than compelling. Certain categories of medical patients may benefit, in some cases because of decreased out-of-hospital time. However, the benefit is more likely due to the enhanced capabilities of the medical team.

The Bottom Line

The medical value and cost-effectiveness of helicopter medical programs are still a debatable issue. A number of well-designed studies have demonstrated the positive impact of air medical programs on mortality and morbidity, but others have shown minimal or no positive impact on outcomes, notably in the area of trauma. Those associated with air medical programs have abundant anecdotal evidence of the worth of the programs but have neglected to produce either quantitative or qualitative research studies to back up their intuitive claims. Much more good-quality, high-number research is needed to clearly demonstrate the areas in which air medical programs have the most (and least) to offer. Until that data is available, programs must remain objective in evaluating their value to the health care system.

Financial Benefits

A helicopter medical program can be a positive financial resource for a sponsoring hospital. While few air medical programs actually make money (or even break even), when viewed as stand-alone cost centers, many do have a net positive impact on the budget of the sponsoring hospital(s). Long-term use of an air medical program can significantly increase the size of a hospital's catchment area. The quicker availability and additional medical equipment and personnel aboard the aircraft often make this mode of transportation more attractive than traditional ground transport, and referring physicians may feel more comfortable with a flight crew when dealing with critical patients. Under certain demographic and geographic conditions, 25 percent or more of the referrals attracted by a flight program may have been lost to competing hospitals if not for the flight program. Considering the fact that each high-acuity emergency or critical-care patient transported has the potential to generate a significant amount of income for the hospital after transport, the cost of the flight program may become incidental.

One recent study evaluated the impact of the closure of an air ambulance service from both medical and financial perspectives.[9] Termination was associated with a 12 percent decrease in trauma admissions over 2 years, as well as a 17 percent decrease in admissions of severely injured patients. From a medical perspective there was no change in mortality in any of the patient subgroups that were investigated. There was a temporary decrease in hospital length of stay.

The public relations value of a flight program cannot be overstated. These aircraft immediately become the center of attention wherever they happen to show up. When used as part of an outreach program, the attendance increases substantially, giving program personnel a unique opportunity to meet and educate administrators, physicians, EMS providers, and nursing staff at potential referral hospitals. These contacts almost certainly lead to increased use of the aircraft. AM programs can be an integral part of a hospital's marketing and outreach program.

It has been suggested that simply displaying a medical helicopter on a hospital campus may increase the number of patients using that hospital. One study concluded the number of new patients rose by 3 percent. Apparently the presence of a helicopter gave observers the impression that the hospital was willing to invest in high technology, which made them more likely to use the facility.

Educational Benefits

Some air medical programs serve as clinical training sites for health care education programs. This is an excellent opportunity for air medical personnel to have a positive impact on the education, beliefs, and practice habits of students. An air medical rotation offers an invaluable experience for paramedic and nursing students and physician residents. Students generally see these rotations as exciting and rare opportunities. They usually hold the flight team in high esteem and are easily influenced by their words and actions.

This is also an excellent way for the air medical program to maintain a presence in the medical community. Students who rotate through eventually graduate and are employed by hospitals and ambulance services that may refer patients to the flight program. From that perspective, serving as a clinical site provides the AM program with a marketing opportunity.

Summary

An air medical program has much to offer the community it serves in terms of medical care and more efficient patient transport and delivery. Although research on air medical transport and patient outcomes is not as complete as it might be, several studies suggest improved outcomes, especially for certain categories of trauma patients. However, not a lot of data is available to support air medicine from a clinical perspective.

catchment area
The geographical area served by an institution or program.

The air medical program may be useful in other areas as well. It can be a valuable marketing tool for a hospital or consortium. It allows hospitals to effectively extend their **catchment area** and attract patients from greater distances. Outreach programs may be an effective means for dispersing medical information from larger teaching facilities to smaller community hospitals. In short, these programs provide medical and humanistic benefits to the residents of the service community and may also offer marketing and financial benefits to their sponsor hospitals.

Notes

1. L. Urdaneta et al. "Role of an Emergency Helicopter Transport Service in Rural Trauma," *Archives of Surgery* 122 (1987): 992–96.
2. Joseph A. Moylan et al. "Factors Improving Survival in Multisystem Trauma Patients," *Annals of Surgery* 207 (1988): 679–85.
3. Stephen H. Thomas et al. "Helicopter Transport and Blunt Trauma Mortality: A Multicenter Trial," *J Trauma* 52 (Jan 2002): 136–45.
4. Collin Braithwaite et al. "A Critical Analysis of On-Scene Helicopter Transport on Survival in a Statewide Trauma System," *J Trauma* 45 (July 1998): 140–46.
5. S. Koury et al. " Air vs. Ground Transport and Outcomes in Trauma Patients Requiring Urgent Operative Interventions," *Prehospital Emergency Care* 2 (Oct–Dec 1998): 289–92.
6. Siem Oppe and Frank De Charro. "The Effect of Medical Care by a Helicopter Trauma Team on the Probability of Survival and the Quality of Life of Hospitalised Victims," *Accident Analysis and Prevention* 33 (2001): 129–38.
7. W. Keit, Y. Kerns, and R. Bissell. "Differences in Mortality Rates Among Trauma Patients Transported by Helicopter and Ambulance in Maryland," *Prehospital and Disaster Medicine* 14 (July–September 1999): 159–64.
8. S. H. Thomas, T. H. Harrison, W. R. Buras et al. "Helicopter Transport and Blunt Trauma Mortality: A Multicenter Trial." *J Trauma* 52 (January 2002): 136–45.
9. V. L. Chappell, W. J. Mileski, et al. "Impact of Discontinuing a Hospital-Based Air Ambulance Service on Trauma Patient Outcomes." *Journal of Trauma-Injury Infection & Critical Care* 52(3)(March 2002): 486–91.

REVIEW QUESTIONS

1. Discuss two studies that have been done that show an improvement in outcomes for those patients transported by air ambulance.

2. Discuss the financial implications of an air medical program.

3. Explain how an air medical program can be a valuable asset for an academic/teaching hospital.

4. The interpersonal skills of members of the flight team are important because:
   a. Programs with team members who are friendly may receive large tips from patients and family members
   b. Patient ratings of medical team members may determine the size of future pay raises
   c. Flight programs are important public relations and educational tools for their sponsoring institutions
   d. None of the above

5. A reasonable form of media involvement with the air medical program may include:
   a. Allowing media representatives to accompany the flight team during patient transports
   b. Allowing media representatives to provide patient care
   c. Allowing media representatives full access to patient medical records
   d. Paying media representatives to present only positive aspects of the program

6. Effective forms of air medical program promotion include all the following except:
   a. Distribution of a newsletter
   b. Offering an active outreach program
   c. Offering an informative website which actively promotes the flight program
   d. Offering cash incentives for using the flight program

Outreach
and Promotional
Activities

Objectives

Upon completing this chapter, the reader should have a
better understanding of the following topics:

* The potential marketing impact of the air medical
  program

* The benefits and risks of working with the media

* The process for establishing and evaluating an outreach
  program

* Newsletters and Web pages as marketing and
  educational tools

Introduction

In this era of tight reimbursement and unprecedented competitive-
ness, health care organizations must use every tool at their disposal
for self-promotion. Air medical programs have tremendous potential
for marketing and public relations. These programs can be very effective at not only marketing themselves, but also at marketing their
sponsoring hospitals or consortia. The importance of self-promotion
may be even greater in the case of for-profit operations. These organizations may be unable to survive without an active marketing and
public relations program. This chapter addresses the marketing and
public relations strategies that may be employed by air medical
programs.

Marketing

Flight programs are often used as public relations and educational tools for their sponsoring institutions (Figure 16-1). Hospital-based programs should visualize each member of their flight team as an ambassador for the hospital who can play a significant role in public relations and marketing. These people frequently visit other hospitals and assume responsibility for patient care from medical personnel at those facilities. As a result they become trusted and respected members of the health care community. Who better to offer on-site educational programs for remote medical facilities?

The flight team can also distribute promotional items for the sponsoring hospital. Cups, pens, calendars, and so on that are inscribed with key telephone numbers can be valuable tools in recruiting new users and new patients.

A website can be an excellent tool for promoting a flight program. Posed and action shots, pictures of personnel, short biographies, and even digital film footage can be integrated into a site. A hit counter allows program managers to monitor the number of users accessing the site. Some sites contain links to outreach and continuing education sites and schedules.

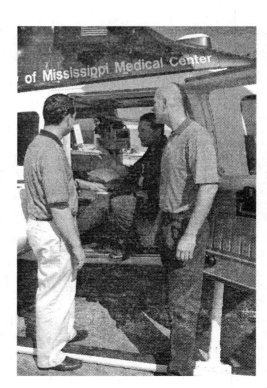

FIGURE 16-1
Flight team member presenting a demonstration to a group of health care professionals
Photo courtesy of Mark Galtelli

Many Internet users access the World Wide Web through dial-up service providers. Those connections transmit and receive information, especially graphics, relatively slowly. For that reason home pages should contain minimal graphics. Pages that are heavy in graphics should be included as optional links.

Importance of Interpersonal Skills

While mass marketing is important, it is only a starting point. It can help a program make initial contacts and project a positive image to potential users. However, following this initial grace period, virtually all interaction between the air medical program and its customers will be on an individual basis. The quality of that interaction will affect the level of customer satisfaction and continued use of the program.

In most programs the flight team responds only when requested by a customer—a hospital, physician, paramedic, nurse, or first responder. Few programs respond to 911 calls as ground ambulances do. Hence there is no automatic demand for AM services. The very existence of an AM program often depends on the relationships its team cultivates with potential customers.

We hear the term "interpersonal skills" a lot. But what does the term mean, and why are these skills so important? Quite simply, interpersonal skills are the tools we use to establish and maintain relationships with others. They consist of the words we speak, the tone in which we speak, the way we listen (or fail to listen), the way we respond to comments from others, and our body language. In most cases, good interpersonal skills are developed over time. They are the result of our observing and learning from others and of our own trial and error.

In the medical setting, interpersonal skills may be divided into two categories: interaction with patients (bedside manner) and interaction with other members of the health care team (interprofessional interaction). Relations with both these groups are very important. While there are similarities between these two relationships, there are also important differences. Members of both groups should be treated with dignity and respect.

Media Involvement

Few things are more exciting to the typical television viewer than watching an air medical helicopter on final approach at the scene of an emergency. Inviting the media to participate in ride-alongs can be an excellent way to gain positive exposure. Reporters are often eager to see firsthand exactly what it is that flight personnel do. They are also eager to bring their cameras along so that their viewers can share in this inside experience.

For programs using larger aircraft, carrying an extra passenger may not be a problem. In smaller aircraft it may not be possible. A media representative can still be taken for a PR flight and allowed to get flight footage and action shots of the crew. Shots of patients at accident sites or being unloaded from the helicopter can be edited in later. The result is often seamless footage.

As with any other area of medicine, patient confidentiality issues must be worked out in advance and medical personnel must agree to abide by any restrictions placed on them. The new HIPPA requirements stipulate that patient medical information be made available only to those with a need to know. That does not include media personnel, who must acquire a written release from each patient.

Dangers of Working with the Media

Media personnel are eager to report on anything likely to attract public interest and provide good ratings, whether or not the stories reflect well on their subjects. It is best to assume that anything said or done in the presence of reporters may appear on television or on the front page of the local newspaper. Flight team members should be properly oriented before working with the media. They should be on their best behavior and consciously control what they say.

Another danger of working with the media is misreporting. EMS personnel are well aware of the mistakes that often show up in the news. Flight team members must make an extra effort to communicate clearly with reporters. It is wise for a senior flight team member to review the material that will be used for the story before the media representative leaves the premises. Although there is no guarantee that the material won't be changed, major mistakes may be caught.

Outreach

Outreach refers to the provision of educational programs at off-site locations. The sponsoring institution is "reaching out" to the medical community. These programs offer health care providers in the community access to educational opportunities that may otherwise be too expensive or difficult to obtain. Outreach may be offered in a number of formats, including classroom lectures, continuing education sessions, seminars, and canned courses. Some outreach courses are provided by distance education or on the Web, but less personal approaches tend to lose some of the value of face-to-face interaction, and the benefits to the sponsoring institution may be diminished.

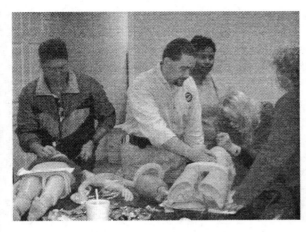

FIGURE 16-2
Flight team member presenting outreach
demonstration

The flight program is often the department of the sponsoring hospital that coordinates and provides outreach activities (Figure 16-2). This is a natural secondary role for the flight team members, who routinely visit other hospitals, assist with stabilization, and transport patients on to referral centers. They have already established a relationship with many of the medical personnel at those facilities. Teaching classes and explaining difficult patient care issues are excellent ways to earn credibility with both existing and potential customers.

The sponsoring hospital also has much to gain from the arrangement. As the connection between the flight team and off-site hospitals grows stronger, the off-site hospitals are more likely to call the flight team for emergency and critical referrals, and, assuming the appropriate resources are available, to refer patients to the sponsoring hospital. An active outreach program may substantially increase the number of referrals a hospital receives.

Program Goals

In conjunction with the program director and others, the outreach coordinator should determine early in the development of the program exactly what the program wants to accomplish through outreach. Generally, the goals of the outreach program should focus on expanding the participants' knowledge and skills in the following areas:

1. Patient assessment
2. Clinical decision making
3. Patient management
4. Quality management/improvement

Program Development

Developing an outreach program is not a complex process. However, it can be time-consuming and may require a significant amount of travel. The first step is to identify a member of the flight team who believes in the program, is willing to coordinate the effort, and has time to do a good job. The person who volunteers for this position will be required to interact extensively with medical personnel at the prospective outreach facilities, so excellent interpersonal skills are a must. Credibility and a strong working knowledge of emergency and flight medicine are also essential.

The format of the program must be determined. The simplest and most effective way to begin a new program is by providing classroom lectures. The only investment required is for a laptop computer and digital projector. Programs with established track records may want to offer Web-based or distance learning courses. Again, that approach may not be as effective as face-to-face presentations.

Once a coordinator has been appointed and all necessary equipment and supplies acquired, the program should be marketed. The ideal target audience is personnel at hospitals where the program would like to increase flight volume. The primary purpose of the outreach program is to share knowledge and improve patient care, but it should also market the flight program and, if the program is hospital based, market the sponsoring hospital as well. Increasing patient volume for both the flight program and the sponsoring hospital helps to justify the expense of an outreach program.

There must be adequate funding for the program. That money typically comes directly out of the flight program's budget. The program director may be able to secure an increase in funding to offset this additional cost. In any case the program will likely pay for itself in a few months' time. The program director should track flight volume to hospitals involved in the outreach activity so that any increase in flight numbers can be noted at budget time.

If more than a few hospitals are located in the target area, the outreach coordinator will need help with presentations. Additional crew members should be involved in this process as time allows and should be chosen according to the same criteria used to select the coordinator. It is important that they understand the sometimes fragile nature of their relationship with outside hospitals and avoid making comments that may undermine any relationships the program has built.

Another sensitive issue involves dealing with patient care errors. During the course of a presentation, a question may be asked regarding the questionable judgment or actions of another health care provider at that hospital. The presenter should be very cautious when responding. One effective way to address this issue is to avoid making any judgment regarding the propriety of the action, but to focus instead on the flight program protocol and its underlying rationale.

Targeting the Right Population

The outreach program will accomplish little if it fails to reach the desired audience. The target audience should be determined first by identifying individuals or groups that will benefit most from the medical content of the outreach program, then by identifying those who might benefit from an air medical program. Ideally these two groups will be identical. If not, the outreach coordinator should focus first on patient-care-related issues and second, on the marketing aspect of the program.

The most common target groups include emergency department and critical-care physicians and registered nurses. But others—LPNs, respiratory therapists, and EMS personnel—should also be encouraged to attend outreach programs.

Members of the lay public should not be overlooked in this process. After all, they are the people most likely to use the AM service. The goal should be to make the flight program a household name. The types of services provided to the lay public are slightly different from those intended for the medical community. Injury prevention programs and anti-drug and -alcohol programs are an excellent means not only for providing a beneficial service to the community but for getting positive media exposure for the program.

Outreach Content

The content of the outreach program should be based on an ongoing needs assessment. This does not need to be a formal pretesting process, which may intimidate potential recipients and undermine the whole effort. Members of the flight team generally interact with medical personnel at referral hospitals frequently enough to know the latter's strengths and weaknesses. That may be a starting point for developing a program for a hospital. However, an outreach program prescribed by the flight team is likely to be short-lived. It is essential to get input from those who will participate in the program. Their stated needs may be different from those perceived by the flight team. In order for the program to be successful, the outreach coordinator should strive to address both sets of needs.

One approach that seems to work well is for the outreach coordinator to periodically mail surveys to referral facilities. These questionnaires serve two functions. First, they help determine the degree of interest of potential participants. Second, they solicit input on topics for presentations and workshops. Over time the outreach coordinator will get a feel for how frequently to contact each facility and who the appropriate contact people are.

Surveys should not be open-ended. They should offer a list of potential topics and ask for a preference. People will often take time to check a box or two but will send something more complicated to the trashcan.

Also, if the choices are not limited, the outreach coordinator may end up with a large volume of suggestions based on individual preferences and of limited interest to others.

Continuing Education

One of the purposes of an outreach program is to provide continuing education credit to health care providers who would otherwise have difficulty attending classes. AM programs associated with teaching institutions generally have an office of continuing education through which the awarding of credit can be arranged. Programs operated by private or public agencies may have more difficulty getting official continuing education credit for the classes they present. The program director or medical director may be able to establish an affiliation with a teaching institution capable of awarding CE credit. An outreach program may attract more participants if credit is awarded.

Evaluation of the Outreach Program

In order to determine if the outreach program is effective, there must be some means of measuring the results. The most common method involves the administration of a pretest and posttest. Any improvement in scores on the posttest can generally be assumed to be the result of the educational activity.

In another, more subjective method, participants complete an evaluation form. Most forms allow for the evaluation of each presenter on a numeric (Likert) scale. Presenters are evaluated on topic content and presentation skills. The disadvantage of these evaluations is that they are generally completed with little conscious thought on the part of the participant. Personality and appearance may be weighed as heavily as instructional performance.

A more useful method involves the use of guided questions that force the participant to provide meaningful feedback. These questions focus on the content of the presentation, the presenter's effectiveness in presenting the material, and suggestions for improvement. Sample questions may include:

1. Did the lecture provide insightful and useful information that will help improve your clinical practices? If so, provide a specific example of what you will use in the clinical setting.
2. Was the speaker knowledgeable about the subject matter?
3. Were you given ample opportunity for open discussion and for asking questions?

4. Did the speaker answer your questions in a knowledgeable and appropriate manner?
5. If you were asked to present the same material, how would you modify the presentation to make it more effective?

Newsletters

Another method for marketing/promoting a flight program is to distribute a periodic newsletter to all hospitals and EMS providers within the flight program's service area. That can be a relatively simple task with any desktop publishing program such as Microsoft® Publisher. Otherwise, with a little more effort and patience, a word processing program such as Microsoft Word or Word Perfect can be used.

The newsletter may include information on current and upcoming events and on selected medical topics. It may even have a continuing education session whereby medical providers submit answers and receive continuing education credit. The newsletter should be used to market the flight program as well. It can describe milestones that have been reached by the program and professional accomplishments of flight team members. Articles about referring hospitals and their personnel should be included in the newsletter whenever possible.

Website

Every flight program should have its own website, which is basically a more dynamic and high-tech version of a newsletter. Flight program websites usually have a high volume of access (hits). A site may contain static pictures and information as well as sections that are updated periodically. The main page should have an action shot of the helicopter and flight team. Linked pages may contain information on the program and its personnel. Some programs include digital video showing an aircraft takeoff or landing or other interesting action.

Web design is generally best left to a professional. A Web-hosting site can provide a Web address and host the site for a nominal fee. This is usually well worth the cost.

Large-Scale Activities

Programs based at universities or teaching hospitals often have the resources to offer larger-scale education programs. Some programs host seminars or conferences centered around a topic related to emergency or critical-care medicine that attract large numbers of participants to a central location.

The air medical team should play a key role in the organization and presentation of the program. Team members who are experienced lecturers may be topic presenters. Others can play support roles. Emergency medicine and specialty care physicians can be recruited to lecture on topics related to their areas of expertise.

A tour of the local facilities and the aircraft may be included in these activities. Program souvenirs such as cups, pens, and T-shirts imprinted with the name of the program may be given to participants. This is an excellent time to point out new and innovative activities in the flight program and in the sponsoring institution. Arrangements should be made in advance with the appropriate agencies so that continuing education credit can be awarded to participants.

Summary

An outreach program can be an excellent means for enhancing knowledge and skills and ultimately improving patient care in the medical community. It can also be an effective way to advertise and market a flight program and its sponsor institution. When developing such a program, the primary emphasis should be on patient care.

REVIEW QUESTIONS

1. Discuss the marketing/public relations potential of the hospital-based air medical program.

2. Marketing is especially important for air medical programs because:
   a. Most programs respond only when requested by a customer to do so
   b. Most programs recieve governmental funding for their marketing activities
   c. Marketing is essential for obtaining permanent licensure in most states
   d. There is no cost associated with marketing activities

3. Allowing a local media representative to ride along on actual patient transports can be beneficial for an air medical program if:
   a. The flight team can be reasonably certain that the media approach will be positive
   b. There is a clear understanding regarding the need for patient confidentiality
   c. The media representative agrees not to smoke aboard the aircraft
   d. a and b

4. The provision of educational programs at off-site locations is known as:
   a. Distance learning
   b. Compressed video instruction
   c. Outreach
   d. Informal education

5. A website can be an excellent method for promoting an air medical program if it:
   a. Is updated on a regular basis
   b. Is maintained by a professional Web-hosting site
   c. Has data that can be downloaded to a Macintosh system
   d. Is viewable in at least 16 colors

6. Discuss two other methods that an air medical program can utilize for publicity and promotion.

CHAPTER 17

Military
Operations

Objectives

Upon completing this chapter, the reader should have a better understanding of the following topics:

* The early years of air medicine (Korean and Vietnam conflicts)

* The role of military air medicine in the post-Vietnam era

* The role of the modern Air Force medical service

* The components of the wartime aeromedical evacuation system

* The military patient classification system

* The contributions of the military to civilian air medicine

Introduction

During the early hours of a cool morning in 2002, Major Deborah Mikita and Colonel Marshall Williams, both flight surgeons, adjusted infusion pumps that maintained a steady intravenous drip of painkillers and antibiotics into a Canadian journalist who, just hours earlier, had been critically injured when a hand grenade was tossed into her lap while she was on a reporting assignment in Afghanistan. The patient had already received immediate care by military forces, and resuscitative care (including hypotensive resuscitation) and surgery by an army forward surgical team (FST). Still in very critical condition, just hours after her injury, she was transported by military aircraft to Turkey. A three-member critical-care air transportation team (CCATT) from Incirlik Air Base, Turkey, coordinated total patient care during an aeromedical evacuation flight to Ramstein Air Base, Germany. Following further stabilization and surgery, the fortunate journalist was transported to her homeland in Canada for rehabilitation and convalescence. She has since returned to work.

On December 5, 2001, a 2000-pound laser-guided bomb (JDAM), dropped from a U.S. Air Force B-52H Stratofortress, fell on a position held by members of American special operations and Afghan freedom fighters north of Kandahar, Afghanistan. Uninjured Special Forces medical personnel immediately began to administer emergency care. Within a short time, a multiagency medical care team was launched to the scene aboard U.S. Army CH-47 helicopters. All injured personnel were evacuated to an established care and treatment site in a secure area. Aeromedical teams from Incirlik Air Base, Turkey, and Wilford Hall Medical Center, Lackland Air Force Base, Texas, provided en route medical care from Turkey to Ramstein Air Base. Fourteen of the soldiers arrived at Ramstein on December 7, aboard a C-141 Starlifter from McGuire Air Force Base, New Jersey, and were transported to nearby Landstuhl Regional Medical Center for treatment.

Following an earthquake of magnitude 7.8 in Izmit, Turkey, in 2001, rescue and recovery efforts were helped by five search-and-rescue dogs from Fairfax County Fire and Rescue Department, Fairfax County, Virginia. The dogs and their handlers were transported to the ruined city via U.S. Air Force C-5 Galaxy. American military medical units based in Turkey provided logistical support to these and other humanitarian efforts.

On February 11, 2000, a three-day-old baby boy, the dependent of a military service member stationed in Okinawa, Japan, was struggling with a life-threatening medical condition requiring specialty surgery and extracorporeal membrane oxygenation, or ECMO. Neither was available in the region. A highly specialized neonatal transport team from Wilford Hall Medical Center, the only long-range team of its kind, delivered the ECMO, assumed total patient care, and transported the patient in stable condition back to a Texas hospital. The duration of the complete mission exceeded 56 hours.

There is little doubt that any of the medical evacuations discussed above could have been as ably performed by an entity other than the military. While the military obviously has priorities that differ from those in the civilian world, there are many similarities between military and civilian air medicine. Many military approaches and techniques have been adapted by the civilian AM community. Significant contributions have been made in the areas of flight physiology, safety, and survival medicine. This chapter will address the basic concepts of military field and transport medicine, including historical, operational, and research perspectives.

Military Medical History

Revolutionary War

Military medicine began with the formation of the Continental Army in Boston in 1775, during the Revolutionary War. Congress approved the building of a hospital to support a 20,000-man army. The staff for the hospital consisted of a director general, who was also the chief physician; 4 surgeons; 20 surgeon's mates (surgical technicians); 2 storekeepers (supply); 1 clerk; 1 nurse for every 10 patients; and laborers. Before this time, prostitutes rendered much of the nonphysician care. Thankfully, the army refrained from continuing that practice.

Of the 1300 physicians who served in the Continental Army, only about 100 actually had a formal degree in medicine. The others were self-taught. It was an acceptable practice for those who wanted to be physicians to acquire a medical text or texts and to study on their own. There were no curriculum standards. When the aspiring physician thought he had mastered the material, he would go out and begin to practice.

Each military unit acted independently in caring for its troops. Medical care in the Continental Army was actually more dependent on the support given by the unit commander than on the skill of its physician. Sanitation, by today's standards, did not exist. Surgical skills were very limited. Surprisingly, there was widespread use of an inoculation against smallpox.

By March 1776, the Army's hospital had cared for over 2700 patients from the total force of 18,500. Later in the year, Congress increased the number of surgeons and expanded their scope to include health and sanitary inspections. Each surgeon was paid $1.66 per day, and the importance of their positions was officially noted within the force. In 1777, as a result of further congressional action, the Army Medical Service was strengthened and ordered to establish and regulate sufficient numbers of hospitals to provide medicine, dressings, bedding, furniture, food, and everything else that was necessary for the proper care of the sick and wounded. Funding for salaries and expenses was included as well. At the conclusion of the Revolutionary War, medical services were reduced significantly and the Army medical corps was reduced to fewer than 100 members. From 1794 to 1800, there were only 12 surgeons and about 30 surgeon's mates in the entire Army.

The year 1818 marked the beginning of a central and formal medical organization in the United States Army. Congress reorganized the Army and established a Medical Department headed by a Surgeon General. Since then, the army has continuously maintained a Medical Department.

The first enlisted medical force was created in 1856 with the appointment of hospital stewards. As noncommissioned officers, these stewards served as pharmacists, record keepers, and ward masters. Other enlisted personnel from line units served as orderlies and attendants. The provision of medical care was considered hazardous duty, and medical personnel received hazardous-duty pay supplements.

Civil War

During the Civil War, treatment delays, infection, and nonbattle-related illness accounted for more deaths than direct combat. However, several important advances were made during this period. Major Jonathan Letterman, a Union Army surgeon, devised a system for evacuating casualties from the battlefield and created the first ambulance corps. His system also included the development and use of field aid stations, field hospitals, hospital trains, general hospitals, and convalescent camps. It was used for the first time at the battle of Antietam in Sharpsburg, Maryland, and worked so well that it was immediately adopted throughout the Army. The basic principles of this evacuation system are still applied today. Other advances in patient care involved the use of anesthesia, wound care, and surgical amputation.

Post-Civil War

Between 1865 and 1898, the Hospital Corps was formally established within the Medical Department. Specialty training for medical attendants was initiated. In 1903, the hospital steward title was eliminated and standard army rank titles were established for all members. The Army Nurse Corps was established in 1901, the Reserve Medical Corps in 1908, the Dental Corps in 1911, and the Veterinary Corps in 1916.

World War I

The origins of the Army Air Corps medical services can be traced back to World War I. A medical Air Corps totaling 34 physicians, officers, and enlisted personnel deployed to France under the command of Major

Robert R. Hampton, the first flight surgeon of the American Expeditionary Forces. In the 1920s, surgeon Malcolm Grow joined the army. Grow had previously gained experience working with the Russian army. As he rose through the ranks, he helped to shape the army's medical operations. He eventually attained the rank of major general and later became the first head of the Air Force Medical Service.

The rapid expansion in the size of the army, the large scale of combat operations, and the remoteness of the battlefields created complex problems for the Medical Department. Two specific entities were created to deal with these problems. Medical services were divided into those within the theater of operations (war zone) and those within the zone of the interior (continental United States). By 1918, the Army had grown to nearly 4 million men and the Medical Department to nearly 100,000. As a result of advances in military medicine, the ratio of death from disease to death from combat dropped to roughly one to one. Casualty evacuation was improved, and mobile hospitals and surgical teams were pioneered. Sick or wounded soldiers got more prompt and improved care. Immediately following the cessation of hostilities, the Medical Department was downsized along with the entire army.

Post–World War I Era

After the war, combat aviation developed into a major field. The potential role of aviation medicine became clear, and it began to develop as a parallel field. A research laboratory was opened at Mitchell Field, New York, and eventually became the School of Aviation Medicine. It was moved to its present home at Brooks Field, Texas, in 1926. Medical researchers, including Dr. Grow and a group of aviation engineers, were instrumental in the development of flight suits, the application of supplemental oxygen, and techniques for carbon monoxide abatement.

World War II

Beginning in 1939 and continuing over the next 6 years, the ranks of the Army swelled to their highest numbers ever: over 8 million, with the Medical Department at over 600,000. The major focus of the Medical Department was to conserve the fighting strength, which included the development of preventive medicine as a new specialty area. Immunizations were developed against typhus, yellow fever, typhoid, cholera, and several other diseases. Water purification techniques were perfected. New drugs, including penicillin, were also developed. For the first time, the number of deaths due to disease were fewer than those from battle-related injuries.

At the outbreak of the war, members of the Medical Department, including Grow, worked with Britain's military medical forces and learned new ways to strengthen the medical services. This collaboration yielded the text *Fit to Fly: A Medical Handbook for Flyers*. In this book, the first of its kind, the authors discussed topics such as the effects of altitude, hypoxia, stresses to the digestive system, and inflammation of the middle ear. They also discussed the anticipated impact of flight fatigue on combat effectiveness. With the assistance of other researchers, the Air Corps medical department invented the G-suit, refined cockpit oxygen equipment, and developed cold-weather flight gear to reduce the stresses of high altitude and long-duration flights. Many other areas in the management of battle injuries were also improved, such as the evacuation system, including ambulances, trains, and hospital ships. By the end of the war, new methods in air evacuation were introduced and became common practice.

During World War II, the number of American casualties was the highest since the Civil War. More than a million casualties were moved by air, most in military cargo aircraft. As the war progressed, aviation medicine continued to evolve, providing injured soldiers with the most prompt and modern medical care available. During one campaign in northern Africa in 1943, the Army Air Forces evacuated over 15,000 patients from Tunisia, with only one death occurring in flight. The same year, a long-range C-54 Skymaster evacuated five injured soldiers from Pakistan to Washington, D.C., proving the feasibility of long-distance aeromedical evacuation and demonstrating the superiority of air evacuation over traditional evacuation by sea. Most evacuations, however, continued to be performed intertheater. For example, following the D-Day invasion, 33 percent of American casualties, about 18,000 soldiers, were evacuated to Great Britain by air. Aviation medicine advanced tremendously over the course of the war. Nearly 6000 physicians completed aviation medical training; over 3000 became "flight surgeons." In 1942, the Nurse Corps was given officer rank. In 1943, the Pharmacy Corps was established. By 1945, the Air Corps had nearly 75,000 hospital beds at over 200 stations, hospitals, and convalescent centers.

Post—World War II

Once again the Medical Department was reduced in size, but it retained its global footprint and responsibility. Training of medical personnel continued, as did research and development of new concepts of medical care and equipment. In the late 1940s, branches were formed for medical administrators, dietitians, physical therapists, and occupational therapists.

Although the Air Force was officially born in September 1947, many of the support functions remained Army responsibilities. It was not until 1949, following the release of Air Force General Order 35, that the Air Force Medical Service was established. A total of 3706 Army personnel were transferred to the Air Force.

The Early Years of Aviation Medicine

Korean War

Even before the first anniversary of the Air Force Medical Service, the United States was involved in the defense of South Korea against communist invaders from the north. During World War I the Medical Department had only 30 physicians, 30 nurses, and 25 medical administrators to provide care for U.S. forces in the Far East. The Korean War was a fast-moving conflict requiring rapid evacuation of casualties from the battlefield. Heavy United Nations casualties quickly overwhelmed Allied medical resources.

During the wartime buildup, the Air Force Medical Service (AFMS) grew substantially, and the aeromedical evacuation lessons learned during World War II were quickly adapted to the Korean conflict. Although poor weather, mountainous terrain, and heavy enemy fire hampered aeromedical operations, Air Force rescue helicopters and propeller-driven airplanes managed to evacuate most of the war's casualties. In 1953, a decision was made to transfer the responsibilities for casualty staging from the Army to the Air Force, even in far forward areas. The first air transportable hospitals (ATHs) were also pioneered. These squadrons, including a hospital with a capacity of at least 36 beds, were designed to be transported completely by air. Following the cease-fire, and with the beginning of the Cold War, the Air Force Medical Service continued to grow and improve technologically.

Vietnam War

During the Vietnam War, the AFMS quickly adapted to combat casualty care and evacuation as it had done in Korea and its predecessors had done in World War II. Long-range aeromedical units ferried casualties from the theater of operations in Vietnam to the Philippines, Hawaii, and the U.S. mainland. While military cargo transport aircraft still performed the majority of aeromedical evacuations, the Air Force recognized the need for a more dedicated medical aircraft. As a result of the extensive casualties and specialized-care needs of soldiers injured in Vietnam, the

Air Force acquired the C-9 Nightingale in 1968. These aircraft are still in service at the time of this publication, but they are scheduled for retirement very soon, and no replacement has yet been selected.

Modern Aviation Medicine

Post-Vietnam War Era (Operational Readiness)

During this period of relative world peace, the AFMS performed numerous training and simulation exercises to test performance assumptions and further prepare the force for wartime operations. Air transportable hospital (ATH) capacity was enlarged to 50 beds. Transporting this unit for deployment required the use of six of the largest Air Force transport aircraft. Aeromedical staging facilities were also placed into operation that could hold a maximum of 250 patients. By 1990, the ATH was the backbone of the U.S. military wartime casualty management system.

Gulf War

Just six days after the Iraqi invasion of Kuwait in 1990, the Air Force deployed medical assets to the Middle East. ATHs from the continental United States quickly followed. Years of planning and numerous training exercises ensured the smooth deployment of medical personnel from active and reserve units and the Air Force National Guard. Within roughly four months, the AFMS had deployed 15 250-bed ATHs, 31 air-transportable clinics, and about 80 percent of total aeromedical evacuation capabilities to the theater of operations. Although this represented the most rapid deployment of any force in military history, there were minimal casualties and little actual medical care was required.

The Modern Air Force Medical Service

Even though its ability to respond and deploy during the Gulf War had been exemplary, the AFMS set about improving its wartime capabilities. It reorganized both ATHs and aeromedical operations to accommodate future deployment scenarios, guided by a vision of much lighter and leaner active and reserve units. Today the force consists of over 48,000 physicians, nurses, administrators, medics, and technicians. This well-trained and highly mobile force responds and adapts quickly to the circumstances and needs of U.S. military personnel anywhere in the world. The mission of the modern Air Force Medical Service is twofold:

1. Its primary mission is to provide medical care to ill or injured military personnel and return them to duty as quickly as possible. If that is not possible, its focus turns to evacuation of casualties from the war zone and the coordination of rehabilitation.

2. The secondary mission involves all the steps required to prepare for execution of the primary mission. In addition to training, this may include providing care for military dependents and retirees and participation in humanitarian operations.

To accomplish this mission, the Air Force Medical Service is continuously evolving. Mobile hospitals that are transportable by air have been designed to allow for quicker mobilization and availability of services in remote areas. Flexibility and responsiveness are further increased through joint training exercises involving both reserve and active duty personnel.

Case Study

The following scenario provides an overview of the aeromedical evacuation system. It offers some insight into the medical resources available to the military and illustrates the inner workings of military air medicine. While specific military aeromedical transports may vary tremendously as scenarios change, the basic elements are designed to easily adapt to virtually any situation. This scenario focuses on the assets and services provided by the air force, but in times of war and conflict, all service branches play a role in the evacuation of the sick and injured.

Evacuation of PFC Henderson

Private First Class Jeffrey Henderson, an infantryman in the 101st Airborne Division, has been deployed with his army unit into combat. While on a night patrol, Henderson's platoon is ambushed by a band of armed guerrillas and he is seriously injured. Arterial bleeding from a gunshot wound (GSW) to the upper thigh is controlled by another soldier who is trained to the level of Combat Lifesaver. Shortly afterward, a medic assumes further stabilizing care, and an army helicopter is already inbound for an emergency extraction. Within 30 minutes Henderson is delivered into the hands of the newest forward medical element, the Forward Surgical Team (FST). This six-member team of surgeons, a nurse anesthetist, and trauma nurses works with equipment carried in backpacks. They are trained to perform life- and limb-saving surgery as far forward as possible, recover the patient, and evacuate rearward for additional care. The FST caring for Henderson inserts two chest tubes for management of a chest wound that has penetrated his body armor, and performs a hemastatic repair of his spleen.

While still sedated, Henderson is transported to the nearest army field hospital for additional care. Shortly after arrival, it is determined that he cannot quickly be returned to duty and requires evacuation for extensive convalescence in the United States. Air force assets (AELT) attached to the army field facility begin to manage the logistics and administrative tasks necessary to transport Henderson out of the theater of operations. AELT ensures that Henderson is in good enough condition to survive the evacuation. Additionally, as the battle line is advancing, the hospital element will soon be expected to pack and redeploy. Henderson and other casualties are "excess baggage" in such a move and will all be moved rearward for additional care.

Arrangements are made to transport Henderson and 12 other soldiers, two of whom are enemy prisoners of war under guard, to a mobile aeromedical staging facility (MASF), located adjacent to a dirt runway about 10 miles from the army hospital. The MASF, a temporary air force holding facility, will triage and assess all these casualties, provide preflight care, and continue the administrative processes as they wait for the arrival of the transport aircraft. Every casualty travels with all the food and medical supplies needed for several days. No more than two hours following the arrival of Henderson and the others, a C-130 Hercules, the mainstay transport aircraft of forward areas, approaches and lands. The aircraft, carrying vital military supplies, taxis to the end of the runway and begins to discharge tons of cargo. Within about 20 minutes, the aircraft is repositioned about 200 feet from the MASF.

Inside the aircraft, a medical crew of five works to convert the flying tractor trailer into an air ambulance, completing this task in only 15 minutes, with the aircraft still running, The medical crew director, standing at the rear of the aircraft, gives the thumbs-up signal, which indicates that they are now ready to accept all patients. First to be onloaded are the walking wounded. Wearing goggles and hearing protection, they follow one of the MASF personnel out to the aircraft and up the rear ramp. They must walk quickly, following hand on shoulder like a line of ducklings through the dust, heat, and exhaust of the jet engines. Another thumbs-up indicates that the flight crew is now ready for litter patients. In the MASF, litter patients have been arranged so that the less seriously ill are loaded first. Loading involves all hands, even the most senior members of the team. At a rate of one patient every 9 seconds, in full military protective gear, Henderson and the other soldiers are carried to the rear of the aircraft. At any point in the on-load, if the aircraft should come under attack, it could choose to depart, leaving some or all patients behind. In times of war, less seriously injured soldiers get the priority for care in some cases. The C-130 in standard aeromedical configuration can carry up to 74 litter-bound patients, to be managed by the crew of five.

Existing agreements allow the air force to lease Boeing 767 airliners from U.S. airlines, including the pilots and flight attendants. The Civil Reserve Air Fleet kit can be installed quickly, and the aircraft can transport large numbers of casualties.

After all the casualties have been loaded, the ramp is raised and the aircraft taxis to the end of the dirt runway for a high-performance takeoff. Inside the cargo compartment, crew members quickly assess all patients, secure any loose equipment, and take their positions for takeoff. Once airborne, they reassess the patients, perform any necessary inflight care, and handle all emergencies (medical and aircraft). Tactical aeromedical evacuation flights usually do not exceed two hours.

Henderson and the other patients are delivered to a rear-area airfield and unloaded from the aircraft. All are transported to either Allied general hospitals or the aeromedical staging facility (ASF). In addition to meeting medical needs, the ASF feeds the patients and their attendants, documents their status and movement precedence, and arranges for follow-on transport. Strategic aircraft arriving into the area of operations are also designed to fill the role of aeromedical platforms for the return trip. These and a limited number of commercially leased airliners are configured from time to time for these missions.

Due to his critical condition, Henderson is transported to a general hospital and placed in the ICU while awaiting transportation back to the United States. Two days later, an air force critical-care aeromedical transport team (CCATT) arrives, takes a thorough medical report, and assumes all care. Comprised of a flight surgeon, a respiratory therapist, and a CCRN, the CCATT has been trained to provide advanced care for up to four seriously ill patients and otherwise assist the standard aeromedical evacuation (A/E) crew. These patients, along with other routine patients, are transported out of the general hospital and ASF and enplaned aboard a long-range military aircraft bound for Wilford Hall Medical Center at Lackland Air Force Base, Texas. Five days after being seriously wounded halfway around the world, PFC Henderson is back on U.S. soil and receives the American standard of medical care.

Importance of Aeromedical Evacuation

While there are many reasons for the military to devote extensive resources to the A/E system, the most commonly recognized is the transport of the seriously injured to places where they can receive life-saving care. The strategic placement of these resources not only improves medical outcomes but also helps to eliminate the "crisis response." Civilian research has clearly shown that early access to medical care leads to shorter hospital stays. Since a major goal of military health care is to conserve the fighting strength, the emphasis is on returning soldiers to duty. Quick and reliable A/E helps in this matter. The present system uses nondedicated aeromedical aircraft in the theater of operations and provides for the effective utilization of all available air force aircraft. A strong, efficient, and effective evacuation plan improves the morale of front-line soldiers. These brave men can perform their hazardous activities with the full knowledge that, if injured, they will be expeditiously evacuated to receive care. Finally, the use of the A/E system has virtually reduced the "front-line census" and allows those assets assigned to and forming an essential part of the army (organic assets) to move lightly and leanly in support of the combat troops.

Service Responsibilities

The army is responsible for all evacuation and immediate care in forward areas. At the basic unit level, soldiers are trained to provide self- and buddy care. Medics assume field care and provide en route care to battalion aid stations or other advanced-care locations. This movement may be accomplished by litter, truck, ambulance, or helicopter. The navy provides many of the services mentioned above for the Marines. In addition, the navy is responsible for evacuation over routes that are of exclusive interest to them. The air force provides a wide range of care services for organic air force assets at both fixed and deployable sites within the theater of operations. Further, the air force provides all domestic and intertheater aeromedical evacuations.

A/E System Responsibilities

Since the air force has been tasked with the dominant role in moving patients both intertheater and domestically, it has identified several major responsibilities necessary to meet this objective. Over the last 20 years, air force medical planners have developed and continuously improved the most sophisticated, centralized patient tracking system in the world. Headquartered at Scott Air Force Base in St. Louis, this system has undergone frequent changes. It is capable of tracking each individual casualty who is in the aeromedical evacuation system at any given time.

Centralized tracking would not be possible without an effective and reliable communications network. In peacetime, this center tracks the movement of all Department of Defense patients being moved worldwide and serves as real practice for wartime scenarios. This communications network, one of the most sophisticated in the military, is an essential element at every step of the evacuation process. A/E radio operators are colocated at the army forward treatment areas as part of the AELT, in the mobile staging facilities, and in all the A/E coordinating centers both inside and outside the theater of operations. All radio communications related to the movement of casualties are encrypted, as information on patient movement could be valuable intelligence for enemies.

Specialized aeromedical crews provide the en route care for all evacuation missions. They are positioned throughout all parts of the Air Force Medical Service and regularly perform peacetime patient movements for the Department of Defense as well as participate in contingency training exercises.

The A/E system would not be complete without a sound infrastructure to support all the essential elements that make the system functional. Command and control, supply and equipment acquisition, aircrew training, and readiness are just some of the functions required to support the system. Lodging, security, food service, and aircraft are not the direct responsibility of aeromedical evacuation operations but are supplied by various civilian or contract sources. Coordination of these resources is the responsibility of command and control elements.

Resource Readiness

The United States is not continuously involved in conflict, and it is therefore not practical to maintain a massive active-duty military force. As with the other branches of the military, the air force maintains aeromedical evacuation readiness within its three major divisions:

1. Active duty A/E units—4
2. Air National Guard A/E units—10
3. Air Force Reserve A/E units—18

The majority of resources responsible for casualty movement in times of war now reside in the guard and reserves. Members of the reserves components maintain considerable depth in clinical care experience, since most work in the health professions and are required to train in military-related duties at higher rates than most other branches of the reserves. During the last 10 years, with the increased tempo of small military deployments worldwide and the simultaneous downsizing of the active-duty element, the reserves have been major players in planning, training, and operations.

Components of the Wartime Aeromedical Evacuation System

Some of the elements of the system highlighted in the evacuation of PFC Henderson will be discussed here, including how the system is designed to function in times of full deployment and how many of the components and concepts employed within the A/E system also apply to civilian transport medicine.

Aeromedical Evacuation Liaison Team (AELT)

The AELT is the most far-forward footprint of the system, and is usually colocated with medical treatment elements of the army and navy. When the medical treatment facility determines that a casualty needs to be moved to another facility by air, the liaison team begins to coordinate the process. These activities are completely customer-driven in that they take their "customer's" product, the casualty, examine the needs for sustained care, and determine the viability of survival following transport by air.

The AELT is composed of six members: a flight nurse, a medical administrator, and four radio operators. The team, operating around the clock, begins radio communication with the other coordinating elements needed to physically move the patient from the forward line. Physicians treating patients at the medical treatment facility are responsible for "certifying" the transport for each casualty and his or her fitness for flight. Clinical coordination with the treating physicians provides the information needed to ensure that moving the patient by air is medically indicated and balanced against other operational concerns. Numerous administrative tasks that must also be done include identifying supplies that must travel with the patient (sufficient for three days), briefing the patient about the upcoming move, preparing the flight manifest, antihijack inspection, and certification. Throughout all activities, from the time of the initial request for aeromedical evacuation until the casualties are delivered to the next medical treatment facility, the radio operators continuously monitor the process.

Mobile Aeromedical Staging Facility (MASF)

The MASF is usually a tent-based, rapidly deployable holding facility at the edge of the far-forward airfield in austere environments. Its primary role is to collect, process, temporarily hold, provide limited care to, and safely transfer casualties onto aircraft. Patients may arrive from several different medical treatment facilities in anticipation of airlift. The MASF staff of 39 personnel, including flight nurses, medical technicians, and radio operators, triages and arranges patients for enplaning. Physicians are not generally assigned to this unit. Numerous additional tasks such as briefing the patients for flight, medical treatment, premedication, and another antihijacking inspection occur during the two-hour holding time.

The standard deployment package includes sufficient supplies for three to five days and is designed for a daily census of approximately 200 casualties. The MASF also contains personnel and equipment to configure an opportune aircraft for aeromedical operations, if necessary. While every effort is made to send a designated flight crew with the in-bound aircraft, the MASF is always prepared to support the mission with its own personnel. When this occurs, the unit must continue operations with five fewer personnel until the contingency crew returns. As the forward line of battle moves, so does the entire medical system.

Aeromedical Evacuation Coordinating Center (AECC)

The AECC is often considered the brain center of the aeromedical evacuation system in theater. Composed of 19 members, including flight nurses, medical administrators, medical technicians, and radio operators, the AECC monitors all aspects of the system and controls the resources. Some of its specific functions are receiving all movement requests, finding appropriate beds, finding airframes for the missions, and alerting and deploying the MASFs. Ordinarily the AECC is colocated near or with the command elements of the tanker and airlift command, since it must work harmoniously in effectively moving casualties to accomplish the end result.

Aeromedical Evacuation Crew (AECM)

The standard tactical aeromedical evacuation crew consists of five personnel—two flight nurses and three medical technicians. The role of the AECM is to configure and deconfigure cargo aircraft for A/E operations, enplane waiting patients, provide emergency and nonemergency care, and safely deliver patients to the next medical treatment facility along the evacuation route. Recent changes to doctrine involve the routine addition to the standard crew to include a flight surgeon and/or the critical-care aeromedical transport team. The AECM must meet strict training and competency guidelines. The team is trained to care for up to 74 patients in flight, loading the litter patients (five levels high), and mitigating numerous aircraft-related emergencies.

Radio Communications

Clear and effective communication among the various A/E elements is essential during operations. The system has adopted and standardized three basic sets of radio transmissions—Alpha, Bravo, and Charlie. All other communications are designed to work in conjunction with these three.

Alpha Message

The Alpha message is sent by the aeromedical evacuation liaison team (AELT) to the aeromedical evacuation coordination center (AECC). The message, a request for movement, identifies the number of patients, classifies them by ambulatory status and general condition, and states the final destination for each. Upon the receipt of this information, the AECC begins to coordinate location of the appropriate flight crew and a suitable airframe, both of which must meet the requirements of the Alpha request.

Bravo Message

When all the necessary details are successfully coordinated and scheduled, the AECC sends a Bravo message to the mobile aeromedical staging facility (MASF) and back to the AELT. In this message the two important pieces of information are the estimated arrival time of the aircraft and the airfield location. Since more than one medical treatment facility may have patients requiring movement, the AECC may schedule the same aircraft to pick up all the patients. The sending unit is responsible for arranging transportation and en route care of all patients repositioned to the MASF. Typically, this occurs by a combination of ambulance, truck, and helicopter. (The navy is proposing the future use of the V-22 variant Osprey VTOL for this type of transport.)

Charlie Message

Following arrival of all patients at the MASF, personnel perform various administrative and health care functions while they await airlift. The communications net remains "up" during this period. If the aircraft fails to arrive or is unreasonably delayed, the sending medical facility must recover its patients and return them to its own facility until the mission can be rescheduled. The MASF is not equipped to provide extended care for these patients. As one might imagine, once the patients arrive at the MASF, it is very difficult to do anything other than keep the patient moving rearward. It is highly possible that a medical treatment facility could have already moved forward in support of active operations. In most cases the airframe arrives as scheduled and all patients are successfully on-loaded. Once the aircraft is airborne, the MASF officer in charge sends the "wheels-up" communication, or the Charlie message. This communicates to both the AECC and AELT the time of takeoff and the final number of patients on-loaded. The AECC continues to follow the progress of the remainder of the mission.

The Patient Classification System

A system designed by the U.S. military and subsequently adopted by the North Atlantic Treaty Organization (NATO) assigns each patient needing transport between medical treatment facilities specific classification criteria. While no similar classification system is necessary in civilian transport medicine, military casualty movements almost always involve numbers of patients with a diverse range of clinical and administrative needs. Often, such classification assists in the preparation of patients for movement and specific placement on board the aircraft, boat, or medically equipped bus (ambus). Classification assignments are made by the sending physician with strong input from nursing. This is important in predetermining the abilities of each patient in the event of an aircraft emergency. While somewhat complex and specific to military issues, the classification system identifies each patient by such needs as litter or ambulatory, psychiatric, and inpatient or outpatient.

Six classifications have been developed:

Category 1   Inpatient psychiatric: This category is subdivided into groups based on safety issues associated with the disease state and observations related to orientation, harm potential, and predictability of behavior.

Category 2   Inpatient litter patient: This category is subdivided into groups that are permitted to get off the litter under specific conditions and those that must remain confined to the litter at all times.

Category 3   Inpatient ambulatory.

Category 4	All infants under three years old.
Category 5	Outpatients (not frequently used in contingency operations).
Category 6	Attendants (medical and nonmedical) assigned to meet the specific needs of particular patients. They take up space in the aircraft, too.

Precedence of Movement

Movement precedence is determined by the certifying physician and helps to determine how quickly a patient should move through the A/E system. VSI, or very seriously ill, are patients potentially at higher risk for deterioration due to clinical status, en route time between medical treatment facilities, or the duration of the mission. Two questions that assist in making this determination are:

1. Is the patient currently stable?
2. Can the crew manage the patient?

    Movement precedence is further classified into three groups:

1. Urgent: requires movement ASAP to save live, limb, or eyesight, or to avoid serious complications
2. Priority: requires prompt movement as appropriate care is not locally available, usually within 24 hours
3. Routine: routine or scheduled movement

Special-care needs of the individual patient are also important considerations in mission coordination and planning. These may include altitude restrictions or other special needs such as burn care or neonatal intensive care. The flight nurse assigned to the AELT and located at the sending facility or the flight clinical coordinator located in the AECC are experienced resources for making both classification and precedence decisions.

Qualifications and Training for the Mission

It has been the practice of the air force that all members of aeromedical evacuation crews must meet specific training and standards that are uniform across the service. In fact, with the exceptions of evolving medical technology and new airframes, little about meeting qualifications has changed in nearly 50 years. The basic framework for this process originated directly from the system used for the pilots and flight engineers. There is a set of basic standards, training, and physiological criteria that all basic aircrew members meet in their initial training. Following this "schoolhouse" training, candidates return to their assigned military unit and enter unit training. During this phase there is both review of the basic elements for their position and additional training related to the specific functions of the military unit. Candidates are observed during training missions before receiving written, oral, and practical examinations. In the final phase, called the "check ride," candidates perform all the functions to meet the standards of the air force. Once fully qualified, they must continue to meet various standards, receive additional training, and fly regularly in a "crew" position to maintain familiarity with the aircraft and the mission. Most crew members are qualified in each specific aircraft in which they are expected to perform.

Aeromedical Evacuation Aircrew Training

Military members assigned to positions that require or may someday require serving on an A/E crew receive their basic schoolhouse training at the U.S. Air Force School of Aerospace Medicine in San Antonio, Texas. Although this institution is operated by the air force, many of its students are from the various branches of the military as well as allied nations. Presently, flight surgeons are not routinely assigned to A/E missions or trained as members of the A/E crew. Nurses and enlisted medical personnel attend joint and combined classes, based on their skill level.

The curriculum is designed for the experienced health care provider and specifically addresses the clinical needs of the airborne patient, limitations and alterations of care in flight, and working in and about the aircraft. All students are prescreened by a flight surgeon for medically disqualifying conditions. Usually, during the first phase of this month-long course, the curriculum focuses on the specific stresses of flight. (These are addressed in Chapter 11.) Students learn to recognize the effects of these stresses on both themselves and their patients. This block of training is reinforced with several "rides" in the school's altitude chamber. While often anxiety-producing at first, this experience quickly teaches students about the signs of hypoxia and the principles of gas expansion. These lessons are not easily forgotten and are invaluable in understanding the effects on patient care.

Nursing fundamentals addressing multiple patient conditions as well as operational considerations such as management of in-flight aircraft emergencies must be committed to memory. Students learn and practice loading, caring for, and off-loading patients on various aircraft simulators.

At each phase of this training program, there is both written and practical examination.

All military members attending the A/E schoolhouse program also attend a week-long survival skills training course. The faculty teaching the SERE (survival, escape, resistance, evasion) course provide an informative and demanding curriculum. Students practice a variety of survival skills such as water ditching, environmental considerations, escape, and enemy avoidance. The course culminates with a multiday survival exercise in an undisclosed location, where the student is encouraged to enjoy all the fine delicacies of the outdoors, if they can find them.

The Contributions of Military Evacuation/Air Medicine

The military's experience in providing and planning for aeromedical evacuation during combat has contributed greatly to these areas of civilian transport medicine:

* **Altitude physiology:** Virtually all theory and knowledge about how altitude affects the human body is a direct result of the work of military aviation pioneers. The efforts of Malcolm Grow and many others are still of tremendous practical value today.

* **Stressors of flight:** The early practitioners identified the basic nine stresses of flight and their practical effects on the flyer and the patient. Most civilian basic curricula have adopted these without change.

* **Crash survival:** Over the last decade or so, there has been an explosion of training programs for civilian air ambulance personnel in the basic principles of survival. In nearly all cases, the content is derived from the military. The military has continually worked toward maximizing the survival potential of aircrew members.

* **Biomedical equipment evaluation:** At the present time, various elements of the military are the only source for unbiased testing of biomedical devices manufactured for direct military use. In recent years, the same organizations have also undertaken the contracted testing of biomedical equipment that has not been designed or selected for A/E use. This equipment is evaluated for its ability to function under simulated normal and abnormal flight conditions and measured against specific military standards.

* **Research:** The military is continually involved in various research initiatives that have improved the outcome of both sick and injured patients. Recent initiatives include investigations into artificial blood

products, hypotensive resuscitation, hemastatic dressings, tourniquet use, and telemedicine. Many of these studies have affected the delivery of transport medicine, and this trend is expected to continue.

Military Air Medical Practices Recommended for Civilian Programs

Despite the contributions described above, there are still many other valuable concepts that should be adopted into civilian transport medicine.

* **Physical standards:** Research and practice related to the physical standards for persons assigned to flying duties have been well described by military authors, but many of these recommendations have not been addressed in civilian programs. Many civilian aircrew members have never been screened by a physician experienced in altitude physiology. Often, issues of medical fitness for duty are related to issues of weight standards and divisions of labor. More specifically, this issue really involves answering the question "Can this flyer reasonably function without deficit while performing aircrew duties?" Underlying medical conditions may not necessarily disqualify the crew member. The screening physician must understand the role of the individual crew member while flying and in the event of an emergency situation. If a care provider becomes incapable of performing his tasks during ground transport, the ambulance can pull over to the roadside and additional assistance summoned. This cannot be done during flight, and attendant incapacitation should never compromise a patient's care.

* **Biomedical preflight:** Prior to any aeromedical operations, crew members are required to review and check all biomedical equipment and medical supplies. Many will state that they "always" check their equipment before operations. Most, however, consider the task accomplished by turning on each device to see if it is fully functional. Military crew members are required to use a standardized checklist. One member reads the printed checklist while another operates the equipment as instructed. This eliminates omissions and shortcuts in equipment checks. Example: What is the operating voltage and battery life of the infusion pump? On most models the start-up screen displays this information.

* **Schoolhouse training:** Schoolhouse training provides all aeromedical crew members with the same basic initial training. While licensure in many states requires that all health care personnel complete the DOT Aircrew Curriculum Training Program, this program is often presented by individuals lacking the qualifications and experience. Requirements for those teaching basic CPR or EMT courses are more stringent.

* **Standardization and evaluation:** There is generally no standardized evaluation of prospective aircrew members prior to assignment or periodically thereafter. Frequently, the assignment of flying positions is driven by organizational politics and the "who you know" system.

* **Aircraft emergency management:** Civilian medical aircrew members are seldom trained to respond to in-flight emergencies. A problem with a door not being secure, a fire, ditching, or a rapid decompression can occur in any type of fixed-wing aircraft. Crew members must be able to respond in all these situations. In 1999, golfer Payne Stewart and others perished while flying in an aircraft type often used for civilian medical transport, because of a slow decompression. Had it been a medical transport, would the crew members have recognized signs of hypoxia?

* **Crew rest:** This is another controversial issue. There are well-established standards (both civilian and military) for pilots and flight engineers concerning crew rest prior to duty time. In civilian aeromedical operations, this issue is frequently ignored. Nurses usually like to "bunch" their work days together and/or work long hours so they can have longer periods of time off. EMTs and paramedics often perform medical flights following their 24-hour shifts. Reasonable standards that ensure sufficient periods of rest prior to duty will increase safety, improve the quality of care, and reduce medical errors. Setting standards will require the elimination of numerous political and economic considerations.

Summary

The history of air medicine is inextricably linked to the military. Civilian programs have benefited greatly from that relationship. It was not until the late 1960s that the first large-scale steps were taken to adapt air medicine to the civilian world. Since then military and civilian services have evolved in a parallel manner, but there continues to be a link between the two. The modern military continues to be a source of new information for the civilian sector.

REVIEW QUESTIONS

1. The origin of military medicine in the United States can be traced back to:
   a. World War I
   b. The Korean War
   c. The Civil War in 1965
   d. Formation of the Continental Army in Boston in 1775

2. Its mission is to provide medical care to ill or injured military personnel and return them to duty as quickly as possible. If that is not possible, its focus turns to evacuation of casualties from the war zone and the coordination of rehabilitation.
   a. Navy Seals
   b. Army portable military intelligence
   c. Air Force Medical Service
   d. Air Force Information Systems Command

3. Since a major goal of military health care is to conserve the fighting strength, the emphasis is on:
   a. Reuniting injured solders with family
   b. Returning soldiers to duty
   c. Finding local sponsors for injured soldiers
   d. Treating injuries as cheaply as possible

4. Discuss the leadership role played by the U.S. air force regarding the movement of military patients.

5. These teams are composed of six members: a flight nurse, a medical administrator, and four radio operators.
   a. Aeromedical Evacuation Liason Team (AELT)
   b. Aeromedical Triage and Sortation Unit (ATSU)
   c. Medical Liason Unit (MLU)
   d. Military Anti Stagnation Unit (MASU)

6. The Mobile Aeromedical Staging Facility is a:
   a. Traveling dance troupe that entertains military personnel
   b. Military support unit that moves from base to support tactical activities
   c. Tent-based aircraft deployment unit
   d. Tent-based, rapidly deployable holding at the edge of the far-forward airfield in austere environments.

7. Discuss the role of the Aeromedical Evacuation Crew.

International
Air Medicine

Attila J. Hertelendy, MHSM, BHSC, CCEMT-P, NREMT-P

Objectives

Upon completing this chapter, the reader should have a better understanding of the following topics:

* The philosophy and approach to air medicine outside the United States

* Air medicine organization and operation in Canada, Europe, South America, and Australia

* Implications of international travel

* The repatriation process

Introduction

The majority of this book was written from a U.S. perspective and in reference to U.S. programs. There are large numbers of programs operating in other countries around the globe as well. Many programs, notably those operating in Canada, Europe, and Australia, have well-trained medical personnel and use aircraft similar to those used in the United States. Other countries have lagged behind in the development of their air medical systems, which resemble the early EMS in the United States. This chapter presents an overview of programs operating in a few of those countries.

Canada

Air medicine in Canada is similar in many ways to that in the United States, with commonalties in aircraft, personnel, and safety requirements. There are also some significant differences. Variations in weather, geography, population density, and access to medical care have led to the development of a flexible air medical system that varies in organization and design across provinces and regions. The result is a variety of fixed-wing and rotor-wing programs, some government operated and others privately owned and operated.

The development of education and service guidelines is the task of a national organization known as the Canadian Aerospace Medicine and Aeromedical Transport Association (CAMATA). Establishing standards for air medical transport is the responsibility of each province or territorial government. Some provinces have established minimum standards through legislation, while others have done so through the terms of their contracts with providers. Northern Canada is expansive and sparsely populated and has extreme weather conditions. Inhospitable terrain, ice, and snow sometimes make access difficult. Health care facilities may be great distances apart and are often staffed by community health nurses with limited medical capabilities. Patients who present to those clinics and require specialized care must be transported to the nearest hospital, which may be hundreds of miles away.

Emergency cases are generally moved by air, a process that may cover hundreds of miles and last several hours. Transports of that distance require specialized patient preparation, transport knowledge, and equipment. The flight team must be prepared for all contingencies and the aircraft must be designed and equipped for all necessary medical treatments.

In the Canadian Arctic, long-distance transports are carried out on a daily basis. People in remote parts of Canada accept some degree of risk by choosing to live there, but they expect reasonably timely access to the health care system. Since there may be no local EMS systems in remote areas, the air ambulance service often makes first contact with emergency patients. The medical team must be prepared to manage all types of emergencies, even when responding to health care clinics. Many nurse-staffed health centers do not have cardiac monitor/defibrillators, laboratory capabilities, and some emergency medications.

The patient population may vary from one extreme to another. One day the patient may be a neonate, the next day a geriatric patient. The medical team must be prepared for any medical situation. Many of the treatments it provides may differ from the norm. For example, the "golden hour" may stretch into the "golden day," and treatments may have to be modified to compensate for prolonged out-of-hospital time.

In contrast to the long-distance transports from remote communities in the Canadian north, air ambulances operating further south in more densely populated areas provide more traditional treatment and transport services. Those programs operate primarily rotor-wing aircraft but may also have fixed-wing aircraft available for longer transports. They respond to scene requests and also provide interfacility transports. Helicopter services are commonly located in larger cities such as Toronto, Calgary, Edmonton, Halifax, and Vancouver. Similar services may be found in some rural settings as well.

Air medical services in Canada vary in the level of medical service provided. The Canadian health care system provides funding to each province for the support of air medical programs. In some cases the government may pay to have residents flown outside the province for medical care.

The province of Ontario has an air medical program that is often viewed as a benchmark for Canada. It was developed in 1977 by the Ontario Ministry of Health to make medical resources more accessible to those in remote areas. The province of Ontario is home to 11 million residents. The majority of the population (approximately 10 million) is clustered in the metropolitan areas of the south. That is also where most of the medical resources are concentrated. The other 1 million people are spread throughout the rest of the province in terrain that varies from that of the Great Lakes to dense forests to the rocky hills of the Canadian Shield. At its inception, the program consisted of five bases with dedicated aircraft. Over the years, the service has expanded and now includes multiple bases strategically placed about the province to better access the residents.

In January 2002 the Ontario Air Ambulance Base Hospital Program (OAABHP) was created to incorporate and standardize the regional air bases and hospitals throughout the province. The current air ambulance system consists of 12 Sikorsky 76 helicopters, 35 fixed-wing aircraft, and approximately 200 certified critical-care, advanced-care, and primary-care flight paramedics. The goals of the OAABHP are to improve patient care during transport, to provide access to all levels of care (primary, advanced, and critical) for all residents of Ontario, and to facilitate flight paramedic mobility and education throughout the province. The OAABHP is now the largest air medical program in North America. The centralized dispatch center dispatches over 20,000 calls per year using medical algorithms to ensure that each patient has prompt access to the appropriate aircraft and medical team.

Ontario is divided into two regions: the northern, extending north of Sudbury and west of Sault Ste. Marie, and the central, comprising the remainder of the province. The head office is located in Toronto. Medical directors representing the regions form the Medical Board of Directors, which is responsible for establishing patient care standards. Program managers and coordinators are strategically located across the province to provide support and direction. Other programs, including quality management, education, and information systems, play key roles in the operation of this system.

A variety of aircraft types are used in Canada. Canadian standards require fixed-wing aircraft to be turboprop or turbine-powered. A majority of rotor-wing aircraft are multiengine turbine-powered. The interior of the aircraft is modified to provide an easy-to-clean, functional environment for patient care. In addition, a minimum inventory of equipment, supplies, and medications is carried on the aircraft. The qualifications of air medical care providers may vary across programs. However, there is an effort to ensure that each patient has access to proper medical personnel.

Europe

Air medical programs in Europe are similar to those in the United States in terms of equipment but significantly different in terms of organizations and personnel. The largest single difference involves staffing. Virtually all programs staff with a physician. Given the European model, that is not considered unusual, as physicians also staff ground ambulances. The concept of physician extenders providing emergency medical care, as in North America, has not caught on in Europe. Generally, the Europeans view emergency medical service and air medicine as an extension of the hospital and as a public service. EMS operations are rarely established with a profit motive as in the United States. A sampling of the approaches used in European countries is provided below.

Norway

Located on the northwestern edge of the European continent, Norway is mostly a high, mountainous plateau covered by bare rock. The northern third of the country is north of the Arctic Circle. Most of the population is located near or along the sea, where warm sea breezes moderate the cold temperatures in winter. Outside the urban areas, the population is scattered in numerous small villages.

The first air medical program was established in 1978 in the capital city of Oslo. Today the Norwegian Air Ambulance is composed of six helicopters, each responding to 300 to 1200 requests annually. Many of these requests are from distant rural areas. Norway's aeromedical system is based on the philosophy of bringing the doctor to the patient. To this end, when an emergency call is received in any of the nurse-staffed "medical emergency communication centers," the dispatcher determines whether an air or ground ambulance is indicated. In many cases both may be dispatched simultaneously until it is determined whether the helicopter is needed. The time from notification to liftoff of the helicopter averages 3 minutes during the day and 15 minutes at night.

Personnel

The flight team consists of a pilot, physician, and rescueman. All flight physicians are anesthesiologists with training in emergency medicine, critical-care medicine, and advanced techniques of pain management. Flight physicians use their skills and experience as anesthesiologists frequently. Patients needing intubation are always given an anesthetic and/or sedative/analgesic. The administration of analgesics for trauma patients is common.

Rescuemen are trained to assist with in-flight navigation and radio communication and are also trained to land the helicopter in an emergency. Professional training generally involves paramedicine or nurse anesthesia. Rescuemen are trained to rappel and perform other basic mountaineering skills, are licensed divers, and assist the physician on the scene. Their training is comparable to that of search-and-rescue technicians.

Pilots must have at least 2000 rotor-wing pilot-in-command hours to qualify for a job with Norwegian Air Ambulance. Most pilots gain their experience in the air force. While most flight physicians work part-time, pilots and rescuemen are full-time paid employees.

The state also operates the ground ambulance system in Norway. These vehicles are staffed by rescuemen, accompanied by flight physicians as necessary. Norway is the only Scandinavian country with a fully integrated ground and physician-staffed air EMS system.

Aircraft

The air ambulance fleet consists of MBB BO-105, MBB BK-117, and Sea King helicopters. These aircraft are owned and maintained by the Norwegian Air Ambulance service. The larger Sea King helicopters are used by the Coast Guard as well as for ambulance missions. The Coast Guard works within an integrated system in which military and civilian aircraft are used for search-and-rescue and medivac missions.

Financing

The government pays roughly half the cost of operating the Norwegian Air Ambulance service. The remainder of the cost is borne by paying members, both individuals and corporations. The program relies on public support for survival. This philosophy is based on the idea of supporting "your own" physician-staffed ambulance helicopter.

Italy

Helicopters are used extensively throughout Italy's network of 20 regional health authorities (RHAs). Fourteen of the RHAs use helicopters to provide both prehospital and interfacility transport services. Aircraft types include the Aloutte III SA 316 and Augusta A109 Max. Systemwide, an average of 17,000 flights are completed in a typical year.

The flight team is composed of a pilot, a physician (generally an anesthesiologist), and one or two nurses. In cases involving mountain rescue, an experienced mountaineer may replace one of the nurses.

Aircraft are dispatched from call centers established by the RHA and accessed via the national emergency telephone number (118). However, the aircraft generally do not fly at night. Night flying is restricted to the armed forces, which provide after-dark coverage for interhospital transfers on request from the emergency medical services.

Fire brigades may operate their own helicopters in Italy. In some regions they may use helicopters for multiple roles, including firefighting and patient transport. There are no privately operated air medical programs.

As in most European models, the helicopter service is paid for by the state. In this case the money is channeled to the RHAs. The service is free to patients and there are no costs to insurers or other third-party payers. In some RHAs the costs associated with providing care to foreign European nationals is billed to the patients' national health care service by means of the E111 European health card, which covers helicopter and other hospital services.

Greece

The health care system in Greece is a mixture of public and private. The national health system provides health services and hospitalization for Greek citizens at no cost. Private health care is available in urban areas and may offer diagnostic and advanced medical services not available from the public system.

Greece is composed of a mainland and over 1000 surrounding islands, many of them inhabited. During the tourist season the population on the islands may increase dramatically. Since few have comprehensive medical care available, medical transportation is of particular importance. The first air medical transport in Greece occurred during World War I. From then until 1979 the air force was responsible for air medical transport. From 1979 to 1984 the responsibility for coordinating air medical transport rested with the Center for Immediate Help, based in Athens. Helicopters from the air force and from Olympic Airways, the official Greek airline, were used. The crew consisted of physicians and nurses who were employees of the public hospital system. Although the service operated 24 hours a day, it was inefficient because all staff were based in Athens.

Unlike Norway and Italy, modern air ambulance service in Greece is provided by a combination of government-operated programs and private providers. Historically the Greek government had borne all expenses for ground and air ambulance transport, but in recent years that policy has changed and today the patient's insurance carrier is expected to bear those expenses. That shift has sparked controversy because the government tends to operate very large and expensive aircraft such as the CH 47D Chinook.

Australia

Australia has a landmass of nearly 3 million square miles (7.7 million square kilometers), and is only slightly smaller than the United States. Most of its population of 17 million is concentrated in cities along the eastern coast, but roughly 325,000 people are scattered across the rest of the continent. This remote population includes indigenous people such as the Australian Aborigines, who are heavily dependent on the world's oldest continuously operating air medical program, the Royal Flying Doctor Service (RFDS). The RFDS operates primarily fixed-wing aircraft because of the great distances that must be covered. In contrast, air ambulances operating in more populated areas such as Melbourne and Sydney consist almost exclusively of rotor-wing aircraft.

The air medical system in Australia was designed to match the population density and demand for medical care. The placement of aircraft is also influenced by the availability of medical care at the local level and the capabilities of the local medical community.

History and Development of the Australian Air Medical Service

In 1917 the Reverend John Flynn, a Presbyterian minister with the Australian Inland Mission, conceived the idea of combining "wireless" radio, aviation, and medicine to produce a mantle of safety in the outback. Over the next 10 years, with the assistance of inventors, radio technicians, physicians, philanthropists, and fellow missionaries, his idea literally took off. Although sporadic medical flights had been occurring for at least a year, the Inland Mission's Aerial Medical Service (AMS) was the first organized program. The first official flight was from Cloncurry in Queensland on May 17, 1928. The aircraft was a deHavilland DH50 biplane on assignment from the fledgling Queensland and Northern Territory Airline Service (now Qantas, Australia's national carrier). The first communications network started out of Cloncurry at the same time, with pedal-powered radios. Without radio dispatch capability the AMS would have been useless. It would be many years before telephone service would become available in the outback.

From the beginning Flynn was in favor of offering a complete health service, not just air ambulance service. Soon routine "clinic flights" were being performed to strategically located airstrips. The advent of the AMS soon led to the development of airstrips in small communities throughout the outback. On occasion local residents had to clear these grass- or dirt-covered strips of livestock, kangaroos, or ant mounds before aircraft arrived. The AMS developed an impressive safety record, in part because pilots were given the freedom to decline high-risk flights.

The fact that the service provided complete medical care and not just emergency transport also contributed to safety margins. Experienced physicians were able to deliver anesthesia and perform surgical procedures in lieu of attempting risky return flights at night or during adverse weather.

Flynn's home state of Victoria was next to introduce the AMS concept. As the smallest mainland state, Victoria was unable to justify its own AMS, so it developed a cooperative with the huge and sparsely populated Kimberly region in the north of Western Australia. The first Victorian AMS base opened at Derby in 1934, followed by the formation of the West Australian section in 1936. By the time of Flynn's death in 1951, he had seen his infant service grow to a federation of six sections and a dozen bases, change its name to the Flying Doctor Service in 1942, and introduce such concepts as the Medical Chest, with numbered oral, topical, and injectable medications administered under radio control, and the School of Air, both utilizing the Flying Doctor radio network. The service's value to the outback was recognized in 1955 with the granting of the "Royal" prefix; it remains a vital part of Australian outback life to this day.

Australia was also a leader in the development of rotary-wing air medical services. In 1972, the same year that Flight for Life commenced at St. Anthony's Hospital in Denver, the Angel of Mercy medical helicopter commenced service in the Mornington Peninsula area of Victoria. The following year, the Sydney branch of the Surf Life Saving Association (SLSA) began the first civilian rescue helicopter service in Australia. The SLSA program was modeled after a similar service introduced in Auckland, New Zealand, the year before. This service also pioneered the concept of corporate sponsorship of rescue helicopters, which offers the sponsor both community involvement and a high media profile. The service expanded its role in the following two years to include attending both medical and trauma patients with a doctor and crewman medic. Patient transport from the scene and between facilities followed. The SLSA Helicopter Rescue Service (HRS) eventually grew to nine programs, all with combined beach patrol/rescue/medivac roles.

Australia's rotary-wing services generally employ dual-role aircraft, unlike their counterparts in the United States and Canada. In Sydney, those who favored a more medically optimized service formed Careflight, the country's first physician-directed, hospital-based, medically dedicated program, and others that have emulated it, but they have found it necessary to retain at least a secondary rescue role. Only one program to date—Child Flight, a dedicated neonatal/pediatric service—does not retain a secondary rescue role. In contrast, the HRS programs have become more medically optimized, as have the police; hence the dual-role services predominate.

Classification of Air Medical Services

There are three broad categories of air medical service in Australia. Aerial health services, typified by the RFDS, cover large distances where air is the travel mode of choice for nonhealth- as well as health-related tasks. These programs provide a broad array of services, including health education, medical consultation, immunizations, routine transport, emergency transport, and the delivery of supplies. When not involved in patient transport, they may use chartered passenger aircraft or scheduled airline services. Similar in concept are aerial ambulance services, most of which are involved in routine transport. Compared to aerial health services, these serve less sparsely populated outlying regions, flying to smaller hospitals rather than individual homesteads and providing access to more specialized services.

At the opposite end of the spectrum are medical retrieval services, which are designed for the timely dispatch of mobile intensive-care teams for stabilization and transport of critically ill patients. This approach to critical-care transport works well for long-distance transports. Most fixed-wing retrievals take 4 to 12 hours to complete. These services are usually hospital-based and physician-staffed and may be run by a major critical-care service.

The third category involves helicopter services that combine rescue and medical roles. The major advantage of the medical rescue model is the ability to provide rescue stabilization, extrication, and medical care simultaneously.

There is considerable overlap among these groups. As an example, the New South Wales Air Ambulance service does mostly routine interhospital transports of ambulant patients but can also perform urgent medical retrievals. While predominantly a helicopter service, Careflight provides rescue and medical retrieval teams by both ground and air.

Air Medical Staffing

Staffing of air medical services in Australia is similar to that in Europe. There is extensive use of physicians rather than paramedics and registered nurses, as typically seen in North America. There are a number of reasons for this. Only two states in Australia have developed paramedic-enabling legislation within their state ambulance services. Paramedics in those states work under protocols without on-line physician control; consequently, their protocols are somewhat limited. The predominance of long-distance transports has fostered the model of "stay and stabilize," with a high level of definitive care being provided preflight and in-flight. Also, the concept of expanded-scope nursing has not caught on. Although nurses are used extensively in Australian air medical services, their function independent of physicians tends to be limited to the provision of basic life support skills and nonemergent transfers. The most common staffing pattern for interhospital air medical transports is physician/nurse. For scene flights the variance is greater, but the physician/ambulance officer (EMT or paramedic) is perhaps the most common combination. There is one exception: In Victoria, industrial and political forces have resulted in nearly exclusive staffing of ambulances by ambulance officers.

The Royal Flying Doctor Service

The RFDS continues to fill the role of an aerial primary health service to the majority of the outback population. It also staffs air ambulances from bases in more populated areas such as Adelaide and Perth. Operated by a federal council, RDFS staffs 14 bases in seven divisions. Services include:

* **Emergency flights:** These tend to be primarily for patients suffering from medical illness rather than for victims of trauma because of the lack of on-site primary medical care. All calls are screened by a doctor, and the medical escort (nurse, doctor, or both) is selected on the basis of the initial physician triage.

* **Medical transfers:** Transfers of patients between hospitals, either arranged or urgent. Again, the level of medical care provided is selected on the basis of the patient's condition.

* **Field clinics:** General medicine and specialty clinics are conducted at remote locations, often under the shade of the aircraft wings. Services include routine health checks, immunizations, children's and women's health programs, and dental, eye, and ear clinics.

* **Medical chests:** Over 2500 "medical chests" containing an extensive range of numbered drugs and medical supplies are located at remote locations across Australia. Each of these sites is equipped with a radio so that an RFDS physician can direct patient treatment. This service is supplied at no cost to the patient.

- **Radio communications:** RFDS physicians and nurses provide consultation services by radio to remote outposts or homesteads. Consultations may result in use of the medical chest or an evacuation flight, as indicated. This aspect of RFDS operations is becoming less important as microwave and fiberoptic technology has extended the normal telephone network farther into the outback.

The RDFS is funded by state and commonwealth governments, assisted by contributions from the corporate and public sectors. It services virtually the entire outback area with the exception of the Northern Territory. There the Northern Territory Aerial Medical Service fills a similar aerial health and air ambulance role from the capital, Darwin, and two rural bases.

South America

Brazil

Brazil, one of the larger countries in South America, covers more than 5.3 million square miles of plains and plateau. The population of 155 million is distributed irregularly across the land, with the population density ranging from 1 person per square mile in the Amazon region to 400 per square mile along the Atlantic coastal strip. Approximately 75 percent of the population is found in urban areas, principally in metropolitan Sao Paulo and Rio de Janeiro. There are 10 other cities with more than 1 million inhabitants.

History of Air Medical Transport in Brazil

Organized civilian air medical transport is a new activity in Brazil. Throughout the 1970s some isolated services were established, with no quality control over training, equipment, or flight crew qualifications. In 1993 professional services emerged as a result of public initiatives in the larger metropolitan areas. The first specialized air transport service was formed in Rio de Janeiro as a branch of the fire brigade. This flight program began operations with an aeromedical version of an AS-350 helicopter. Today, with the surge in new services and the growth of existing ones, discussion and implementation of specific legislation regulating these activities are occurring on a national level today.

Air Medical Staffing

Crew configuration is identical in all services, with only small variations in staffing allowed. The law requires that a physician be a member of every air medical team. Other team members are typically nurses or nurse technicians. Paramedics, emergency medical technicians, and respiratory therapists are not recognized by the government and are nonexistent. Flight physicians and flight nurses receive no special recognition as specialists in the civilian sector. However, they are recognized as having specialized knowledge and skills by the Ministry of the Air Force.

Present Situation

Economic stability and technological innovation have forced both public and private investments in air medical transport systems. Activity still remains concentrated in the larger cities, where all current services are situated. Although Brazil has the world's fifth-largest fleet of air medical aircraft, there is no effective integration among the various public and private transport services.

The military sector has several rotary-wing aircraft (Super Puma, Bell 205, and AS-350) capable of executing air medical transport missions. However, these missions are not directed toward civilian assistance. The armed services lend these resources to the civilian population only in cases of public calamity or large-scale disasters, in conjunction with other regional emergency response.

Prospects

With the growing importance of the commercial health care industry, the privatization of important highways, and the recognition of the usefulness of air medical transport in a nation as vast as Brazil, the future looks positive. However, there are still obstacles to overcome. There is still no comprehensive specialty organization to unite emergency medicine physicians and there are no emergency medicine residency training programs with rotations in air medicine.

Argentina

Argentina is a large country located along the Atlantic Coast in the southeastern area of South America. It has a relatively small population of 39 million. The country has both public and private paramedic emergency services. The private services are operated by a variety of trade unions, private hospitals, and social security organizations.

A polio epidemic occurred in Argentina in the early 1950s, during the first term of President Juan Peron. In the years after World War II, Argentina was a rich country, with a strong air force and a healthy aeronautical industry that designed and produced its own aircraft. It was in that context that the first air medical transports took place. Chest ventilators were installed in military aircraft, and patients with respiratory problems were flown to Buenos Aires from the interior of the country. The South Atlantic conflict between Argentina and Great Britain in 1982 resulted in a large volume of air medical transports, primarily with Hercules C-130 aircraft.

However, the country's economy has deteriorated significantly over the past two decades. Despite the enormous transport distances within the country and the lack of adequate health services, there has been limited government interest in developing a nationwide air medical transport system. Unstable economic and political conditions, punctuated with periods of hyperinflation, have made for-profit ventures very risky.

The development of an organized air transport system is further hampered by antiquated air traffic regulations that have little relevance to modern aircraft. The poor quality of airports is a further barrier. Only 11 airports throughout the entire country are open 24 hours a day.

At present there are two government-sponsored air medical transport services. The most significant is operated by the Buenos Aires province and is headquartered in the city of La Plata. That program uses a variety of aircraft, including the C-441 Conquest, C-241 Golden Eagle, and BO-105 Helicopter. The program completes 600 to 1000 missions per year, averaging 600 hours of total flight time. The second service is attached to the Ministry of Social Welfare, which operates two fixed-wing aircraft (Metro II, Guarani) and three helicopters (two BO-105's and a Bell UH-1). Their activity level is kept low by budget constraints. The Coast Guard also makes their AS 365 Dauphin helicopters available for medical transports.

Two private companies offer the aircraft, equipment, and personnel for critical-care transports. They operate a total of two dedicated fixed-wing air ambulances (Merlin II and Chieftain). The plane to be used is determined by the distance of the transport, the patient's condition, and weather conditions. Flight costs are a major limiting factor in the use of these aircraft.

One private company operates an air medical helicopter, a piston-engine Hiller. It is used primarily to promote the company's ground ambulance operation. The Hiller was used in the United States during the very early years of air medical development and is now considered an obsolete aircraft for that purpose.

Many towns in the interior of the country have air clubs that make aircraft available for the transport of emergency patients. These aircraft are not configured as ambulances and may not have medical personnel or equipment aboard during transport.

Future Prospects

The economy has shown some evidence of improvement. However, it remains in a precarious state. There does not appear to be adequate government interest or financial incentive for the development of an air ambulance system. Public hospitals are also ill equipped to manage serious medical or traumatic conditions. The public hospital system, which serves the majority of patients, is in a deep financial crisis and often lacks the most basic equipment for the management of trauma patients. The development of an organized air medical system will likely not occur until emergency medicine physicians have become better organized.

International Travel and Repatriation

Over the past two decades, international travel has become a common phenomenon. The residents of economically well-developed nations have become more comfortable with the concept of international travel for business and leisure. For many businesses, international travel is a requirement for success. Regardless of the purpose of travel, a portion of international travelers become ill or injured while out of their home countries.

Some international travelers are at increased risk for illness or injury: the elderly, those with chronic medical conditions, the obese, and those who live sedentary lifestyles. They may be at increased risk for decompensation of existing medical conditions and of acute illness because of the greater emotional and physical stressors associated with long-distance travel. In many cases they walk and otherwise exert themselves at a pace they are not accustomed to.

The physical aspect of prolonged travel alone may have medical implications. Sitting in one position for longer than four hours may cause an increased incidence of emboli. While still a controversial issue in the medical community, it seems plausible that prolonged immobility could have negative health implications. Other common causes of illness include exposure to unfamiliar microorganisms.

Regrettably, many travelers are not prepared for illness in a foreign country and are often left totally dependent on the health care system of that country. The medical system in many countries lacks the basic capabilities that we take for granted. Certain surgical skills or medications may not be available. Also, medical insurance plans often exclude coverage during international travel. In any case, many of those who become ill or injured out of country are transported home by air ambulance. That process is known as *repatriation*.

The return home may be prompted by the policies of an insurance company or managed care plan. In other cases the patient simply prefers to be at or nearer to their home while they recover. Repatriation may involve transporting a patient within a province or country, or it may involve crossing one or more international boundaries. The international transport of patients can become a complicated process, especially for the inexperienced. The pilot(s) and air medical personnel accompanying the patient must be knowledgeable and prepared concerning the requirements for international travel. Factors to be considered when planning for repatriation flights include:

1. Distance of transport and estimated time in flight
2. Availability of ground transport at departure and arrival airports
3. Patient condition and anticipated medical needs
4. Types of air medical personnel needed during transport
5. Refueling stops
6. Customs clearance and documentation requirements
7. Family member(s) accompanying the patient and the potential impact of their presence

Transport by Air Ambulance

Repatriation flights may be arranged directly by the patient or a family member. The request may also come from a state or provincial authority or from an insurance company. It is often most effective to deal directly with an insurance or managed care provider. Then both logistical and financial arrangements can be made simultaneously. Because of the significant cost of such flights, many private providers require payment or guarantee of payment by an insurance company before the flight can take place.

The mode of transport may vary according to the patient's medical condition and ongoing medical needs. A patient who is grossly stable may be transported aboard a commercial airline, while a critical-care patient will obviously require a dedicated medical aircraft and medical team. Since these flights often cover great distances and there may be no way to retrieve records and other patient information left behind, the medical team must be thorough and unrushed at the facility where the patient is being acquired. A complete evaluation of patient records will also help to ensure that all necessary equipment and medications are available for treatment during the flight. Because the transport may be significantly longer than typical interfacility transports, special consideration should be given to maintaining fluid status and nutritional needs.

After obtaining the history and all medical records, a thorough physical examination should be performed without regard for the apparent stability of the patient. It is better to perform a thorough exam and find nothing than to be surprised by an unrecognized condition in midflight. While repatriation flights are rarely emergencies, chronic medical conditions may become acute and new conditions unrelated to the condition for which the patient has been treated may appear. It is better to be safe than sorry.

The flight team should double-check to make sure that arrangements have been made for ground ambulance support at the destination airport. They should carry contact names and numbers in case someone else fails to follow up on making these arrangements. All members of the flight team, patients, and family members should be in compliance with customs requirements. Although this is generally the responsibility of the aviation crew, the medical team should double-check so as to avoid unnecessary complications on arrival. Pilots may be required to prepare in-depth flight plans prior to departure. That process may include acquiring navigation approach plates for each airport at which the flight team will be landing.

The medical team should carefully explain the repatriation process to any patient who is lucid and capable of comprehending. The family should be a part of that discussion as well. The patient and family should also be questioned about the patient's medical history, medications, and current condition. They may remember important details that have been overlooked by the referring medical team.

Patients who are ventilator-dependent or who have invasive monitoring will require extra time at the referring facility. Ventilator settings should be obtained and documented. If there is any doubt as to tube placement or ventilator efficiency, blood gases should be obtained. The potential impact of altitude physiology and the need for changes in ventilator settings should be carefully weighed and discussed with referring medical personnel. If the patient is at risk for deterioration at altitude, special precautions may need to be taken. Baseline readings should be obtained from all invasive monitoring devices and the influence of altitude must be considered again. These types of patients may require almost continuous reassessment during flight.

Ongoing medications should be discussed and a determination made regarding whether those medications are to be discontinued at some point or continued indefinitely. An assessment must be made to ensure that there are adequate quantities of needed medications aboard the aircraft. If time zones will be crossed, the medical team must remember to administer medications according to the time at the point of departure.

Upon arrival at the receiving facility, the medical team should relay all pertinent patient information and all medical records to receiving medical personnel. A copy of the patient care record should be completed and left at the receiving facility.

Transport by Commercial Airline

Transport of a medical patient by commercial airline requires a slightly different approach. Special permission is required from the airline before any medical patient may be brought aboard. Most airlines have a representative knowledgeable in this area who can provide information regarding requirements, special fees, and so on. Special equipment such as oxygen and a special diet may also be arranged through this agent.

When a patient travels by commercial airline, the company providing the medical attendant should make arrangements for ground ambulance transport to and from the airport. Arrangements must be made well in advance of the flight for ambulance support at departure and arrival points. If there are long delays between connecting flights, the patient may have to be transported to a nearby hospital until the flight is due to depart. The patient and attending medical personnel should arrive at the airport at least one hour before departure time. Medical patients may be boarded before other passengers. Flight attendants are generally experienced in dealing with medical patients and will be very helpful.

During the flight, monitoring and care of the patient must be continued. If requested in advance, flight attendants may be able to erect a privacy curtain and provide other amenities not typically available to healthier passengers. While airlines are hesitant to allow significantly ill patients aboard commercial passenger aircraft, the likelihood of a medical emergency is generally low. However, if a medical emergency should occur, pilots typically divert to the nearest airport so the patient can be transported to a hospital. Upon arrival at the destination airport, medical patients are disembarked after all other passengers.

Checklist for Repatriation Flights

The following are valuable guidelines for preparing for a repatriation mission:

- Plan and organize the trip in as much detail as possible.
- Itinerary, tickets, passport/visa, contact telephone numbers, hotel registration, air carrier telephone number, and ambulance telephone numbers should be readily available.
- Ensure the equipment is ready for the transport—batteries are fully charged, etc.
- Luggage: Organize all carry-on items, including medical equipment, in as few bags as possible. Enough personal items should be included to last one or two days beyond the anticipated stay.
- On long flights, request aisle seating (gives more room to stretch legs). Review aircraft type and location of rest room.
- Take along snacks, as restaurants may be closed when you arrive.
- Wear loose, nonrestrictive clothing for comfort—you may be sitting for long periods—but dress appropriately and professionally.

- Wear glasses rather than contact lenses.
- Eat properly and get adequate rest prior to departure.
- Avoid coffee, tea, soft drinks, and alcohol during the flight. Water and juices are preferable to maintain adequate hydration.
- Avoid taking any unnecessary medications, especially those that may cause drowsiness.
- If traveling to a foreign country, take time to obtain information regarding language, culture, and customs.
- Obtain an atlas so you are familiar with the destination.

It is suggested that air medical personnel have medical and liability insurance coverage before traveling into a foreign country. Many domestic policies exclude care received during international travel. Air medical providers should have their policies checked carefully and, if necessary, a rider or supplemental policy purchased to cover international travel. Similarly, malpractice insurance policies may not cover cases occurring out of country. A supplemental policy provides a safety net in case a legal case is filed in another country.

Safety During International Flights

While flight safety is basically the same whether flying domestically or internationally, a few extra precautions may be helpful.

- Keep seat belts fastened as much as possible, even during high-altitude cruise. Unexpected turbulence may occur at any time.
- Be familiar with all safety equipment aboard the aircraft. This is especially important if the medical team is flying aboard an unfamiliar aircraft. A safety check should be performed long before the patient is loaded.
- Be familiar with safety exits and the mechanisms for opening them.
- Never try to pressure aviation personnel into flying in inclement weather. Let them make the decision without such influences.
- Safety should always be the primary consideration. If there are any unresolved safety issues, do not make the flight.

Long-distance air medical transport requires attention to detail and careful planning. International transports may subject the patient and flight team to as much as 30 hours of flight time. On the medical side, the patient's history and physical condition must be thoroughly explored prior to transport. Sometimes patients do not speak the same language as members of the flight team, and an interpreter may be required. Other factors that must be taken into consideration include:

- *Patient's ability to tolerate a trip of the proposed length.*
- *Patient's needs during transport:* For example, even large reserves of oxygen rarely last 20-plus hours. If a patient is potentially unstable, the stressors of flight must be considered and compensated for (this may require a collaborative effort between the medical team and the airplane crew).
- *Patient's nutritional needs:* Food should be available for the flight crew and for family members traveling with the patient. Cultural and religious beliefs should be taken into consideration when preparing meals for the trip.
- *Necessary equipment and supplies.*
- *Passenger and storage space:* This may be a limiting factor. Family members may not be able to accompany the patient because of space limitations. Baggage may also have to be limited.
- *Composition of the medical team:* This must be adequate to meet the patient's needs during the flight.
- *Rest for the medical team:* The emphasis on "duty day" for pilots often overshadows the needs of the medical staff.
- *Ground ambulance service:* Making arrangements is typically the responsibility of the air ambulance service. The quality of EMS enjoyed in most urban areas in North America should not be expected in many other parts of the world. In some areas an ambulance will consist of little more than a van with a stretcher thrown in.
- *Special international considerations:* In some countries, meeting the treating physician may require special arrangements. Specific immunizations may be required, and consulates or other authorities may need to be involved.

Aviation considerations are also significant, especially in areas of the world where there is anti-American sentiment. Limiting potential conflicts and delays associated with border crossings is critical. Aviation considerations include:

- Some of the international considerations described above apply to the aviation crews.

- Flight planning can be challenging, particularly outside of North America. It may be necessary to consult with professionals familiar with optimal routings and other aspects of flying into and over different countries.

- Careful planning includes assessments of weather and airport facilities. Patient transport should not begin unless aviation experts can ensure that the trip will be uneventful.

* Selection of ground support services at each destination, including refueling capability, is key. Selection of an airport with poor ground support can threaten the viability of the mission.

* Flying internationally requires expertise in dealing with customs and immigration officials at each stop on the way. During some long flights, this may involve several different countries, each of which has different information needs and customs. The aircraft and all passengers must have appropriate documentation.

* Obtaining the necessary permits to land, overfly, arrive, and depart are essential to the smooth orchestration of a long-range transport. Failure to anticipate these needs can result in delays and possibly uncomfortable confrontations with officials.

* Having appropriate currency is essential. In some countries cash is required for financial transactions. There should be enough cash on hand to pay for fuel, permits, ambulance transports, phone calls, and other services. Credit cards may be taken in some areas, but a tip may be expected along with the credit card payment.

* Communications are challenging in many countries. Satellite communications may be especially helpful in maintaining contact with the base of operation and in making contact with necessary parties in the destination country.

* The trip should accommodate crew duty days and provide for appropriate rest. This may include having relief pilots available at key stopover points and flying crews to locations via commercial airline.

* Catering—getting safe food and ordering appropriate types of food for long-distance transports—is an important part of the plan.

Summary

International air travel can be significantly more complicated than domestic travel. Flights may be of long duration and require a great deal of preparation. Oxygen, IV fluids, medications, and other supplies may need to be increased. It may be necessary to prepare meals during flight. Rest time for pilots and medical crew members must be planned in advance. Arrangements may have to be made for stopover points.

Pilots, crew members, patients, and passengers may need passports and other documentation. Approach plates may have to be prepared by pilots prior to departure. Fuel stops will have to be arranged. In short, international travel can be a demanding process requiring extensive planning.

REVIEW QUESTIONS

1. Air medical transport in northern Canada is characterized by:
   a. Long-distance responses over inhospitable terrain and under weather conditions.
   b. Occasional requirement for refueling during a transport
   c. A highway system that is open year round
   d. a and b

2. The Canadian province that has played a leadership role in developing air medicine is:
   a. Manitoba
   b. Toronto
   c. Ontario
   d. Saskatchewan

3. Air medical programs in Europe are similar to those in the United States in terms of equipment but significantly different in terms of:
   a. Governmental oversight
   b. Communications capabilities
   c. Organization and medical practice
   d. Organization and personnel

4. Air medical transport teams in what country are composed of a pilot, a physician, and one or two nurses? In cases involving mountain rescue, an experienced mountaineer may replace one of the nurses.
   a. Norway
   b. Italy
   c. France
   d. Spain

5. The world's oldest continuously operating air medical program is:
   a. Australia's Royal Flying Doctor Service
   b. Norway's Central Oslo Service
   c. France's C'est Médical
   d. The U.S.'s MAST program

6. Compare and contrast the U.S. air medical system with that of two other countries.

7. Explain some of the requirements of international patient flights that are not encountered during domestic transports.

Fixed-Wing
Operations

Attila J. Hertelendy, MHSM, BHSC, CCEMT-P, NREMT-P

Objectives

Upon completing this chapter, the reader should have a better understanding of the following topics:

* The pros and cons of FW aircraft compared to RW aircraft

* The roles of the FW air ambulance

* The FW transport process

Introduction

The majority of this text addresses rotor-wing operations, but there are a large number of fixed-wing (FW) programs operating in the United States and around the world as well. This book would be incomplete without some discussion of those operations.

Fixed-wing aircraft (FWA) offer a number of advantages over rotor-wing aircraft (RWA). Most notably, they are faster and have greater range. Although RWA are more flexible in their requirements for landing space, their speed and range are generally limited, and most RW flight programs have relatively small service areas. A typical one-way response range for an RW program may be 150 miles. FWA, on the other hand, are capable of speeds of 400 miles per hour or greater and may have a range of 1200 miles or more. In areas where population densities are very low and transport distances are great, FWA are the desired mode of air transport.

However, FWA have one significant limitation: They require an airport for takeoff and landing. Some smaller planes may be able to land and take off from grass or dirt landing strips, but most turboprop and jet-type aircraft require a concrete runway several thousand feet long. While most cities and towns have an airport in their general vicinity, there is not an airport on every corner. Airports, especially in major urban areas, are generally remotely located, and moving a patient to or from an airport may take a great deal of time and require the use of a ground ambulance. Coordinating a fixed-wing transport, including ground transportation on both ends, can be a relatively complicated process.

FW programs are typically concentrated in areas where long-distance transports are the norm and in urban areas where specialty-care transports are routine. The following variables influence the volume of fixed-wing operations in a given area:

1. Geography of service area
2. Population distribution and density
3. Location and capabilities of medical facilities
4. Alternate means of patient transport/backup systems
5. Airport/runway conditions and helipad access

KEY TERMS

advanced life
support (ALS),
p. 300

basic life support
(BLS), p. 300

Roles of Fixed-Wing Air Ambulances

Just as ground ambulances and rotor-wing ambulances can have multiple roles, so too can FW craft. They can be used to bring medical treatment to a patient in a very rural or otherwise inaccessible area, move a patient from a primary care hospital to a referral center, or move a patient over a long distance for a variety of reasons. FW craft are also frequently used for repatriation.

Patient Access

Sometimes an FW ambulance is the most appropriate mode of transport in a medical or traumatic emergency. Granted, FW craft are rarely able to land at the residence of a patient or the scene of crash site, but the medical team can be brought within reasonable distance by air and then transported by ground the rest of the way. Some rural areas in the United States and Canada are so sparsely populated that FW transport is the only practical means for accessing and transporting patients. In the northern United States and Canada, weather conditions are another factor. Ground transport may not be an option in the winter. In very rural areas volunteer teams may ferry FW-based medical teams from the airport to the site of the illness or injury and then back to the airport with the patient. While this arrangement may not provide an ideal response time, it may be all that is available.

Interfacility Transport

This is one of the most common uses for FW ambulances. Patients are transported from a smaller or less specialized hospital to a referral or tertiary-care facility that offers a level of care or specialized services not available at the referral facility. FW transport is most practical and cost-effective when the two facilities are a significant distance apart. Some of the medical conditions more commonly associated with FW transport in this context are:

* Patients being transported for specialized surgical services
* Neonatal patients being transported for NICU level care
* Patients being transported for organ donation (donors or recipients)
* Patients needing critical-care services not available at the local hospital

Conversely, patients may be transported from a higher level of care to a local or community hospital following advanced treatment and stabilization. This practice, known as repatriation, may be common in areas with well-developed trauma systems. During the acute stages of management these patients may require a Level I or II trauma center. Once they have been definitively stabilized, they may be transported back to a community hospital for continued recovery and rehabilitation. This practice ensures that patient needs are matched with medical resources. In areas with few trauma centers that are spread far apart, FW transport systems may play a key role in this process.

Convenience Transports

In some cases a patient may simply wish to be closer to home—for instance, a traveler involved in a motor vehicle crash while out of town, or a terminal patient who wishes to spend his or her remaining time at home. FW ambulances may also be used to move a patient from a hospital to an extended care facility. Families of elderly patients sometimes prefer to move their relatives closer to home when they must be moved to one of these facilities.

Medical Preparedness Levels of FW Air Ambulances

The medical capabilities of FW air ambulances may vary dramatically. In some cases an FW air ambulance is nothing more than a passenger plane with a few seats removed so as to accommodate a stretcher. In other cases it may be a well-equipped flying intensive-care unit used exclusively for AM transport. While both may be useful, the first example is of value only to a patient flying strictly for convenience—although even a completely stable patient has some chance of deteriorating unexpectedly. Any patient requiring, or potentially requiring, advanced-level medical care should be transported only by competent and experienced medical personnel who have access to a full complement of advanced and critical-care medical equipment and supplies.

The Shared Mission Air Ambulance

The requirements for licensure for air ambulances vary from state to state; some are considerably more lenient than others. With the high cost of purchasing and maintaining a plane and the relatively low call volume in many areas, many licensed FW air ambulances are dual-purpose vehicles. They are used primarily as standard passenger transport vehicles but are also advertised for air ambulance use. The operator generally has an on-call agreement with medical personnel who respond when needed. Since air ambulance transports are unscheduled and those called may be working at other jobs, there is often a large pool of medical personnel. While that may be reasonable from a business perspective, the experience and credibility of team members is often lower than that of a dedicated team.

As the role of these aircraft may change frequently, there should be a reliable process for reconfiguring the aircraft in a reasonable amount of time. Ideally, the equipment and medical care available aboard a shared-mission aircraft should be equal to that on a dedicated aircraft. In reality, that may be a difficult goal to achieve.

Shared-mission programs often use a compact, slide-in medical interior such as that offered by Lifeport Systems. These interiors are often quite good, offering all the basic and advanced equipment necessary for a critical-care transport. This may include a built-in stretcher, loading system, oxygen tank, power inverter, suction device, and IV poles. As long as the medical team is qualified and performs enough transports to remain competent, this can be a cost-effective way of offering FW air medical transport.

However, shared-mission programs are sometimes thrown together for the sole purpose of financial gain. The medical team may lack the knowledge and experience to ensure the well-being of their patients. As with RW operations, each member of the medical team should receive extensive training in flight physiology, flight safety, and emergency preparedness before being allowed to serve as an independent team member and as part of a recurrent training program thereafter.

The Dedicated Air Ambulance

An FWA that is used exclusively for air medical transportation is likely to offer more consistent and better quality service. It can be permanently configured with the specialty care equipment typically needed for emergency and critical-care transport. Medical lighting and IV hooks can be installed in the ceiling. Storage cabinets can be affixed to the walls or floor for more efficient access. Mounting brackets for monitoring equipment can be permanently mounted to provide easier viewing and quicker access. The intracabin communication system can be tailored to meet the needs of a medical team. Although a shared-mission aircraft has the potential to offer good-quality service, the fact that medical equipment is continually being moved in and out of the aircraft can be problematic. With a dedicated air ambulance, everything stays put. If medical care is the sole focus of the program, related activities, including training and quality management, are likely to be elevated to a higher status. Another advantage of a dedicated air ambulance is availability and response time.

FW Aircraft Types

A variety of fixed-wing aircraft may be converted for air medical transport. The ideal vehicle has a cabin large enough for one or two patients, two or three attendants, all necessary medical equipment and supplies, and one or two family members. The aircraft should be capable of a cruise speed in excess of 350 knots (400 mph or 182 kph) and have all avionics equipment required for IFR flight conditions and international travel. Unlike RW aircraft, FW aircraft may be available that nearly reach the ideal. When FWA are powered by turbine engines, weight becomes less of a limiting factor, so the cabin can be larger and hold more passengers, equipment, and baggage.

Over 70 different aircraft types and models are used for air medical transport. Of these, a few are particularly popular. The ten fixed-wing aircraft most commonly used as dedicated air ambulances are:

Beach KingAir 200
Dehavilland Twin Otter
Cessna 421
Lear 35
Beech KingAir 100
Dehavilland DHC6-300
Lear 25
Lear 35A
Piper Navajo
Cessna 441

The Transport Process

Planning Phase

All medical transports should begin with an evaluation of the mode of transport that will be most beneficial to the patient. Medical considerations must be the single most important factor, although cost and cost-effectiveness must also be taken into account, especially when the cost differences between alternatives are considerable. The options may include private vehicle, ground ambulance, RW air ambulance, or FW air ambulance. Over shorter distances, ground ambulance or RW transport is generally most appropriate. For intermediate distances, RW or FW transport may be considered. For long-distance transports FW is generally the most efficient.

The following variables should be considered:

1. Distance: Ground ambulances are generally most appropriate for shorter-distance transports. Rarely is it beneficial to use an aircraft for a transport of less than 30 miles. One exception may be during times when traffic congestion may impede ground transport. However, as distance increases, so do the benefits of air transport. The typical distance at which FW air transport becomes the better choice is approximately 300 miles. Such a transport would require 4 to 5 hours of riding time in the back of an often-bumpy ground ambulance but can take as little as one hour in an FW ambulance. An RW ambulance may also be capable of performing a transport of that distance but will require more time.

2. Time: Patients being transported distances of 300 miles or more and whose medical conditions require minimal out-of-hospital time should be considered prime candidates for FW transport. Some factors that must be evaluated include response time to sending facility, downtime at airports on both ends, and availability of ground ambulance to deliver the patient to the sending airport and pick up at the receiving one. All those time intervals must be added together to arrive at an accurate estimate of total time in transit.

3. Weather: Certain weather conditions may prohibit the use of aircraft. The options are to delay transport until the weather improves or complete the transport by ground ambulance.

4. Space: The transporting ambulance, whether air or ground, must have enough room to accommodate the patient and all necessary medical equipment and personnel. Specialty-care patients may require bulky equipment such as a neonatal isolette or an intraaortic balloon pump. FWA come in a variety of sizes, but most are small or medium-sized. However, there is often more space in an FWA than in a helicopter. A Type I or Type III ground ambulance usually has the most room. In rare cases equipment demands are so great that the only practical way to move a patient is by large FWA or ground ambulance.

5. Family: A family member may ask to accompany a patient during transport. That may be appropriate if there is adequate room, the patient is relatively stable, and the medical team is comfortable that the family member will not become a distraction during the flight. The presence of the family member may have a clinically significant calming effect on the patient. In addition, the family member may be able to provide medical history or other needed information that may not otherwise be available. In any case, the medical team must have the authority to determine what is best for the patient in this regard.

6. Emergency diversion: In the event a patient rapidly deteriorates, ground or RW teams may easily divert to the nearest appropriate facility for stabilization before continuing the transport. An FW ambulance doesn't have that capability. Once a flight is under way, it is more difficult to divert. The medical team must have available all supplies and equipment they anticipate needing during the flight.

Legal Considerations

The transport process should begin with an assessment of what is best for the patient. The goal is to anticipate the patient's needs during transport and to have resources available to meet those needs. Two considerations must be addressed: mode of transport and capability of attending medical personnel. Ideally, these two options could be selected independently, but in reality that rarely occurs. Because of specialized equipment and liability issues, ambulance operators are often hesitant to allow inexperienced and unsupervised medical personnel in their vehicles. Ground ambulance operators generally allow supplemental medical personnel to accompany their core medical team during transport, but air ambulance operators are often stricter in this regard.

In the United States, interfacility transports are regulated by federal legislation. The Emergency Medical Treatment and Active Labor Act (EMTALA) sets forth specific requirements regarding the assessment and treatment of patients presenting at emergency departments and requesting medical care. EMTALA stipulates that the attending physician must perform a medical screening of each patient prior to discharge or transfer. It also states that the patient must be stabilized as much as possible before beginning the transport process. The physician must certify in writing that the patient's need for referral outweighs the risks associated with the transport. The American College of Emergency Physicians (ACEP) has developed guidelines to help clarify this process.

Once it has been determined that a patient meets the criteria for appropriate transfer, the mode of transfer must be determined. The following variables should be considered:

1. **Level of treatment needed during transport:**
   a. **Basic life support (BLS):** The patient is grossly stable and will not require IVs, medications, cardiac monitoring, or any other complex monitoring or treatment during transport.
   b. **Advanced life support (ALS):** The patient may or may not be stable and will require cardiac monitoring, IV administration, medications, or other advanced-level medical care during transport.
   c. **Critical care:** The patient may or may not be stable and will require a complex combination of advanced medical observations and/or treatments during transport. In most urban and many rural areas of the United States, ground ambulances are staffed with ALS-level personnel capable of managing virtually all prehospital emergencies and the vast majority of interfacility transports. Nearly all RW air ambulances are staffed with medical teams, most of which include a specially trained registered nurse and a specially trained paramedic. FW services are less predictable in

basic life support (BLS)
A certification level for ambulances. It implies that personnel are capable of performing cardiopulmonary resuscitation and other basic emergency skills.

advanced life support (ALS)
A certification or licensure level for ambulances. The term implies that personnel possess the knowledge and skills necessary to assess and manage patients with complex medical conditions in the prehospital setting.

their staffing. Almost all dedicated services have appropriately trained personnel at whatever medical level is required for the transport. Shared-mission programs generally, but not always, provide appropriately trained staff.

2. Most appropriate mode of transport: Whether the patient will require ground, RW air ambulance, or FW air ambulance depends primarily on the length of the transport. However, other factors may come into play. For example, a patient requiring critical care during transport may be transported by air over a shorter distance simply because that level of care is not available from the local ground ambulance service. This category may include:

a. Patients who require a cardiac intensive care unit not available at the referring facility

b. Patients who require cardiac catheterization not available at the referring facility

c. Patients in cardiogenic shock requiring transport with the support of an intraaortic balloon pump or mechanical assist device

d. Patients who require transport for organ transplantation

e. Patients requiring experimental medications or medications outside the scope of practice of ALS providers during transport

f. Patients requiring extracorporeal membranous oxygenation (ECMO)

3. Patient and/or family preference: Some patients may prefer not to fly or may be terrified of flying, especially in a helicopter. They may insist on ground transport even if the distance is great. Another factor is cost—air transport is generally much more expensive than ground transport. In any case a lucid and mentally competent patient may selectively refuse any or all medical treatment, including a particular mode of transportation.

Consent for transport of an ill patient must be obtained unless the consent is implied. Implied consent is only given in an emergency situation when the patient is incapacitated and unable to consent and the situation is life-threatening. A family member may be able to consent to transport. The consent should be written, if possible. Most institutions have formal "Consent to Transfer" forms.

Patient Assessment

Upon arrival at the referral center, the medical team should learn as much as possible about the patients and their medical condition. This should be done face to face, unless prevented by unusual circumstances. In rare cases it is appropriate for a patient to be sent to the airport to meet the flight team, such as when a badly injured trauma patient is being moved to a trauma center for urgent intervention. The need for timely intervention may outweigh the medical team's need to gain complete medical information on the patient. However, in nearly all medical cases it is in the patient's best interest that the medical team go to the referring hospital and interact directly with the medical personnel who have been treating the patient. That interaction minimizes the risk that important information will be overlooked. Information should include:

1. Reason for transfer: chief complaint/diagnosis, services required but not available at referral center, or other
2. Treatments the patient has already received
3. Patient's condition before and after treatment
4. Pertinent history, both HPI and PMH
5. Laboratory results
6. Medical imaging studies (X ray, CT, MRI, and ultrasound films)
7. Medications and treatments that will be continued during transport
8. Name of transferring physician
9. Name of receiving facility and receiving physician
10. Possible Do Not Attempt Resuscitation (DNAR/DNR) orders for critical patients

After the information has been obtained, and before accepting or moving the patient, the medical team should perform a physical exam. For clinical and legal reasons, it is essential that the flight team conduct its own examination, regardless of information provided by referring personnel. If questioned about the need for this assessment, the flight team should explain to the referring personnel that the exam is a necessary part of the patient acceptance process. Sometimes the exam may lead to a new diagnosis based on missed signs or symptoms, or complications of the initial diagnosis may have developed (such as a tamponade resulting from purulent pericarditis).

The assessment performed by the FW medical team may vary in complexity according to patient type. If a patient is flying strictly for convenience, the exam may be brief. For patients being transported by a critical-care team, it will obviously be more detailed. The physical assessment should include an initial exam (primary survey), a focused exam, a detailed exam (secondary survey), and an ongoing assessment. The primary survey includes airway, breathing, circulation, and disability (AVPU). As patient problems are identified, critical interventions should be initiated. During the focused examination, specific details related to the chief complaint are gathered. This includes a focused examination of the systems involved with the chief complaint. It also includes basic assessment tools such as vital signs, monitor, pulse ox, and glucometer. The detailed exam (secondary survey) is a head-to-toe examination. The ongoing assessment is a continuous monitoring of the patient's ABCs, mental status, vital signs, and effectiveness of interventions.

At this stage the medical transport team should also make certain it has all the necessary equipment, supplies, and working knowledge necessary to meet the patient's medical needs during flight. Otherwise, other options should be considered. For example, an adult transport team that arrives on scene to find a neonatal patient in distress may not be equipped or possess the knowledge to complete the transport, and alternative arrangements may need to be made.

Preparing the Patient for Transport

Patient preparation for transport is based on the patient's existing medical condition(s) and anticipated needs, which are determined from the history and physical examination. Other variables include the size and type of aircraft, the altitude of the flight, whether or not the cabin is pressurized, and the expected in-flight time. One other factor is the weather. If the flight will be done under IFR conditions, alternate landing sites must be identified and the medical team must be prepared to manage the patient until the most remote of the alternate landing sites can be reached and the patient moved by ground to the nearest appropriate medical facility. For example, if a patient is being flown to a city 400 miles away but one of the alternate landing sites is 600 miles away, the crew should have adequate supplies on board to complete the 600-mile trip. Ground ambulance time to and from airports should be included in this calculation. The same calculation applies to compressed air.

The medical team should make certain the patient has adequate intravenous access, that medications are running at the appropriate dosage, and that there are no medication incompatibilities. The patency of each IV line should be checked. Transporting a patient by air without an IV line should be reserved only for the absolutely stable patient (convenience transport). Patients being transported secondary to cardiovascular conditions have the potential to decompensate quickly, and immediate access for drug administration is essential. The senior member of the medical transport team must determine if the team has enough people to manage any reasonably foreseeable emergency that may develop during flight, including cardiac arrest.

If any of the medications in use are not familiar to the flight team, they should perform a quick study before accepting the patient. A pocket-sized critical-care pharmacology book is an invaluable tool that flight team members should routinely carry.

Oxygen needs should be determined. Flow rates should be converted into total flight consumption to determine if the on-hand oxygen supply will be adequate to meet those needs. If not, supplemental tanks will have to be acquired. While some FW ambulances have larger, permanently mounted oxygen tanks or liquid oxygen, many rely solely on a supply of smaller portable tanks.

There should be an adequate supply of intravenous fluids aboard the aircraft, especially when the flow rate is high (burns, for example). Most flight programs restrict the quantity of IV fluids carried because of weight limitations. If that is the case extra bags may need to be acquired before the flight.

Portable medical equipment that runs on batteries should also be evaluated. The crew should be satisfied that batteries are adequately charged and that battery life will extend beyond the span of the transport. Most medically configured aircraft have AC/DC inverters so these devices can be plugged in during flight. The inverter should be checked for proper operation, although there is always a chance of inverter failure.

Once in the aircraft, the patient and all medical equipment must be secured prior to transport. The patient stretcher must be locked into place and the patient strapped to the stretcher. Large equipment such as intraaortic balloon pumps and ventilators may cause serious injuries if not secured properly, according to FAA guidelines. Some medical aircraft have permanently mounted floor tracks for this purpose. Straps that lock into the tracks may be used on an occasional basis, but permanent mounts affixed to the airframe for each piece of equipment are preferable.

Psychological Preparation of the Patient and Family Members

Some people are very uncomfortable about flying. It is worth taking a few minutes to determine if there is any anxiety and dispel any misconceptions. If the patient's anxiety is so intense as to have clinical significance, the flight crew should explain the transport process and reassure the patient (Figure 19-1). If that fails and there are no contraindications, anxiolytic medications should be considered.

The same steps should be taken with accompanying family members. Anxiety is contagious, and an anxious family member may lead to an anxious patient. However, since family members are not patients, the administration of an anxiolytic agent should be considered only in extreme cases and only after a patient evaluation and consultation with the appropriate physician.

Once aboard the aircraft, each step of the transport process, from starting the engines to takeoff, should be explained in advance. The goal

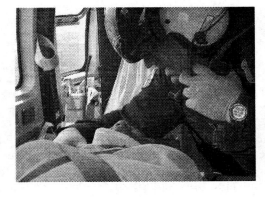

Flight team calming and reassuring patient
Courtesy of MIEMSS, Dept. of Public Information and Media Service

is to avoid surprises that may rekindle the anxiety. Similarly, advance notice should be given before beginning the descent, final approach, and touchdown.

In-Flight Activities

In the aircraft the patient should be reassessed and one last check made to ensure that all necessary equipment, supplies, and medications are readily available and everything is working properly. Once in the air the patient should be monitored carefully for altitude-related changes in status. This may be a particular concern for any patient with pneumothorax or any other condition compromising respiratory status. The pressure in endotracheal tube cuffs should be evaluated to ensure that there is no overinflation. Tubes with higher pressure may expand as altitude increases and impossibly lead to laryngeal ischemia. This is less of an issue in pressurized aircraft, which generally have cabin pressure limits equivalent to 6000 feet AGL. Limiting the cabin altitude pressure to that level has been shown to virtually eliminate altitude-related problems for people with cardiovascular disease. However, if a patient is at high risk for deterioration and an unpressurized aircraft is being used, the medical crew should ask the pilot to maintain altitude as low as is acceptable. Significant physiologic changes are usually not likely at altitudes below 10,000 feet. FAA controllers are generally as accommodating as possible when assigning altitudes to medical craft. The downside to flying at lower altitudes is often increased turbulence.

As with any other mode of transport, the patient should be monitored carefully for changes in condition and corrective actions should be taken if decompensation is noted. Pulse oximetry should be monitored continuously and any trends noted. Vital signs should be reassessed every 10 to 15 minutes for critical patients and for those with a high risk of deterioration. Grossly stable patients should have vital signs taken at least every hour during flight. Hydration status should be monitored. While it may be difficult to auscultate breath sounds in an FWA in flight, other parameters, such as the presence of edema, JVD, and hepatojugular reflux, may be assessed. Some dedicated air ambulances have Doppler devices integrated into the intracabin communications system, allowing breath sounds that are auscultated via the Doppler stethoscope head to be heard through the headset or helmet ear cups.

The medical team should be prepared to deal with patients at high risk for developing cardiac arrest during flight. Each member of the medical team should have a predetermined role in cardiac arrest management. Defibrillation pads should be placed on the patient prior to transport. Intubation equipment, a suction device, and all ACLS medications should be at the ready. The patient's head must be easily accessible so that endotracheal intubation can be performed. The patient's torso should be easily accessible to allow for cardiac compressions. That may be a problem in aircraft with very low ceilings.

Cardiac arrest during flight may raise a host of questions regarding patient management. If the patient dies on a flight that involves crossing several states (or countries), in which state did he die? If it is a very long flight and the medical team runs out of resuscitation drugs, what should be done? Should the crew divert to the nearest airport, return to the point of departure, or continue with the transport? When should a resuscitation effort be terminated during flight? The ambulance service's medical control plan should address each of these issues in advance.

Communication with the Receiving Facility

For interhospital transports, flight planning must extend all the way to the receiving medical facility. This becomes more important as patient acuity increases. Receiving medical personnel should have adequate time to prepare for the patient's arrival. Arrangements must also be made to have a ground ambulance waiting at the destination airport to transport the patient on to the final destination.

A call should typically be made to the receiving facility and to the ground ambulance provider before the aircraft leaves the ground to make certain that all arrangements have been made and to give an estimated time of arrival. If the aircraft has a FliteFone or similar radio telephone system, the call may be made from the aircraft after liftoff. It should be remembered that cell phones cannot legally be used in flight. An early call to the receiving facility will allow them to begin making necessary arrangements for ventilators, IV pumps, anesthesia, or operating room preparation. The receiving physician can also be notified so she can be prepared as well.

Arrival at the Destination

Proper planning is also necessary to ensure that everything goes smoothly at the destination. Nothing is worse than arriving at the destination airport with a critical patient to find that there is no ground ambulance waiting. Such a blunder may have both clinical and legal ramifications. It is essential that the ground ambulance be equipped with all necessary equipment and supplies and that the crew be familiar with the hospital or other destination where the patient is being taken.

Upon arrival at the destination hospital, the AM team should provide a thorough report to the receiving physician and/or nurse. All necessary paperwork should be delivered as well. It is a good idea to have the receiving physician or nurse sign an acknowledgment that the patient was conveyed to them and that they accepted responsibility for the patient.

The medical report should be written at the earliest opportunity, ideally before the team leaves the point of patient delivery. That way all necessary medical information is readily available and a copy of the completed report can be left with the receiving medical facility.

SUMMARY

While there are similarities between FW and RW transport of patients, there are also some important differences. The fact that FW ambulances require an airport is the most significant difference. The use of an airport requires the coordination of ground transport on both ends and can significantly complicate the process. It may also limit options in the event of an unanticipated in-flight emergency. For that reason the medical team should be fully prepared to manage any emergency that may occur during flight. FWA tend to fly higher than RWA, increasing the potential for altitude-related decompensation among susceptible patients. The medical team must maintain a strong working knowledge of altitude physiology and be prepared to manage any related complications accordingly.

REVIEW QUESTIONS

1. Some of the circumstances in which use of a fixed-wing aircraft would be appropriate include patients:
   a. Being transported long distances
   b. With cardiovascular conditions
   c. Who are dependent on Medicaid
   d. With conditions making them sensitive to altitude changes

2. Repatriation involves:
   a. Returning a patient who previously required specialty care to a community hospital for recuperation/rehabilitation
   b. Returning a patient to the hospital where he was initially seen for his illness or injury
   c. Moving a patient with burns to a local burn unit
   d. Moving a cardiac patient from a cardiac care unit to a less specialized area of the hospital

3. Transports made due to the wish of a patient to be closer to home are known as _____ transports.
   a. Nuisance   c. Repatriation
   b. Fee for service   d. Convenience

4. A fixed-wing aircraft that is used as an air ambulance and also for some other purpose is known as a _____ air ambulance:
   a. Dual standard   c. Fee for service
   b. Shared mission   d. Repatriation

5. List and discuss two advantages and two disadvantages of fixed-wing patient transport, as compared to rotor-wing transport.

Starting a New Air Medical Program

Objectives

Upon completing this chapter, the reader should have a better understanding of the following topics:

* Assessing the need for a new air medical program
* The planning process for a new program
* The 24 steps of assembling a new program

Introduction

Starting a new air medical program can be a challenging task. It involves assembling a set of unique components in a prescribed manner. Air operations are regulated by a number of government agencies, each with its own rules and regulations. It is essential that the person(s) setting up the program are familiar with these requirements. This is one area where the early involvement of an expert can save a significant amount of time and money. Whether or not outside help is used, the process is essentially the same and consists of 24 distinct steps.

1. Needs Assessment

Given the extensive financial and human resources necessary to start and maintain an air medical program, a needs assessment must be performed before any commitment is made. The purpose of the needs assessment is to determine objectively if a new air medical program would be of significant value to the service population or the sponsoring institution. In an ideal world only the former category would be assessed. In the real world a new program must contribute something of value to the sponsoring institution as well.

The key variables are the number of competing programs in the area, the population base, and the catchment area. Other factors include demographics, geography and accessibility, and the relative capabilities of hospitals in the area. Historically, a number of formulas have been applied in an effort to predict flight volume. However, these estimations are rarely accurate and should be used with caution. The marketing and public relations value of the flight program should also be considered. Evidence suggests that simply parking a medical helicopter on the premises of a hospital may attract new patients. Prestige may be another variable. A high-profile hospital with a well-known emergency and critical-care service may gain prestige through the addition of a flight program.

2. Feasibility Assessment

If projections indicate that a new program will have a positive impact on patient care and that there will be enough volume to justify its existence, the next step is to determine financial feasibility. A new air medical program started by a hospital will likely be required to attain financial independence, either directly or indirectly. While the income directly generated by the air program cost center is rarely enough to break even, when other program benefits are factored in, the net impact of the program is often positive. For example, the catchment area may be expanded, new patients may be generated by marketing efforts spearheaded by the program, and prehospital providers may call on the program for air support when needed. All these factors serve to increase patient numbers and gross revenue for the sponsoring institution. Programs started by consortia or government entities may have more leeway in their financial performance.

A proposed budget should be prepared based on the available projections.

3. Commitment

Starting an air medical program requires a significant amount of money and labor. Planners should be absolutely certain that the necessary financial and human resources are forthcoming before committing to the program. This commitment should extend all the way to the top executive. Those in decision-making positions should understand the complexity of the program and the up-front and ongoing operating expenses before committing prematurely.

4. Hiring the Program Director

This should be the first step once the institution(s) have committed to forming an air medical program. The program director will have a tremendous impact on shaping and administering the program and should be carefully selected. This person will generally be responsible for assembling the flight program and directing it once it is in operation. It is essential that she have experience in both air medicine and management.

Although it is not an absolute prerequisite, most program directors have a background in health care. This experience provides valuable insight into many aspects of the program and may make the director more credible to the medical flight team early in program development.

5. Hiring the Medical Director

The medical director influences the shaping of the program's medical policies and protocols and serves as the focal point for medical activities within the program. This person should be experienced in emergency and critical-care medicine and should have a basic understanding of prehospital care and air medicine. Ideally this person has completed an emergency medicine residency and a prehospital preceptorship. Board certification in emergency medicine or another closely related area should be a prerequisite.

It is essential that the person hired as medical director not only meet educational and certification requirements but also have a personality and attitude that are conducive to good relations with members of the health care community and the general public. The medical director will work very closely with all members of the medical flight team, especially in the early stages of program development, and will have significant influence on their attitudes and behaviors. Any bad habits that the medical director brings to the program may quickly rub off on other personnel. Excellent interpersonal skills are an absolute prerequisite. (The role and qualifications of the medical director are discussed in Chapter 12.)

Medical Control Plan

The medical director will play a key role in writing, reviewing, and editing the *medical control plan*. This document specifies exactly how the program will operate from a medical perspective. It details the roles and responsibilities of key personnel, including the medical director and the quality assurance officer. It also includes medical policies, procedures, protocols, and standing orders. Many states require a completed medical control plan before they will consider licensing a new program. In addition to the information listed above, they may also require staffing qualifications and staffing patterns for all medical employees.

6. Determining Organizational Structure

The air medical program may be set up along a continuum. At one end is a turnkey program, which assigns responsibility for startup and operational activities to a vendor or vendors. Vendors provide the aircraft, mechanics, pilots, all support services, and sometimes even the medical team.

The turnkey program is by far the simplest to implement and requires the least amount of time and effort on the part of the sponsoring institution. However, it is typically the most expensive option. Vendors are willing to assume responsibility for starting and managing a new program, but they expect to be paid for assuming that responsibility. There is always the danger of unscheduled maintenance, catastrophic equipment failure, and so on. Each of these risks has a financial price that the sponsoring institution must be willing to pay.

At the other end of the continuum is the program set up and operated entirely by the sponsoring institution. The program hires its own people, buys its own equipment and supplies, and assumes total risk for any unanticipated expenses. While this option is cheaper in the long run, the institution must have the financial reserves to pay for unexpected repairs. For example, if an engine develops mechanical problems and requires replacement, the cost may easily exceed $100,000. Those funds must be immediately available.

In between these two options is a hybrid program in which the sponsoring institution owns and manages the program but a vendor provides certain key services. One common scenario has the vendor providing pilots, aviation technicians, maintenance services, and sometimes the required FAA certification.

When choosing the best option, the sponsoring institution must decide how much time and effort it is willing to put into the flight program. If money is no object and time and people are in short supply, it may make sense to enter into a turnkey operation. If, on the other hand, money is tight and people and time are not an issue, the best option is to self-manage.

7. Preparing Requests for Proposals (RFPs)

At this point program planners are probably still uncertain of the final shape the program will take. Vendors' proposals will likely provide the information that planners need to make that determination. However, RFPs should be specific enough to eliminate options that will obviously not be considered. For example, if planners are fairly certain that the program will use a midsize twin-engine aircraft, that aircraft type should be specified in the RFP. Vendors will still have the freedom to propose various aircraft models that meet the general requirement. The vendor's degree of involvement should be stipulated as well.

8. Reviewing Proposals

A committee of principals should be assembled to review proposals and formulate comprehensive recommendations. The committee should be composed of administrators, the program director, the medical director, and others with knowledge and experience that may be beneficial to the process. Proposals should be reviewed in depth, and current and past customers should be contacted.

Site visits are an integral part of the proposal review process, particularly with respect to aircraft and medical interiors. The vendor's base of operation should be visited and meetings scheduled with key personnel. Any aircraft that is being seriously considered should be viewed. Test flights are also recommended. If a medically configured aircraft is not available for viewing at the vendor site, a trip to an air medical program that has that aircraft is recommended. A site visit also allows planners to ask questions regarding custom modifications and designs. There are so few medically equipped aircraft in operation that significant travel may be required for an on-site inspection of a particular aircraft type.

9. Determining If a Vendor Should Be Used

Most new programs elect to use a vendor. This arrangement takes some of the workload off the sponsoring institution and ensures that at least some members of the start-up team have aviation experience. The most cost-effective arrangement is for the program to purchase its own aircraft and to contract with a vendor for pilots, aircraft technicians, maintenance, and all necessary FAA certifications.

As the program grows and matures and program personnel become more knowledgeable and experienced, it may no longer be beneficial to contract with a vendor. The program may decide to hire its own operational personnel and to work directly with the FAA regarding certification issues.

10. Hiring the Chief Flight Nurse

The chief flight nurse (CFN) plays a significant role in the air medical program. This person is generally responsible for the quality improvement plan, for day-to-day personnel matters, and for serving as liaison between the medical flight team and the medical director. The CFN is the management representative who most consistently interacts with the flight team and has more influence on the behaviors of its members than anyone else.

The CFN should be competent and credible. Flight experience is strongly recommended. In rare cases an extraordinary candidate may be able to fill this role without experience, in which case there should be a mandatory preceptorship with a CFN at an already established flight program before the new program is implemented. The preceptorship should be completed before the rest of the flight team is hired.

11. Hiring the Chief Pilot

The chief pilot is the primary link between the aviation side and the medical side of the program. This person generally represents the pilots and aviation mechanics and is the go-to person regarding aircraft and aircraft operation issues. He or she will be responsible for scheduling, training, disciplinary action, and other matters for the pilots and technicians. In some larger companies, pilots and technicians may answer directly to a division chief and not to the chief pilot. Regardless of the organizational structure, the chief pilot should be considered a key member of the air medical management team.

The person who fills this slot should be much more than just an experienced pilot. The chief pilot plays an important leadership role and will serve as an ambassador for the sponsoring institution. He should have extensive flight time under all operating conditions and preferably EMS experience as well. IFR certification is a must, even for a program that operates only under VFR conditions. An ATP rating demonstrates a willingness to excel and is desirable. At some point in program development all pilots should be required to attain that rating.

If the program elects to operate its program without the involvement of a vendor, it will need its own FAA Air Carrier Certificate. Once hired, the chief pilot should immediately begin that process. Although some of the requirements cannot be met until an aircraft is available, parts of the process can be completed at this time. Any person or organization operating an air ambulance must obtain air operator certification. The certification process ensures that air operators provide the safest air transport possible. Satisfactory completion of the process is an indication that the program is in compliance with the requirements of the Federal Aviation Act.

There are five phases in the certification process: preapplication, formal application, document compliance, and certification. This in-depth process involves a great deal of paperwork, meetings, and on-site inspections by the FAA. It is important for the AM program to establish and maintain good working relations with FAA representatives.

12. Selecting and Ordering Aircraft and Interior

The Aircraft

Medical personnel often assume that buying a helicopter is similar to buying an automobile. It is dramatically different. Buying a new helicopter has been compared to having a new home built by a contractor. In both cases a long list of equipment, options, and accessories has to be agreed upon by both buyer and manufacturer. Unsold helicopters are usually equipped in a bare-bones way. Once a buyer is found, the aircraft is configured according to the buyer's individual preferences. That process often requires that the aircraft be dismantled and rebuilt, incorporating the custom equipment and amenities desired by the buyer, and can take several months. Each air medical helicopter is unique in terms of avionics and medical interior.

The aircraft selected should reflect the mission of the program. It is often a compromise between the ideal aircraft and what is affordable and practical. Most air medical programs now use midsized twin-engine turbine aircraft, because a second engine provides some degree of redundancy, in case of failure of one engine, as well as additional horsepower, which allows for a higher payload. That is not to say that a single-engine aircraft is not as safe as a twin (see Chapter 5). In any case the second engine is a source of reassurance for most passengers, and the added power allows for a larger cabin with increased capacities.

Medical Interior

The medical interior of the aircraft is generally purchased separately from the aircraft itself. Only a few companies specialize in that type of work. Program personnel should review proposals for the medical interior carefully. A medical conversion may cost $200,000 or more, and once the work is done, it is done. A list of past customers should be requested and contact made to see if they are satisfied with the product. Even programs that are satisfied will generally offer some suggestions for improvement.

Each conversion is a custom project. The vendor should be receptive to program-specific modifications such as mounting brackets and built-in chargers for specific equipment.

13. Determining a Base of Operations for the Aircraft

This step involves selecting office space for the pilots, aviation technicians, and medical team. It also involves choosing a location at which to base the aircraft. This process can be more difficult than one might think. The landing zone must be separated from people and automobiles, in an area where public access is restricted. This may be accomplished by:

* Having 24-hour surveillance
* Building a fence according to FAA guidelines
* Building a rooftop helideck, ideally above the acute-care area of a hospital, with the guidance of an architect experienced in helideck design

14. Purchasing Medical Equipment

Medical equipment used aboard the aircraft is similar to that used in the emergency department or critical-care unit of a hospital, only lighter and more compact. The equipment should be compatible with the aircraft and acceptable to the medical team. Several companies provide equipment for the ambulance industry that can easily be adapted for aircraft use.

The FAA requires that any item that may become a projectile in case of turbulence or crash be secured to the aircraft in such a way as to withstand 8 Gs of force. Mounting brackets must be attached to a structural component of the aircraft. This means that it may not always be possible to mount medical equipment at the desired location within the aircraft cabin, and the crew may have to make some compromises on the configuration of the medical compartment.

15. Determining Communications Arrangement

Communication is an integral part of the flight program. Any breakdown in this process can be disastrous. The two basic options are to set up and operate a communications center or contract with an existing agency for those services. There are pros and cons to either option.

Setting up a Program-Specific Communications Center

This option allows the program to establish and operate the communications center according to its own strict guidelines. Every aspect of the program can be custom designed and implemented. Communications specialists have only one responsibility, to dispatch and maintain communications with their own personnel.

A program-specific operation provides more direct oversight and control, but at a substantial cost. Equipment is expensive, a base station must be purchased and installed, and tower space for transmitters and repeaters must be leased. The cost of purchasing and installing the base station alone may exceed $100,000.

Contracting for Communications Services

There are often ambulance services or law enforcement agencies operating in the area that already have a functional communications system. It is much simpler and cheaper to sign a contract with one of these agencies to use their personnel and equipment for dispatching and flight following. The trade-off is that there may be less direct oversight and control. However, in most cases that potential problem can be managed in advance by writing strict performance guidelines into the contract. This is often the best option for a new AM program.

16. Hiring Medical Crew

The recruitment and selection process should be carefully planned and strictly followed. Standards should not be limited to medical knowledge and skills. Interpersonal skills, attitude, and professionalism should all be factored into the screening process. If the new program is located close to other air medical programs, the hiring process may be somewhat easier since there will likely be applicants with flight experience. However, hiring decisions should not be based on flight experience alone. Inexperienced personnel can make excellent flight team members if they are oriented, educated, and trained properly. The most important factor in this process is to demand excellence in every aspect of their performance. As in any field, people tend to perform to the standards that have been set for them. The bar should be set high from the very beginning.

Evaluating Applicants

Each program should have a set of predetermined criteria with which to rate applicants. It should not be an arbitrary process. A quantitative evaluation tool is preferable so that each applicant ends up with a total score that can be compared to those of other candidates. Some of the categories in which candidates should be evaluated are:

* **Education:**   Registered nurses and EMT-paramedics should be graduates of accredited programs. Minimum degree requirements may be specified. If physicians are part of the AM team, completion of a specific residency may be required.

* **Emergency and/or critical-care experience:**   Flight medicine is an extension of emergency and critical-care medicine. It is essential that anyone considered for a position with a flight team have emergency and/or critical-care experience. This applies to other areas of practice as well. For example, if a program transports primarily pediatric patients, applicants should have some minimum level of pediatric emergency and/or critical-care experience.

* **Specialty certifications:**   Some programs require that personnel pass certain certification examinations. For example, nurses may be required to pass the CFRN exam in order to qualify for an interview. Paramedics may be required to pass the FP-C examination. Physicians may be required to have board certification.

* **Interpersonal and interprofessional skills:**   Applicants lacking good interpersonal skills should not be considered for an AM position. Since applicants are on their best behavior during the interview process, job history should be checked to verify their past performance in this area.

* **Past accomplishments:**   These include instructional activities and participation in clinical ladder or similar professional development programs.

* **Flight experience:** If all other criteria are equal, the person with flight experience has a competitive edge. But other pertinent criteria sometimes outweigh flight experience, and it may be appropriate to hire a very strong and inexperienced candidate over another candidate who has flight experience but is less qualified otherwise.

* **Prehospital experience:** For programs that will make scene flights, prehospital experience should be an absolute requirement. An exception may be made when hiring a team that has one member who is a paramedic. The paramedic can assume the leadership role during scene responses.

* **Physical characteristics:** Each crew member must be physically capable of lifting patients and other potentially heavy objects. Minimum standards should be established for all physical performance categories. Most Human Resources offices have standard forms for this process.

Most programs have strict weight limitations for applicants to ensure that the aircraft can transport heavy patients without exceeding maximum gross weight limitations. Those doing the hiring should strive to communicate the fact that weight limits address safety issues and are not intended to discriminate against larger or heavier people.

Height restrictions may also apply at some programs that use helicopters with a relatively low ceiling in the patient compartment. Other physical restrictions may be necessary depending on the specific aircraft and operating parameters of the program.

17. Hiring Pilots and Aviation Technicians

The roles and responsibilities of air medical pilots are not duplicated elsewhere in aviation. In addition to their aircraft-related activities, they are expected to serve as ambassadors of the sponsoring institution and must possess the interpersonal skills necessary to perform well in that role. Pilots are often the most visible members of the flight program. When the medical team is in a hospital securing a patient, the pilot frequently interacts with physicians, nurses, and administrators, and may be asked questions about the aircraft and the program.

Aviation technicians are arguably the most important members of an air medical program. It is important that flight personnel recognize and appreciate the role they play. A mistake by a technician may result in catastrophe. Aviation technicians are much more than glorified automobile mechanics. They must be accepted as bona fide members of the air medical team and treated with the same dignity and respect as other members.

18. Orientation

At this phase the aircraft is generally not on site yet. All members of the air medical program should take part in a comprehensive orientation. This is a time for gaining new knowledge and skills, for team building, for becoming comfortable with other team members, and for developing mutual respect. Orientation should cover all phases of air medicine, with specific emphasis on safety and patient care.

Safety

As discussed in Chapter 5, safety must always be the highest priority of the entire air medical operation. The management team should consistently promote safety above all other program considerations. Flight team members must internalize that value and must feel comfortable expressing any concerns about safety without fear of repercussion or reprimand. Safety procedures should be presented and discussed in detail. Later, when the aircraft is put into service, these procedures must be practiced as realistically as possible.

Medical

Orientation is the time to present lectures and laboratory sessions in all areas of flight medicine. A thorough course in flight physiology is a prerequisite for all flight team members. Nothing should be assumed at this point. Review courses should be taught in pharmacology, patient assessment, and emergency management. More in-depth courses should be taught in areas involving expanded scope of practice such as rapid-sequence intubation, invasive airway techniques, insertion of chest tubes, and escharotomy. Every crew member should be required to demonstrate competency in each didactic and clinical area during this phase.

Aviation

Pilots and aviation technicians can use this time to familiarize themselves with policies and procedures, pertinent aviation directives, and so on. Pilots can begin learning the local flight area and making contacts with local FAA and flight control personnel. Establishing these relationships early on can be very important once the program is up and operating and when problems arise. This is also a good time to begin studying for certification examinations that may be required by the program. The airline transport pilot certification, recommended for all air medical pilots, requires a strong working knowledge beyond what the typical pilot considers essential for standard duty.

Pilots can also make site visits to hospitals where the program will likely be acquiring or delivering patients. They can meet with administrative and physical facilities personnel and make suggestions regarding proposed landing areas. Obstructions should be identified and recommendations made regarding their removal or modification.

Communications

Communications personnel should understand that they are an integral part of the flight program and be actively involved in the orientation phase. They should attend classes with the pilots and medical team members. During this phase, simulated flights can help communications personnel practice flight following and problem solving. Frequent emergency drills simulating unscheduled landings and crashes will quickly identify weaknesses that need to be corrected before the program goes on-line. Once the aircraft become available, these drills can be continued in a more realistic manner.

First Responders

Pilots should make contact with all agencies that may serve as first responders for the flight program—ambulance services, paid and volunteer fire department personnel, and any other groups that may be involved in coordinating flights for the program. Formal classes should be organized for each of these agencies. By the time the air medical program begins operations, there should be a strong infrastructure of support personnel throughout the service area.

19. On-Site Inspection of Aircraft and Interior

The conversion of a helicopter is not a standardized process; each aircraft includes custom-designed features. Some of the options may be one-of-a-kind, being done for the first time, and the buyer has no way of knowing what the final product will look like until it has been completed and installed in the aircraft. To avoid disappointing surprises, there should be at least one site visit during aircraft configuration to make sure the customization is proceeding as the customer intends. The first site visit should be made long enough into the process that the buyer can appreciate what the final product will look like, but it should not be delayed until the aircraft is nearly complete. At that point it may be too late to correct any customer concerns. Customer and vendor should work closely to determine the ideal time for a site visit.

20. Final Inspection and Acceptance of Aircraft and Interior

Once the aircraft and interior are substantially complete, the buyer should make a final inspection of the aircraft before accepting delivery. This may take place at the vendor's facility or at the point of delivery. It is generally more practical at the vendor's facility, where any problems can be taken care of more quickly and easily. The buyer should never sign to accept the aircraft until all discrepancies have been resolved. The final release form states that the customer has accepted the aircraft according to the terms of the contract.

21. Flight Training

Once all the components of the program have been assembled, and before the program becomes operational, some time should be allotted to training and orientation.

Medical

Flight training allows the medical flight team to become accustomed to the aircraft, communications equipment and operations, and the medical equipment within the aircraft. Providing medical care in a helicopter is very different from providing care in an emergency department or critical-care unit. The medical flight team should be aboard the aircraft for as many training flights as possible during this phase. Mock patients should be used to allow the medical crew to become familiar with the stretcher and loading system, patient access in the aircraft, positioning of the ventilator and tubing, and use of all medical equipment.

Aviation

Pilots need time to become comfortable with the aircraft before the program begins transporting patients. The amount of time depends on the individual pilot's helicopter flight experience, experience in the particular aircraft type, and learning curve. The program director should not force new pilots into operation before they are ready.

Each program typically has an area referred to as the local flying area, which is the geographical area in which most flights will be made. Each pilot should practice approaches into as many of the local landing zones as is practically possible. It is often helpful to take pictures of each landing zone and store them in a book in the aircraft for reference during actual responses. Notes can be added informing pilots of hazards and other unusual circumstances at each landing area.

Referring Medical Personnel

Ideally, hospital personnel at all potential referral sites should be oriented to the aircraft before it is placed in service. They can approach the aircraft and look inside, and the flight team can answer their questions and perhaps demonstrate some procedures. Later, when patients are involved, the team's concentration will be on patient care, and nonessential personnel are likely to be kept away from the aircraft. As discussed in Chapter 16, the establishment of positive working relationships with the medical community is one of the keys to a successful program.

First Responders

First responders are better prepared if they have realistic experience dealing with the aircraft and flight team. Simulated patient scenarios involving the preparation of landing sites and actual aircraft touchdowns allow pilots to identify weaknesses in the operation so that corrective action can be taken before real patients are involved.

22. Program Announcement/Press Conference

Air medical programs—especially the helicopter itself—are attention getters, and attention getters are always of interest to the media. Air medical stories offer high technology, expensive and complicated machinery, an element of danger, and life-or-death scenarios.

A new program is even more attractive because information is being released to the community for the first time. Media turnout for a press conference announcing a new program is generally very high. It is even higher if the program can keep the aircraft away from TV and newspaper cameras until the date of the media event.

23. Marketing/PR

With careful planning, marketing and public relations can be incorporated into the flight-training phase of program development. With a little advance notice, local media representatives will likely turn out for visits to potential referral sites. Their coverage provides invaluable exposure.

A site visit is one of the best ways to gain an audience with hospital administrators, physicians, and others and educate potential users about the benefits of using the new program. Brochures, cups, pens, and other items printed with dispatch telephone numbers should be handed out, as well as materials describing the benefits of referring patients to the flight program's sponsor hospital(s).

24. Program Implementation

An implementation date should be announced at the press conference. On that date the air medical program will become fully operational and available for responses. The first few days will be filled with excitement and anxiety. All eyes will be on the program. Ideally, the senior members of the flight team will be assigned to duty those first few days to ensure that everything proceeds smoothly.

The quality assurance/quality improvement process should be implemented as soon as the program begins operation. The goal is to identify actual and potential problems at the earliest practical point and to take corrective action. This process should include interpersonal as well as medical issues. Referring physicians generally have no obligation to use a particular air medical program, and the flight team's interpersonal skills are often a determining factor in repeat use.

Summary

There are 24 distinct steps in the process of starting a new program, from needs assessment to program implementation. (Table 20-1) Starting a new air medical program can be a complicated process. The key to success is to involve planners who are knowledgeable and experienced and to have a well-defined plan of action. Before any formal action is

Table 20-1 Start-up Activities and Timetable

Task	Responsible Party	Week of Completion
Needs assessment	Consultant	4
Feasibility assessment	Consultant/administrators	6
Commitment	Administrators/politicians	10
Hiring program director	Administrators	10
Hiring medical director	Administrators/program director	14
Determining organizational structure	Administrators/program director	15
Preparing RFPs	Program director/consultant	16
Reviewing proposals	Committee	20
Determining if a vendor should be used	Committee	20
Hiring CFN	Program director/medical director	22
Hiring chief pilot	Program director/medical director/CFN	24
Selecting and ordering aircraft and interior	Program director/chief pilot/medical director/CFN	26
Determining base of operations	Administrators/program director	26
Purchasing medical equipment	Program director/medical director/CFN	28
Determining communications arrangement	Program director/medical director/CFN	30
Hiring medical crew	Program director/medical director/CFN	30
Hiring pilots and aviation technicians	Program director/CFN	30
Orientation	Program director/medical director/CFN	32
On-site inspection of aircraft and interior	Program director/medical director/CFN/ chief pilot	32
Final inspection and acceptance of aircraft/interior	Program director/chief pilot/medical director/CFN	36
Flight training	Chief pilot/CFN	38
Program announcement/ press conference	Administrators/program director/ medical director	
Marketing/PR	Program director/medical director/CFN	38
Program implementation	All	40

Note: Time frames are estimates only. Aircraft preparation and delivery time depend on aircraft type, availability, and terms of contract. Pilot training time depends on aircraft, avionics, and pilot experience.

taken, a needs assessment must be performed to make sure there will be adequate volume to justify the program's existence. It should also be determined whether or not adequate financial support will be available.

REVIEW QUESTIONS

1. The first step to starting a new air medical program should be to:
   a. Hire a program director
   b. Hire a medical director
   c. Perform a needs assessment
   d. Perform a feasibility assessment

2. A turnkey operation is often the simplest and quickest way to set up a new air medical program. It is also the _____.
   a. Highest quality
   b. Most expensive
   c. Easiest to have accredited
   d. Safest

3. The most cost-effective option for a new program is often to:
   a. Purchase the aircraft and contract with a vendor for pilots and service
   b. Lease the aircraft and contract with a vendor for pilots and service
   c. Lease the aircraft and hire the pilots and aviation technicians
   d. Purchase the aircraft, lease medical equipment, and contract with a temporary agency for medical personnel

4. The person who will be responsible for the quality improvement program and day-to-day personnel matters is the:
   a. Program director
   b. Medical director
   c. Chief flight nurse
   d. Chief pilot

5. The person who will serve as the primary link between aviation and medical components of the program is the:
   a. Program director
   b. Medical director
   c. Chief flight nurse
   d. Chief pilot

6. The type of aircraft utilized by most air medical programs is a:
   a. Small single reciprocating engine
   b. Medium single-engine turbine
   c. Large single-engine turbine
   d. Medium twin-engine turbine

7. Some of the criteria that should be utilized when screening applicants for medical team positions include:
   a. Education, experience, religion
   b. Education, experience, certifications
   c. Education, experience, IQ
   d. Experience, IQ, military service

Setting Up
a Landing Zone

The landing zone is the environment in which an aircraft operates as it approaches and makes contact with the ground. For scene responses the options for a landing zone may be limited. Unimproved landing sites can present hazards that must be overcome before the site can be safely used.

The responsibility for identifying and marking a landing zone falls to ground personnel who arrive prior to the helicopter, such as first responders, EMS personnel, or law enforcement personnel. Anyone who may be called on to secure a landing zone must be instructed on how to do it, through outreach programs or EMS classes. Many programs distribute brochures or laminated cards with instructions for preparing a landing zone and approaching the aircraft. These provide valuable information for first responders and also serve to market the program.

Providing Directions

The simplest and most preferable method for giving directions is to provide GPS coordinates, which are now accurate to less than 20 feet. GPS units have made helicopter responses quicker and more efficient than ever. Basic handheld units can be purchased for less than $200 at discount stores. The first responder simply turns the unit on, reads the coordinates on the screen, and radios the coordinates to the dispatch center. The pilot plugs the coordinates into the aircraft GPS unit and follows a straight line to the landing zone.

Older methods still in use in some areas include the use of grid maps. The first responder identifies the location on the map and provides grid coordinates to the pilot. This gives the pilot a general idea of the location. However, grids can be large and pinpointing a landing area can still be difficult, especially during daylight hours. Other landmarks may need to be provided in order to narrow down the location.

The last method is to provide directions in relation to ground-based landmarks. A pilot viewing the ground from more than 1000 feet in the air may not be able to spot smaller landmarks such as street signs and house numbers. But larger structures such as water towers, large buildings, a school bus, construction sites, and so on may be easily spotted from the air. Major highways are generally easy to spot and make good starting points.

Selection and Preparation of the Landing Zone

The area selected for the landing zone should be large enough for the aircraft to enter and exit with a reasonable margin of safety. For a medium twin aircraft, at least 60' × 60' for daylight hours and 100' × 100' during periods of darkness is recommended. The area must be clear of trees, utility poles, and utility wires. The ground should be as level as possible, generally with no slopes of more than 6 to 8 degrees. There should be no areas of elevation or depression within the zone.

The surface should be firm enough to support the weight of the aircraft without allowing skids or wheels to sink into the ground more than a few inches. The area should be free of easily removed debris such as limbs or trash. Areas consisting primarily of dry loose soil should be avoided because of the risk of brownout.

In some areas first responders use portable helipads, which are light and compact enough to be carried aboard a fire or rescue truck and open up to a size sufficient to hold a medium-sized helicopter. The advantage of these devices is that they minimize concerns about the surface of the landing zone and significantly decrease the surface stirring effect. They may be particularly desirable in large, sandy areas or in areas of loose, dry soil.

Communications

Once the flight crew is airborne and within radio range, communications should be established with the ground crew. The ground crew should repeat GPS coordinates and describe the landing zone, any potential hazards, wind direction and speed if possible, and a description of the number and type of patients and any treatment given.

Lighting

During daytime hours, lighting is generally not a concern. At night it can be a significant issue. Ideally, marker lights or flares are placed around the periphery—at each corner of the landing area at a minimum—allowing the pilot to clearly identify a square or rectangular area in which to land. Flares should not be used in very dry conditions because of the risk of fire. If marker lights are not available, the landing zone may be identified by shining portable spotlights onto and across the area from three or more directions, forming an X. These lights must be aimed down on the pad, never upward toward the approaching aircraft.

If neither marker lights nor portable spotlights are available, vehicle lights may be used in the same manner. Vehicles should always be parked well outside the landing zone. Lights should be aimed upwind or crosswind to allow the pilot to land without lights aimed at the nose of the aircraft. Most medical helicopters have a landing light, and vehicle lights should be turned off once the pilot has identified and begun the final approach to the landing zone.

Approach and Landing

As the helicopter approaches, law enforcement or other responsible personnel should make sure all ground personnel are clear of the landing zone. One person should be assigned the task of communicating with the pilot. Others should keep the frequency clear until the aircraft has landed. Anyone near the landing zone should be instructed to turn away from the approaching aircraft or to stand behind a vehicle or structure of some type to avoid flying debris.

Generally, the aircraft should not be approached until the rotor blades have completely stopped. If immediate transport is indicated, the flight team may elect to load hot (not shut down). Ground personnel should be instructed to stay away from the aircraft until motioned to approach by a member of the flight team.

Aircraft Photography

Helicopters and airplanes are wondrous machines. There is a certain mystique associated with flying machines, especially the sleek and fast ones—design marvels with cutting-edge technology, aerodynamic design, and flashy paint schemes. They almost cry out to have their pictures taken.

However, taking pictures of aircraft, especially moving aircraft, can be both difficult and dangerous. As in all other areas of air medicine, safety is the most important consideration. The following suggestions will improve your odds of getting a good picture of an aircraft without compromising your safety or that of the flight team.

* Always get permission before approaching an aircraft for picture taking. In the post-9/11 era, aircraft operators are leery of strangers approaching their machinery. If an aircraft is inside a fenced enclosure, entering that space without permission may provoke an aggressive response. Many programs now either lock their aircraft behind fences or provide continuous closed-circuit monitoring by security or police personnel.

* *Never* use a flash or any other type of lighting device near an approaching or departing aircraft, especially at night. These bright lights may temporarily blind the pilot, making it difficult for him to identify hazards or judge distance and potentially resulting in a crash. Moving helicopters should be photographed during daytime hours when auxiliary lighting is not necessary. If you need to take flash pictures at night, take them only when the helicopter is on the ground and only with the permission of the aircraft operator.

* When photographing a moving helicopter, stay as far away as possible to avoid flying debris. Cameras are vulnerable devices. A speck of dust in the wrong place can make a camera inoperable.

Glass lenses are easily scratched or broken, and impact or exposure to the elements disturbs their electronic mechanisms. A telephoto lens allows you to take good shots while remaining a safe distance from the aircraft.

Camera Types

There are two basic types of cameras: film and digital. Each has advantages and disadvantages. Film cameras typically produce better-quality images, and digital cameras give nearly instant results and allow for easier editing and sharing. The specific situation and desired output will determine which one is preferable for a given job. Many amateur photographers use both types.

Film Cameras

A film camera is basically a lightproof box with a small opening through which light passes. The amount of light is controlled by a shutter that opens for a fraction of a second at the direction of the photographer. When the shutter opens, light enters through the lens and strikes a section of film. The film is a polymeric material coated with chemicals that react in a certain predictable manner when exposed to light. After a picture has been taken, the film is then developed, that is, chemically stabilized to prevent further changes in the captured image. The developed film is known as a negative. Next, a light is shone through the negative and the picture is transferred onto a sheet of photographic paper. The image on the paper is then coated to make it more durable.

Film

For the most part the quality of a picture produced by a film camera is dependent on the film size, film type, lens quality, and amount of available light. Remember that the film size is very small and that the image is spread over a much larger surface area when it is transferred to photographic paper. The larger the picture size becomes, the lower the resolution. Hence, as picture size increases, picture quality decreases. For example, a 5″ × 7″ picture has better color and resolution than an 11″ × 16″ picture made from the same negative. Larger film size provides better resolution—the more film surface area you have to start with, the less distortion there will be as the picture is enlarged.

Film speed—the speed with which a film captures an image—also influences picture quality. Faster film captures an image in less time than does a relatively slower film. However, as speed increases, picture quality generally decreases. When there is adequate light, a slower film will produce a better-quality picture than a faster film. But lighting conditions are often less than ideal, and faster film is required. Film speeds up to 400 are generally of very good quality. Some of the newer 800-speed films are now very good as well. As film speed exceeds 1000, there is a notable decrease in picture quality, especially when larger print sizes are used.

Many single lens reflex (SLR) cameras allow for prolonged exposure times and produce good-quality pictures even in near darkness. Both the camera and the object being photographed must remain still during the entire exposure time. Holding the camera is not an option; the camera must be seated on a nonmoving surface such as a tripod, a three-legged stand that attaches to the camera and locks it in place. Most tripods are adjustable vertically and have a flexible head that may be rotated in any direction.

Lenses

The other important variable in picture quality is the lens. Most SLR cameras have easily removable lenses. That feature allows the photographer to remove and replace the lens as the photographic environment changes. For example, to photograph a group of people in a small room, a wide-angle lens may be used. For distant objects a telephoto lens will make the subject appear closer.

Zoom lenses are more expensive but allow greater flexibility in photographing objects at different distances. These lenses have adjustable magnification. For example, a 35–105 mm zoom lens will zoom out to 35 mm (wide angle) and zoom in to 105 mm (telephoto). The photographer may use the same lens to photograph a group of people up close and a helicopter in flight some distance away. The trade-off is that these types of lenses are typically more expensive, and the complexity of the lens elements increases the likelihood of distortion.

Flashes

Flashes are most commonly used to brighten a subject in a dark environment. They may also be used to provide accent lighting even in well-lit conditions. For example, a person who is photographed at noon when the sun is directly overhead may appear to have shadows under the eyes unless a flash is used to "fill in" the dark spots.

Digital Cameras

Digital cameras take pictures in a slightly different manner. They capture pictures on a light-sensitive diode and then convert the picture to digital format. There is no film involved in this process; each picture is saved as a file on a storage card inserted into the camera. Digital cameras eliminate the inconvenience of loading and unloading film and the delay associated with getting the film developed and processed. They allow for almost instant viewing of shots. Digital pictures can be easily downloaded to a PC or laptop for editing and storage and can be transmitted via the Internet to virtually anywhere in the world in minutes. Some high-end cameras even offer in-camera editing, and printers have been specifically designed to print digital photos.

The negative aspects of digital cameras are expense and picture quality. For $700 you can acquire a 5-megapixel digital camera, or, for $1,500, a 6-megapixel camera. However, a 35-mm SLR camera for less than $200 is capable of producing the equivalent of 20 megapixels of resolution. The trade-off is convenience versus picture quality. The digital camera is clearly more convenient and efficient, but the SLR offers superior picture quality. As camera technology continues to improve, digital quality will almost certainly surpass that of film cameras.

Most of the rules of photography that apply to film cameras also apply to digital cameras. Lighting and the use of a flash are just as important in digital photography. Digital cameras may produce less than ideal color reproduction when used under low-light conditions.

Air-to-Air Photography

One of the best ways to photograph an aircraft in flight is from another aircraft flying alongside. This sounds far simpler than it really is. The two aircraft must remain far enough apart to avoid any potential of collision. The weather is an important variable. On a windy day, aircraft movements may make getting a good picture difficult. Pictures should be taken when the weather is calm and there is little **haze** in the air. Time of day also plays a role. The sun should be in a position that maximizes lighting but does not cause glare. The background must also be considered. If the photographer wants a hospital or other structure in the background, it may take several passes in front of the structure to get the right shot.

haze
Any atmospheric condition that interferes with light transmission; generally caused by high moisture content, smoke, or dust particles in the air.

The aircraft in which the photographer will ride should be carefully chosen. It should have an access port through which the camera can be pointed. Aircraft windows are rarely translucent enough for picture taking. Even unscratched windows often produce glare and make pictures appear hazy. The aircraft should be capable of slow cruise. Some fixed-wing aircraft may not be able to fly slowly enough to make picture taking practical. The desired picture and background will appear and disappear so quickly that the photographer has little time to compose and shoot. Ideally, when the target of the camera is a helicopter, a second helicopter should be used to transport the photographer.

Specialty Certifications (CFRN/FP-C)

Over the past two decades air medicine has developed into a specialty-care area with its own unique body of knowledge, which has developed primarily as a result of research being done in the field. A number of journals now routinely publish articles related to air medicine, in particular the *Journal of Air Medicine, Annals of Emergency Medicine,* and the *Journal of Emergency Nursing.*

As knowledge has grown, so has the standard of care. A standard of care requires that there be some measurement tool to assess competence related to that standard. In recent years two such tools have been developed. The Certified Flight Registered Nurse (CFRN) examination was written specifically for flight nurses and is modeled after other nurse specialty examinations such as Critical Care Registered Nurse (CCRN) and Certified Emergency Nurse (CEN). The unique components of the CFRN examination relate to safety, flight physiology, and the stressors of flight.

As the paramedic curriculum has expanded in breadth and depth, the capabilities of flight nurses and flight paramedics have begun to converge. The Flight Paramedic Certification (FP-C) exam is very similar to the CFRN exam.

For nurses and paramedics who are already members of a flight team or who wish to be, these specialty certification examinations are the best way to demonstrate knowledge of air medicine. The CFRN exam is open to any registered nurse willing to pay the registration fee. Similarly, the FP-C exam is open to any paramedic. Preparing for, taking, and passing one of these exams demonstrates a level of commitment that program directors like to see on job applications and improves the applicant's chances of at least getting an interview.

Taking these examinations can be a relatively expensive venture. The registration fee for the CFRN examination ranges from $210 to

$370 based on whether the exam is being taken for the first time and whether the examinee is a member of the Emergency Nurses Association and/or the Air Surface Transport Nurses Association. The fee for taking the FP-C examination is $175 for members of the International Association of Flight Paramedics and $275 for non-members. What are the benefits of passing these exams? Some air medical programs use successful completion as the minimum knowledge level for potential employees. Others encourage their existing employees to complete these tests as part of their QA/QI programs.

Ground Transport
Systems

The purpose of this book is to introduce the reader to the concept of air medicine. However, the introduction would be incomplete without some discussion of ground transport as well. When both air and ground critical-care options are available, the two complement each other. An integrated transport system allows for a more ideal matching of patient care needs with mode of transportation and level of medical care.

Ground transport can also serve as backup for the air medical program when the aircraft is not available or is unable to fly. For single-aircraft operations, flights are also lost due to maintenance or repairs. The availability of a ground component ensures that critical-care transport is available even when the aircraft isn't.

The addition of a ground service also offers a more cost-effective option for short-distance transports, such as moving critical patients between hospitals in a metropolitan area. It may also be a good way to capture new patients in areas where competing hospitals offer similar inpatient care options.

Critical-care ground transport is somewhat simpler than air transport. The flight physiology, flight communications, and flight safety components are removed from the equation. However, ground transport has its own, unique problems. The vehicles move more slowly, and the patient may be out of a hospital environment for a longer period of time. In some areas of the country road quality can be a significant factor. Patients with illness or injury sensitive to motion may be compromised by ambulance movement over rough areas or when cornering.

Vehicles

Ground ambulances are most commonly used to respond to prehospital emergencies and for the routine transport of nonambulatory patients. These vehicles are trucks or vans that have been configured for medical use. All ambulances must adhere to strict federal guidelines (Federal Specification KKK-A-1822D), commonly referred to as "KKK specs," that specify dimensions, construction technology, safety devices, minimum electrical capabilities, and so on. Contrary to popular belief, ambulances are not designed or intended to be driven at high speed. They are typically top heavy and, compared to standard passenger vehicles, handle poorly. The purpose of these vehicles is to convey trained medical personnel to the scene of an emergency so that stabilization can be accomplished prior to and during transport of the patient. A high-speed, careening ride is not conducive to accomplishing that goal. Employees who drive ambulances must receive special training.

Vehicle Types

Ambulances come in three basic varieties. A *Type I* vehicle is composed of a truck chassis with a box-type patient compartment mounted on the rear frame (Figure D-1). There is generally no access between the patient compartment and the driver's compartment. Communication is possible only through some type of intercom system.

A *Type II* ambulance is a converted van with a higher ceiling and integrated cabinetry (Figure D-2). The cargo area is often longer than in a typical van. The patient and driver compartments are contained within the same structure, generally separated by some type of barrier but connected by an aisle. This type of ambulance is the most similar to a typical passenger vehicle in its driving and handling characteristics.

Type III ambulances are similar to Type I but have some connection between the patient and driver compartments (Figure D-3). This connection may be large enough to walk through or may consist of no more

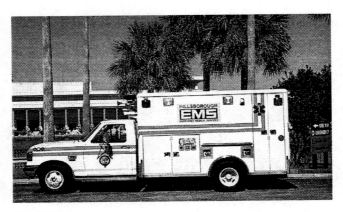

FIGURE D-1
A Type I ambulance

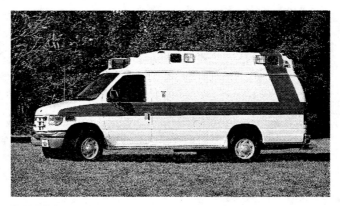

A Type II ambulance

than a small window through which to communicate and pass small items. Type III ambulances are often constructed from modified cutaway van chassis. Vehicle configuration may range from simple (cheap) to elaborate (expensive). Options include everything from refrigerators to miniature laboratory workstations.

While any of these three ambulance types may be used for critical-care transportation, Type I and Type III ambulances are generally preferred because of their larger patient compartments and greater weight-carrying capacity. The downside is that larger trucks have a higher purchase price and higher operating costs. Their larger size may also make them less maneuverable. Although Type II ambulances are used less frequently, they are much cheaper to purchase and configure and may prove more cost-effective, particularly for systems that do relatively few ground transports.

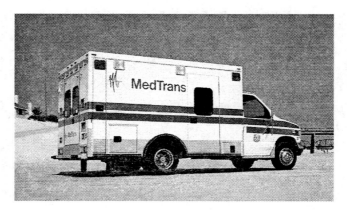

FIGURE D-3
A Type III ambulance

Personnel

First Responders/EMT-Basics

The medical capabilities of ambulance personnel may vary by state and even by area within a state. In some areas medical attendants are First Responders or EMT-Basics with limited training. At that level, patient care consists of first aid, limited use of airway adjuncts, and the use of automatic defibrillators. Prompt patient transport may assume greater importance than in other systems. In other areas, EMT-Basic providers are taught select advanced life-support skills such as IV insertion or endotracheal intubation.

Given the ever tighter reimbursement restrictions being placed on ambulance services by Centers for Medicare and Medicaid Services (CMS) and other groups, basic-level ambulance services are likely to become more common as communities are less able to afford advanced life-support care. For-profit companies will bear the brunt of these cost-cutting efforts, although not-for-profits will eventually suffer as well.

EMT-Paramedics

In most highly populated areas of the United States, ambulances are staffed by EMT-paramedics. These health care professionals generally have at least 1 year of formal education based on the Department of Transportation EMT-Paramedic curriculum. In many areas paramedics complete 2 years of education with a curriculum parallel to that completed by registered nurses but focused more on acute conditions. Paramedics may evaluate patients and determine the need for a variety of advanced treatments, including ECG interpretation and management, intubation, insertion of invasive airways, placement of various tubes and catheters, and pharmacological management of all common medical emergencies.

Paramedics are uniquely qualified to manage patients in the prehospital setting. However, their training in the area of critical-care transport management is limited. Paramedics who will be involved with critical-care patient transports should be required to complete a critical-care orientation program that includes a clinical component. In the absence of that training, a knowledgeable and experienced critical-care nurse should be included in the transport team. The University of Maryland offers a Critical Care Paramedic program that includes 80 hours of classroom instruction. Combined with a clinical component of at least equal duration, that program provides adequate introductory knowledge for a paramedic participating in critical-care transports.

Critical-Care Transport Nurses

Many ambulance systems that provide ground critical-care transportation employ registered nurses. An RN with a strong background in critical-care nursing brings much to the program. However, the ambulance environment is very different from that of a hospital critical-care unit. There are no support personnel in the ambulance setting, no physician to confirm diagnostic impressions and treatment decisions. The nurse often works as a semi-independent practitioner who makes complex medical decisions and implements medical treatments based on a combination of protocols and personal judgment.

Registered nurses who are hired to provide patient care during interfacility transports should be cautious about agreeing to make prehospital responses. The standard of care is significantly different for prehospital care. Medical equipment and supplies are different, and there are important medical and legal implications for nurses in this environment. Many of the skills required to function effectively in the prehospital setting are not taught in nursing programs. It is essential that these knowledge gaps be filled before an RN responds to prehospital calls.

Search and Rescue

The term *search and rescue* (SAR) refers to the process of seeking out and recovering persons who are lost, injured, or otherwise inaccessible, and who are presumably in need of help. The process often involves difficult terrain and difficult access. Disentanglement and high/low angle rescue may also be required. SAR requires specialized equipment and personnel.

The helicopter is often an ideal tool for SAR. It is quickly mobilized and gives the pilot a broad view of large geographic areas. Aircraft equipped with infrared devices may detect even victims who are obscured by trees or bushes or are partially submerged. Once a victim has been located, the helicopter delivers rescue and medical personnel and equipment. Where surface access is difficult, the helicopter may be used to lower a rescue harness or stretcher. If helicopter approach is not feasible due to terrain, the crew can **hover** over the site or provide GPS coordinates and visual cues to ground responders.

In mountainous areas of the country, any program that may be participating in SAR activities should choose its aircraft carefully. The helicopter should be capable of high-altitude, warm-weather flight and of maintaining an out-of-ground-effect hover at the highest point where a rescue is likely to be required. The aircraft must be able to land in rugged terrain on small, unimproved helspots.

Since there is often an element of danger in using helicopters for SAR operations, they must be used judiciously. The safety of an SAR mission depends to a large extent on the knowledge and skill of the pilot and others aboard the aircraft.

While few air medical programs regularly participate in SAR activities, there is always the possibility of a mass casualty incident. All programs should have basic-level training in SAR techniques, and those

hovering
When a helicopter maintains a constant position at a selected point, usually a few feet above the ground.

that participate more frequently in SAR should have even more training. Several courses have been developed to provide training in SAR approaches and techniques. Three are outlined below. (Since these courses contain sections of interest to air medical providers but also a good deal of extraneous information, the best approach may be for an AM program to design its own course. The instructor should be experienced in SAR operations and very familiar with the role of the helicopter and the air medical team in those operations.)

Introduction to Search and Rescue

This course is the first step toward higher-level courses for emergency personnel. It includes a common starting point for those who are new to SAR. The course requires 16 hours to complete and covers the following topics:

* Components of SAR
* SAR management system
* Land navigation and orienteering
* SAR resources
* Search philosophy and probability theory
* Search tactics
* Clue consciousness
* Search operations
* Lost person behavior
* Helicopter operations in SAR (including a section on helicopter safety)
* Communications

Search and Rescue Medical Responder Course

While this course is intended for first responders and others with limited medical knowledge, the principles may easily be adapted to the advanced level. The course addresses common medical and traumatic conditions associated with patients rescued from difficult-to-access environments. For AM programs this course may double as a survival course, as it covers wilderness medicine and survival. The course was developed for SAR responders, EMS responders, and disaster workers who may be called on to provide prolonged prehospital patient care.

Fundamentals of Search and Rescue

This course is designed for persons interested in becoming involved or who have just become involved with SAR, including AM members who have a special interest in SAR and wish to get involved at the community level. Course content is very similar to the Introduction to Search and Rescue course.

Frequently Asked
Questions

This chapter was written for those who are curious about air medicine. They may turn to this page, find the answers to some common questions, and, it is hoped, decide to read the rest of the book.

How fast do air medical helicopters fly?

A variety of helicopters are used for air medical service, and the cruise speed depends on the helicopter type and model. For example, the Bell 206 has a cruise speed of 110 knots. The Sikorsky S-76 C+, a larger and more expensive aircraft, has a cruise speed of 155 knots.

Why does it take so long for a helicopter to start up?

A turbine engine has to be started and allowed to run at idle for a short time until its core temperature reaches a certain level and it can be turned to full throttle. Helicopters with two engines have to go through that process twice and sometimes have to wait for the battery to recharge after starting the first engine before starting the second.

Since helicopters are so expensive to operate, what are the advantages of transporting a patient by air rather than ground ambulance?

Ground ambulances provide a valuable service to their patients. Paramedics are highly trained medical care providers capable of managing the vast majority of medical conditions. However, a helicopter can cut transport time by more than half. Also, most air medical personnel have additional training and may be able to perform specialized medical treatments that ground ambulance paramedics cannot.

Why do air medical programs have weight limits for their crew members?

All aircraft have maximum weight limits. Generally, the smaller the aircraft, the more sensitive it is to weight. Air medical programs limit the weight of their crews in order to transport heavy or multiple patients without exceeding the maximum gross weight limits of the aircraft.

What are the training requirements for an air medical helicopter pilot?

Training requirements for pilots vary from state to state and program to program. Generally, pilots must complete an acceptable training program, possess a valid license, and have a specified amount of experience. Each program sets minimum requirements for total flight time, time in aircraft type, nighttime flying, and flight time in the local service area. Some more progressive programs require airline transport pilot (ATP) certification.

Why do air medical team members wear helmets?

Individual program policy determines whether or not personnel wear helmets. Equipment mounted in the patient compartment of medical aircraft may cause serious head trauma in the event of turbulence. Helmets may protect wearers from head strikes as well as bird strikes. Flight helmets contain sound-deadening material to reduce aircraft noise and integrated ear cups and a microphone for communication. Most models also contain two shields that may be extended and retracted as needed—a clear shield that serves as a biological barrier and a tinted shield that protects the eyes from the sun.

What is Nomex, and why are flight suits made from it?

Nomex is a fire-resistant material designed to protect wearers from being burned in case of cockpit fire or crash. The flame-retardant effects of this material last only a few minutes, and the intent is to give crew members time to escape a burning aircraft.

How do air medical helicopters navigate?

visual omnidirectional aid (VOR)
A radio transmission beacon. Using the transmission from this beacon, a pilot can simply and accurately navigate from point to point.

Pilots have several methods of navigation available to them. The most modern involves use of an aircraft-mounted GPS (global positioning satellite) system that allows the pilot to fly directly from one point to another and provides such information as distance to destination, time to destination, airspeed, and ground speed. An older but still reliable method of navigation uses a **visual omnidirectional aid (VOR)** and compass.

How much space does a helicopter require to land?

A 100′ × 100′ area that is level, firm, and cleared of all obstructions and debris is ideal. However, a helicopter can land in a smaller area whose dimensions are twice the length of the aircraft, as long as the approach and departure path are clear of obstructions.

What is the purpose of the tail rotor?

The tail rotor produces lateral thrust to counteract the torque generated by the main rotor. Without a tail rotor a helicopter would begin to spin as soon as it lifted off the ground. The tail rotor also performs the same function as the rudder of a fixed-wing craft, which is to change the direction of the aircraft.

What do air medical team members do when they are not on a flight?

That depends on individual program policies. Some flight personnel have no additional duties but are expected to read, study, and complete activities related to quality improvement. Hospital-based programs often have additional responsibilities for their flight teams, such as working in the emergency department.

How many flights do air medical programs make?

That varies from program to program. Some programs are busier than others. Generally, a program completing fewer than 15 or 20 flights per month may be viewed as performing well below its capacity. A typical single-ship program may complete 60 flights per month or more without missing a significant number of requests.

Why do some helicopters have wheels and others have skids?

It is a matter of personal preference. Skids create drag and slightly reduce the airspeed of a helicopter. Wheels are retractable and eliminate that drag. They also allow for easier moving of the helicopter on the ground. However, wheels add weight to the helicopter, and the cavity into which they retract often replaces fuel space and decreases the range of the aircraft. Wheels have less surface area than skids and may sink into soft or moist soil.

How far can an air medical helicopter fly without refueling?

It depends on the aircraft type and the size of the fuel tank(s). A typical range for a midsized twin-engine aircraft is 225 to 350 miles.

How many pilots are required to operate an air medical helicopter?

Most small and midsized helicopters require only one pilot. Some of the larger helicopters, such as the Sikorsky S-76, Bell 214, or Bell 412, may require two pilots.

Are flight team members required to pass any special certification examinations?

That varies by program. Many programs do not require specialty certification. Some encourage their personnel to take these exams, and others require certification as a prerequisite for employment. The two most commonly required certifications are for the CFRN (nurses) and CF-P (paramedics).

Are air medical pilots required to pass any special certification examinations?

Some programs require their pilots to complete all requirements for airline transport pilot (ATP) certification. Most do not.

How does an air medical helicopter locate an accident site in a rural area?

In many cases GPS coordinates are provided by first responders. If GPS coordinates are not available, the pilot may have to rely on compass directions, highways, and other ground landmarks.

How high do medical helicopters fly?

Different helicopters have different altitude limitations. Most air medical pilots fly at altitudes of less than 3000 feet AGL (above ground level). In mountainous areas the cruise altitude may be increased. When flying under IFR conditions, the pilot flies at the altitude assigned by the flight controller. That may be as much as 10,000 feet AGL or more.

What happens if an engine goes out in a helicopter?

If the helicopter has only one engine, the pilot must immediately begin an autorotation. A twin-engine helicopter can continue to fly until a suitable landing site can be found.

What is an autorotation?

If a helicopter loses its engine, it can continue to glide. The air moving up through the main rotor keeps it spinning and continues to provide lift. The pilot can vary the pitch on the main rotor to increase or slow the rotation speed so that it stays in the normal range. As the helicopter nears the ground, the pilot increases pitch on the main rotor and slows the descent enough to make a safe landing.

How many blades does the rotor on an air medical helicopter have?

That depends on the make and model of aircraft. Some helicopters, such as the Bell 206, 222, 230, and 214, have two blades. Others, such as the Eurocopter A-Star, have three blades. The Bell 430 and 412 have four blades. Other aircraft may have five or more blades.

What is the difference between VFR and IFR?

VFR refers to flights in which the pilot can visualize the ground and surroundings for a reasonable distance. VFR rules prohibit intentional flight into the clouds or in any other low-visibility condition.

How does a helicopter pilot see to fly at night?

When flying under VFR flight conditions, the pilot uses ground references and instruments to maintain altitude and navigate. Vehicles, highways with traffic, and lighted buildings are easily seen from the air.

How many patients can an air medical helicopter transport at one time?

It depends on the aircraft. Smaller helicopters may be capable of single-patient transport only. Midsized twins typically have two-stretcher capability. A few larger aircraft, such as the Bell 214, can transport up to six patients.

Who is responsible for patient care when the flight team arrives at a referral hospital to acquire a patient?

This is determined by state law and local policy. Generally, the treating physician retains responsibility as long as the patient remains in the referral hospital. The referring physician may retain some degree of responsibility for patient care until the patient is delivered to the receiving facility. In most cases the responsibility is transferred to the flight team at some stipulated point. If the flight team is employed by a hospital or a state-approved medical control plan is in effect, responsibility for patient care is transferred to the flight team and its medical director as the patient leaves the referring facility and enters the aircraft.

What physician provides medical direction to the flight team?

The program's off-line medical director is ultimately responsible for the medical performance of the flight team. However, in some systems a referring physician may be allowed to give orders to the flight team during the course of interfacility transports. This varies by state and by program. Most programs operate under a set of protocols and standing orders that allow the flight team a great deal of autonomy. The off-line medical director is responsible for writing protocols and determining whom the flight team may accept medical orders from.

How much is a patient billed for an air medical transport?

Billing specifics vary from program to program. A typical rotor-wing transport can cost $6,000 or more, depending on the treatments provided and the distance of the transport.

Are family members allowed to ride with patients who are transported by air?

Policies vary from program to program. Most rotor-wing programs do not routinely allow family members to accompany patients but may consider it under unusual circumstances. Allowing a family member to ride along may be beneficial when the patient is a small child or is extremely anxious about flying. Family members are more commonly allowed on long-distance transport by fixed-wing aircraft.

How many medical attendants staff a typical air medical program?

It depends on the size of the aircraft and program policy. Most programs operate midsize twin-engine aircraft and have a medical team of two, usually one nurse and one paramedic. Programs using smaller aircraft typically staff with one paramedic *or* one nurse.

I am interested in becoming a flight nurse/flight paramedic. What can I do to improve my chances of landing a position?

Education and professionalism are extremely important. Paramedics and nurses should educate themselves beyond the minimum requirements of their professions. Certification in ACLS, PALS, neonatal resuscitation, and a trauma course is a must. Nurses should consider taking the CFRN examination, as a passing score suggests ambition and self-discipline. Similarly, paramedics should take the flight paramedic certification exam. A degree in emergency health sciences or a related field will help a paramedic applicant stand out from the crowd.

Answers to
Review Questions

Chapter 1
1. d   2. d   3. a   4. a   5. c   6. b   7. c   8. d

Chapter 2
1. d   2. a   3. d   4. d   5. a   6. a   7. b   8. c

Chapter 3
1. b   2. c   3. d   4. a   5. d   6. d

Chapter 4
1. c
2. a
3. When a patient is seriously ill or injured and when traffic is heavy and movement of ground ambulances is impeded.
4. d
5. b
6. d
7. a

Chapter 5
1. b
2. d
3. In cases where a patient is critical and where time is of the essence. It may also be appropriate in cases where an additional response is holding, or when the aircraft has experienced battery or starter problems making restarting the aircraft difficult or uncertain.
4. a
5. c
6. d

7. The area surrounding a passenger or crew member that could potentially be impacted by the head during a sudden or violent movement of the aircraft.
8. b
9. c

Chapter 6

1. a
2. d
3. The dispatch center coordinates all communications to and from the flight crew. It is the hub of all communications activity related to the flight program.
4. c
5. d
6. b

Chapter 7

1. a
2. d
3. Nurses should be graduates of an accredited school of nursing and should have passed the National League of Nursing Boards examination. A degree at the associate or bachelor's level indicates completion of a well-rounded curriculum and is preferred. Paramedics should be graduates of a CAHEP-accredited school of emergency medical technology and should have passed the National Registry of Emergency Medical Technicians Board examination. In states not requiring the National Registry examination, passage of a designated state examination may demonstrate equivalent knowledge.
   Some degree of experience is often required also. Completion of Advanced Cardiac Life Support (ACLS), Pediatric Advanced Life Support (PALS), and a trauma course such as Trauma Nurse Core Curriculum (TNCC), Basic Trauma Life Support (BTLS), or Prehospital Trauma Life Support (PHTLS) is often required. For programs that transport pediatric patients, pediatric Advanced Life Support (PALS) and a Neonatal Resuscitation course may be required as well.
4. a
5. b

Chapter 8

1. Large patient compartment, instrument rated, fast cruise speed, economical, minimal maintenance, long range

2. d

3. b

4. d

5.

Augusta	
A-109	Economical, fast
A-119	Very large for a single engine, fast
American Eurocopter	
AS-350	Economical, fast, good power, long range
BK-117	Economical, large patient compartment
BO-105	Economical
Bell	
206L	Economical, low maintenance requirements
212	Very large patient comartment
214	Very large patient comartment
430	Large patient compartment, very fast
Sikorsky	
S-76	Very large patient comartment, very fast

Chapter 9

1. a

2. d

3. c

4. Maintain visual reference outside the aircraft, sit facing forward when possible, avoid eating before a flight, utilize prophylactic antiemetics if necessary.

5. c

Chapter 10

1. b

2. a

3. d

4. a

5. d

6. Increases in altitude may aggravate existing pulmonary problems. For example, the size of a pneumothorax may increase as altitude increases. Also, the partial pressure of oxygen decreases as altitude increases, increasing the probability of hypoxia for susceptible patients.

Chapter 11

1. It is important fot the medical team to have a clear and thorough understanding of the patient and his or her medical condition prior to assuming responsibility for that patient. Gaining the necessary information allows the medical team to better prepare for management of the patient during transport.
2. d
3. Family members are often anxious and confused when a loved one becomes acutely ill or injured. They may be easily frustrated and angered. Providing an update regarding the patient's condition, directions to the receiving hospital, and any other necessary and beneficial information goes a long way toward easing the anxiety.
4. b
5. d
6. a
7.

    1. Every patient should have an IV.
    2. Collection bags should be emptied.
    3. The patient's airway should be secured in a definitive manner.
    4. Medicate patients who are nauseated.
    5. IV lines should be shortened or looped and secured.
    6. Oxygen supply tubing should be looped and secured.
    7. If the patient is intubated, one person should be assigned to keep the tube secured and ensure that patient ventilation is uninterrupted.
    8. All equipment should be secured to the stretcher.
    9. The patient should be moved to the aircraft in a slow and controlled manner.
    10. A reliable assistant should carry items that cannot be secured to the stretcher.
    11. Anyone not essential to the move should be kept at a safe distance.
    12. Only members of the flight team should open aircraft doors.
    13. The patient should be loaded into the aircraft by the flight crew.
    14. Only flight team members should close aircraft doors.
    15. Crew members should make certain that all bystanders are at a safe distance from the aircraft durin g start-up and preparation for departure.

8. a

Chapter 12

1. b   2. a   3. c   4. c   5. d

Chapter 13

1. c   2. a   3. a   4. d   5. c   6. d   7. b

Chapter 14

1. a
2. d
3. a
4. d
5. In the short term it is cheaper to purchase fuel from a vendor. However, over a longer period of time significant savings can be realized by purchasing a fuel handling system and buying fuel directly from a distributor.

Chapter 15

1. Numerous studies including those authored by Moylan, Thomas, Siem and Decharro, Braithwaite, Kerr, Koury, and others have demonstrated benefits for select air medical patients.
2. These programs rarely ever produce a profit as a cost center. However, they do have the potential to generate new patients for a sponsor hospital. They do have the potential to be profitable as part of a comprehensive transportation program.
3. The flight program can serve to generate the specialty care patients required by residency programs. They may also offer tremendous learning opportunities for residents and fellows.
4. c
5. a
6. d

Chapter 16

1. The outreach program may benefit the sponsoring hospital in a number of ways. These programs offer health care providers in the community access to educational opportunities that may otherwise be too expensive or difficult to obtain. Teaching classes and explaining difficult patient care issues are excellent ways to earn credibility with both existing and potential customers. As the connection between the flight team and off-site hospitals grows stronger, the off-site hospitals are more likely to call the flight team for emergency and critical referrals, and, assuming the appropriate resources are available, to refer patients to the sponsoring hospital. An active outreach program may substantially increase the number of referrals a hospital receives.
2. a
3. d
4. c
5. a

6. Air medical programs may utilize numerous techniques for publicity and promotion including outreach, distribution of institutional pens, cups, and key chains, free continuing education, a monthly or quarterly newsletter, and even utilizing the aircraft itself as a banner.

Chapter 17

1. d
2. c
3. b
4. The AFMS has played a leadership role in developing out of hospital care since 1949. During the Korean and Vietnam wars the AFMS developed into an innovative and productive arm of the air force.
5. a
6. d
7. The role of the AECM is to configure and deconfigure cargo aircraft for A/E operations, enplane waiting patients, provide emergency and nonemergency care, and safely deliver patients to the next medical treatment facility along the evacuation route.

Chapter 18

1. a
2. c
3. d
4. b
5. a
6. Generally, the U.S. system is very similar to the Canadian system in terms of staffing and equipment. Staffing is somewhat different in the European countries. Most staff their aircrafts with physicians and some combination of nurses and rescuemen. Australia utilizes rotor-wing aircraft in developed areas and fixed-wing aircraft for trips to remote portions of the continent.
7. Passports may be required, pilots may require approach plates not routinely available, there may need to be multiple refueling stops during the trip, it may be necessary to bring food and drink for patients and crew members, the medical team may have to stock additional IV fluids and medications.

Chapter 19

1. a
2. a

3. d

4. b

5. Advantages: Fixed-wing aircraft are generally faster and travel much farther without having to refuel. The cost per mile is often lower than for a rotor-wing aircraft. Disadvantages: Fixed-wing aircraft must use an airport for takeoff and landing, they are unable to fly directly to a hospital, they require a ground ambulance both at the departure and arrival point for patient movement.

Chapter 20

1. c   2. b   3. a   4. c   5. d   6. d   7. b

References

Air and Surface Patient Transport Principles and Practices, 3d ed. Air and Surface Transport Nurses Association. Edited by Renee Semonin Holleran. St. Louis: Mosby. 2003.

"Appropriateness of Air Medical Transport in Acute Coronary Syndromes." Position Statement of the Air Medical Physicians Association. *Air Medical Journal* 22 (July-Aug 2003): 11.

Baker, Judith J., and R. W. Baker. *Health Care Finance.* Gaithersburg, MD: Aspen Publishers, Inc. 2000.

Bird, Mark, and Tracey Stover-Wall. "Air Transport: Preparing a Patient for Transport." *American Journal of Nursing* 12 (Dec 2004): 49–53.

Bowers, Wilson R., and Polly L. Wyrick. "Extracorporeal Life Support: A Transcontinental Transport Experience." *Air Medical Journal* 22 (March-April 2003): 8–11.

Braithwaite, Collin, et al. "A Critical Analysis of On-Scene Helicopter Transport on Survival in a Statewide Trauma System," *J Trauma* 45 (July 1998): 140–46.

Chappell, Vicky L., et. al. "Impact of Discontinuing a Hospital-Based Air Ambulance Service on Trauma Patient Outcomes." *J Trauma* 52(3) (March 2002): 486–91.

Clayton H., et. al. "The Utility of Helicopter Transport of Trauma Patients from the Injury Scene in an Urban Trauma System." *J Trauma* 53 (Nov 2002): 817–22.

Collett, Howard and Annette Mikat. "Two Engines vs. One." *AirMed* 3 (Mar-Apr 1997): 16–21.

De Lorenzo, Robert A., and Robert S. Porter. *Tactical Emergency Care: Military and Operational Out-of-Hospital Medicine.* Upper Saddle River, NJ: Pearson/Prentice-Hall, 1999.

Deschamp, Clyde, et. al. "The Bispectral Index Monitor. A New Tool for Air Medical Personnel." *Air Medical Journal* 20 (Sept-Oct 2001): 38–39.

Deschamp, Clyde. "Hospital-based Air Medical Programs: Surviving Managed Care." *AirMed* (Jul-Aug 1998): 28–30.

Fitch, Joseph J., *Prehospital Care Administration,* 2d ed. San Diego, CA: JEMS Communications/Elsevier, 2004.

Frakes, Michael A., and Wendy R. Lord. "EMS Certification Requirements for Flight Nurses." *Air Medical Journal* 23 (Sept-Oct 2004): 38–40.

Fultz, Julia A., et. al. "Air Medical Referring Customer Satisfaction: A Valuable Insight." *Air Medical Journal* 17 (April-June 1998): 51–56.

Gardner, Bob. *Say Again, Please: Guide to Radio Communications*, 2d ed. Newcastle, Washington: Aviation Supplies and Academics, Inc. 2002.

Heegaard, William, et. al. "Ultrasound for the Air Medical Clinician." *Air Medical Journal* 23 (Mar-Apr 2004): 20–23.

Katz, Lawrence C. "Stress and the Medical Aircrew Member." *AirMed* 5 (July-Aug 1999): 31–34.

Kerr, W., T. Kerns, and R. Bissell. "Differences in Mortality Rates Among Trauma Patients Transported by Helicopter and Ambulance in Maryland." *Prehospital and Disaster Medicine* 14 (July-September 1999): 159–64.

Kettles, Jon. "The EMS Pilot's Standard of Care." *AirMed* 6 (Mar-Apr 2000): 20–21.

Koury, S., et al. "Air vs. Ground Transport and Outcomes in Trauma Patients Requiring Urgent Operative Interventions," *Prehospital Emergency Care* 2 (Oct-Dec 1998): 289–92.

McMullan, Paul, et. al. "The Use of Chemical Restraint in Helicopter Transport." *Air Medical Journal* 18 (Oct-Dec 1999): 136–39.

McNab, Andrew C. "The Cost of Family Oriented Communication Before Air Medical Interfacility Transport." *Air Medical Journal* 20 (July-Aug 2001): 20–22.

Medical Condition List and Appropriate Use of Air Medical Transport. Position Statement of the Air Medical Physicians Association. *Air Medical Journal* 22 (May-June 2003): 14–19.

Moore, Kirsten Johnson. "Strategies for Successful Management." *AirMed* 5 (July-Aug 1999): 28–30.

Nowicki, Michael. *The Financial Management of Hospitals and Healthcare Organizations*, 3d ed. Chicago, IL: Health Administration Press, 2004.

Perez, Leanne, Derek Alexander, and Lowell Wise. "Interfacility Transport of Patient Admitted to the ICU: Perceived Needs of Family Members." *Air Medical Journal* 22 (Sept-Oct 2003): 44–48.

Reinhart, Richard O. *Fit for Flight: Flight Physiology and Human Factors for Aircrew.* 2d ed. Ames, IA: Iowa State University Press, 1999.

Medical Direction and Medical Control of Air Medical Services. Position Statement of the Air Medical Physician Association. *Air Medical Journal* 22 (Jan-Feb 2003): 14–15.

Moy, Mark M. *The EMTALA Answer Book.* Gaithersburg, MD: Aspen Publishers, Inc., 1999.

Moylan, Joseph A., et al. "Factors Improving Survival in Multisystem Trauma Patients," *Annals of Surgery* 207 (1988): 679–85.

Nichols, Kathy, Michael Williams, and David T. Overton. "A Flight Orientation Curriculum for Emergency Medicine Resident Physicians." *AirMed* 22 (March-April 2003): 26–28.

Oppe, Siem and Frank De Charro. "The Effect of Medical Care by a Helicopter Trauma Team on the Probability of Survival and the Quality of Life of Hospitalised Victims," *Accident Analysis and Prevention* 33(2001): 129–38.

Plummer, Dave, et. al. "Ultrasound in HEMS: Its Role in Differentiating Shock States." *Air Medical Journal* 22 (March-April 2003): 33–36.

Shelton, Ray and Jack Kelly. *EMS Stress.* Carlsbad, CA: JEMS Communications, 1995.

Smith, R. P., and B. H. McArdle. "Pressure in the Cuffs of Tracheal Tubes at Altitude." *Anaesthesia* 57(4) (April 2002): 374–78.

Thomas, Stephen H., et al. "Helicopter Transport and Blunt Trauma Mortality: A Multicenter Trial," *J Trauma* 52 (Jan 2002): 136–45.

Urdaneta, L., et al. "Role of an Emergency Helicopter Transport Service in Rural Trauma," *Archives of Surgery* 122 (1987): 992–96.

Glossary

ADCUS   Advise customs.

advanced life support (ALS)   A certification or licensure level for ambulances. The term implies that personnel possess the knowledge and skills necessary to assess and manage patients with complex medical conditions in the prehospital setting. It also implies that personnel are capable of providing care for the medical condition that brought about the need for the transport.

AGL   Above ground level. Vertical elevation above the ground.

air medicine (aeromedicine)   A medical subspecialty that incorporates elements of emergency medicine, critical-care medicine, paramedicine, nursing, and public safety into the treatment and transport of patients by air.

airsickness   Motion sickness that occurs as a result of the movements associated with flight. Similar in pathophysiology to the motion sickness sometimes experienced by those who travel by car or boat.

alternate (alternate airport)   When flying under IFR regulations, a pilot must have at least one alternate airport at which to land in case the weather becomes unacceptable at the primary landing site.

altitude   Distance above sea level (ASL) or above ground level (AGL). Generally measured in feet or meters.

angle of attack   The angle between the direction of the cord of the blades and the relative direction of the wind.

anxiety   An emotional state precipitated by a stressful situation. Many patients become anxious when they learn they are about to fly in a helicopter. Anxiety may increase catecholamine levels, which may in turn lead to increases in blood pressure, pulse rate, and, in certain types of patients, to decompensation.

ASL   Above sea level.

ATC   Air traffic control or air traffic controller.

atmosphere   The gaseous envelope of air that surrounds the earth. The atmosphere extends to roughly 25,000 feet above sea level. Air temperature and density decrease as altitude increases.

automatic direction finding (ADF)   A basic guidance mode which provides lateral guidance to a radio station. A tool for navigating by using a radio frequency to determine position and direction.

autorotation   The process of landing a helicopter without engine power. As the helicopter glides toward the ground, the movement of air across the rotor disk maintains rotor speed. The pilot pulls up on the collective and uses the centrifugal force stored in the moving rotor blades to make a soft landing. The pilot must maintain rotor rpm precisely and must be accurate in estimating altitude at the time he or she begins preparing for landing.

aviation medical examiner (AME)   A physician who is designated by the FAA to examine and certify airworthiness for pilots. AMEs must follow FAA guidelines in making this determination.

avionics   The electronic equipment and systems applied to aeronautics and used in aircraft navigation. The electronic devices a pilot utilizes to set and maintain altitude and direction during flight.

barodontalgia   Toothache that results from increased or decreased pressure due to a change in altitude. May be caused by air expansion in the root area of the tooth or may be referred pain from one of the adjacent sinuses.

barosinusitis   Sinus discomfort secondary to air trapping and air expansion within one or more sinuses.

barotitis media (ear block)   Trapping of air in the middle ear. As one moves to a higher altitude and atmospheric pressure decreases, the volume of air within the middle ear expands, pushing the tympanic membrane outward and creating a sensation of fullness and discomfort. Normally the increased volume of air escapes through the eustachian tubes and the discomfort is relieved (until there is a further change in altitude).

basic life support (BLS)   A certification level for ambulances. It implies that personnel are capable of performing cardiopulmonary resuscitation and other basic emergency skills, and that advanced life-support capabilities are not available.

boom strike   Occurs when the main rotor dips so low as to strike the tail boom. It is generally caused by a very hard landing and most commonly results when an inexperienced pilot descends too rapidly during landing.

Boyle's Law   The volume of a gas is directly proportional to the pressure exerted on that gas (e.g., as pressure decreases, volume increases, and vice versa).

brownout   A condition that may occur when a pilot attempts to land a helicopter in an area of loose soil or sand, which mixes with the rotor wash and produces a dark cloud around the aircraft, reducing the pilot's visibility and potentially resulting in a crash.

catchment area   The geographical area served by an institution or program.

center of gravity (CG)   The fore-to-aft point in the aircraft at which there is exact weight balance. Aircraft are designed to operate most effectively when CG is at a designated point. It falls to the pilot to ensure that the aircraft is loaded in such a way that the CG is at the appropriate point.

ceiling   Height of the lowest cloud layer above ground. The vertical point at which visibility is blocked.

clear air turbulence (CAT)   Erratic air currents that occur in cloudless air and constitute a hazard to aircraft. More likely to occur at higher altitudes and in mountainous areas.

collective   The control that adjusts the pitch of the rotor blades and regulates the rate of ascent and descent of the helicopter. Generally in the form of a lever to the left of the pilot's seat. When the collective is raised, the angle of attack increases. When lowered, it decreases. Sometimes referred to as the "house size adjuster," i.e., when the collective is pulled up, houses get smaller; when it is pushed down, houses get larger.

crew resource management (CRM)   A comprehensive plan whereby human resources are used effectively and efficiently during all phases of flight. Its intended purpose is to reduce the probability of human error.

critical-care transport   Caring for the critically ill or injured patient in an aeromedical environment through the use of available knowledge and skills by a competent health care professional who has received extensive training specific to air medicine. This designation implies that transporting personnel possess a minimum level of knowledge and skills to manage complicated medical patients. Critical-care transports often involve complex physiologic monitoring, the use of ventilators, and the administration of multiple medications.

cyclic ("the stick")   The control that adjusts the horizontal attitude of the helicopter. Movement of the cyclic in one direction decreases the pitch of the rotor in that direction and increases it in the other direction, thus increasing lift on one side and decreasing it on the other. If the cyclic is pushed right, the helicopter rolls right.

decibel   The standard unit of measure of sound intensity. A whisper produces 20 decibels, a car at cruise speed on the highway 70 decibels, a turbine engine 130 to 150 decibels. The human ear is very susceptible to damage from exposure to excessive sound levels. The level of risk is determined by both decibel level and period of exposure.

decongestants   Pharmaceutical agents that, when taken as directed, may result in shrinkage of mucous membranes and a reduction of nasal and pharyngeal congestion. When taken prior to flight, they may reduce the incidence of sinus and ear block.

directional disorientation   The sensation that one is traveling in a direction other than the one being traveled in. Loss of directional awareness.

dissymmetry of lift   As a helicopter gains speed, the advancing side of the rotor disk moves faster through the air and provides more lift than does the retreating side. The pilot must compensate for this by increasing blade pitch on the retreating side. If speed continues to increase, eventually the imbalance cannot be overcome and the aircraft will roll toward the retreating blade side (see *velocity to never exceed*).

drag   The wind force (resistance) exerted against an aircraft as it attempts to move through the air. As speed increases, so does drag.

ear block   See *barotitis*.

emergency locator transmitter   A transmitter maintained in an aircraft that can be activated automatically or manually in the event of a crash to allow rescuers to more easily locate the aircraft.

EMTALA   The Emergency Medical Treatment and Active Labor Act. Passed in 1986, this law defines requirements for participating hospitals to treat emergency patients. A portion of this act stipulates the minimum requirements for medical personnel handling interfacility transport of emergency patients.

estimated time of arrival (ETA)   Approximate time at which an aircraft will reach an intermediary point or final destination.

eustachian tube   A tube lined with mucous membrane that connects the nasopharynx to the middle ear cavity. It is normally closed but opens during yawning, chewing, and swallowing to equalize air pressure in the middle ear with atmospheric pressure.

FAA medical certificate   Evidence of a satisfactory medical evaluation performed by an aviation medical examiner (AME). A prerequisite for licensure as a pilot.

Federal Aviation Administration (FAA)   The federal agency charged with promulgating and enforcing rules and regulations concerning the operation of aircraft.

Federal Aviation Regulations (FARs)   The federal regulations governing the operation of aircraft in the United States.

flameout   Occurs when fuel ignition ceases during flight. Although rare, it may be caused by flying in air with low oxygen concentration (e.g., over a forest fire) or by flying in very heavy rain.

flicker vertigo   A variety of symptoms that may be caused by exposure to flickering or flashing light, such as sunlight shining through rotating main rotor blades on a helicopter. Symptoms may include fatigue, headache, dizziness, nausea, and vomiting. In rare cases it may result in neurological manifestations such as seizures.

flight following   The process of maintaining constant or intermittent contact with an aircraft for the purpose of tracking its location and condition. An integral component of the air medical safety program.

flight physical   Periodic physical examination by a physician. All pilots are required by the FAA to undergo flight physicals to maintain their pilot certificate.

The purpose is to identify problems that may result in medical emergencies or otherwise compromise the pilot's ability to operate an aircraft safely.

flight surgeon Generally, the equivalent of a military aviation medical examiner. Flight surgeons often have more extensive training than do civilian AMEs.

global positioning satellite (GPS) An electronic device that receives signals from orbiting satellites. It uses an advanced form of triangulation to calculate and display an exact location in the form of numbers indicating latitude and longitude. Some more advanced units also display location on a map display.

Graham's Law A gas of high pressure exerts a force toward a region of lower pressure. If a semipermeable membrane separates these two regions of unequal pressure, the gas of higher pressure will pass or diffuse through the membrane toward the region of lower pressure.

ground effect The increased lift gained from hovering or flying close to the ground. The air bouncing upward from the ground provides additional lift.

haze Any atmospheric condition that interferes with light transmission; generally caused by high moisture content, smoke, or dust particles in the air. Haze may distort perceptions of distance and attitude and hasten onset of fatigue.

head strike envelope Inside the aircraft, the area within which the head may contact structures and equipment in the event of turbulence or a hard landing.

helipad A temporary landing site, built to enable a helicopter to land safely. Generally not a permanent structure.

heliport (helideck) A permanent helicopter landing site that conforms to FAA and other government regulations.

helispot An open area that has been cleared of obstacles on which a helicopter can land safely. Generally used for scene flights.

hot load To load (or unload) a patient while the rotors are turning.

hot start Occurs when too much fuel enters the engine and passes through to the exhaust system during start-up. When the fuel is ignited, flames erupt from the exhaust pipes, causing overheating and potential damage to the engine.

hovering When a helicopter maintains a constant position at a selected point, usually a few feet above the ground. Helicopters may be capable of hovering at high altitudes if they have sufficient power. As altitude increases and air density decreases, more power is required to maintain a hover.

in-ground effect (IGE) Apparent increase in aerodynamic lift experienced by an aircraft flying close to the ground.

instrument flight rule (IFR) A set of rules governing the conduct of flight under instrument meteorological conditions.

Jesus bolts   The bolts that hold the main mast to the frame, and the head to the main mast. Most helicopters have two of these bolts. If you lose either one, the rotor head will separate from the helicopter. (They are called "Jesus bolts" because if one breaks, the pilot and crew are on their way to see Jesus.)

jet lag   A form of circadian dysrhythmia caused by moving from one time zone to another. Typically characterized by disrupted sleep cycle, fatigue, and difficulty concentrating.

knot(s) (kt)   Unit used to measure aircraft speed. One knot equals approximately 1.15 mph. For example, a 120-knot airspeed would be approximately 138 mph.

medical direction (medical control)   A process whereby knowledgeable physicians provide guidelines and oversee the practice of paramedics, nurses, and other nonphysician members of a health care team, generally in the out-of-hospital setting.

medivac (or medevac)   Air medical evacuation. Term sometimes applied to helicopters utilized for air medical purposes.

motion sickness   A condition that results from prolonged exposure to erratic or rhythmic movement in any combination of directions. May be associated with riding in a boat, aircraft, or car. Nausea, vomiting, headache, and vertigo characterize severe cases (see *airsickness*).

myopia   Nearsightedness.

National Transportation Safety Board (NTSB)   The federal organization charged with investigating the causes of aircraft accidents. The data provided by the NTSB often lead to changes in operational policies and procedures involving AM programs.

night vision   Ability to see during relative darkness.

night vision goggles (NVG)   Electronic device that magnifies radiated light and increases the wearer's ability to discern objects during relative darkness.

partial pressure   The pressure exerted by any one gas in a mixture of gases or in a liquid, with the pressure directly related to the concentration of that gas to the total pressure of the mixture.

physical fitness   The ability to withstand stress and persevere under difficult circumstances in which an unfit person would quit. An indicator of general health. Persons with a high level of physical fitness may have increased longevity and a decreased incidence of illness compared to those who are less fit.

pilot error   A generic term for any mistake made by a pilot. Generally applied when referring to the cause of an incident or accident. Pilot error is often singled out as the most preventable element of air crashes. Approximately 80 percent of all accidents are attributed to pilot error.

pilot in command (PIC)   The pilot responsible for the operation and safety of an aircraft during flight. The PIC is the ultimate authority concerning all activities occurring within the aircraft during flight.

position report   An exact description of an aircraft's location as transmitted to the ATC or other flight following center. Many rotor-wing programs require that flight following updates be transmitted every 10 to 15 minutes (see *flight following*).

post-accident/incident plan (PAIP)   An action guide for dispatchers outlining a course of action in the event that a pilot declares an in-flight emergency or fails to provide a position report at the designated time. Generally includes step-by-step instructions and all necessary telephone numbers.

postural disorientation (attitude disorientation)   The sensation that one's person (or aircraft) is in a posture other than that in which it actually is. For example, one may "feel" that the aircraft is in a bank when in reality it is flying straight and level.

pseudoephedrine   An over-the-counter decongestant. An alpha-receptor agonist. May decrease the incidence of sinus and ear block when taken prior to flight. Side effects may include tachycardia, ectopic beats, and anxiety/restlessness.

quality assurance (QA)/quality improvement (QI)/quality management (QM) Ongoing programs designed to monitor and improve the performance level of employees and systems. The quality of medical care provided by an AM program is strongly influenced by its quality management program.

retreating blade stall   During fast flight a helicopter may reach a speed at which it is moving so fast that the retreating blade is unable to maintain lift on that side of the aircraft. The aircraft rolls toward the retreating blade side, potentially causing the pilot to lose control of the aircraft. Aircraft manufacturers determine this speed when the aircraft is designed and post a warning accordingly (see *velocity never to exceed*).

rotation   The point during takeoff of a fixed-wing aircraft when the pilot pulls back on the yoke and the front of the aircraft rotates upward, leaving the runway.

search and rescue (SAR)   Mission in which an aircraft is used to search for a person or persons who may be lost on the ground. May follow a suspected plane crash, overdue campers, and so on.

settling with power   A condition in which the helicopter settles into its own downwash. The aircraft continues to descend even though the collective is elevated. Conditions conducive to settling with power are a vertical or nearly vertical descent of at least 300 feet per minute and low forward airspeed. The rotor system must also be using some degree of available engine power (from 20 to 100 percent), leaving insufficient power to retard the sink rate. These conditions occur during approaches with a tailwind or during formation approaches when one aircraft is flying through the turbulence produced by another.

sinus block   See *barosinusitis*.

spatial disorientation   Illusions that sometimes occur as a result of unusual relative motion.

sunburn   A skin injury (burn) resulting from prolonged exposure to sunlight radiation. Characterized by redness, tenderness, and, in severe cases, blistering. Sun damage is cumulative and significantly increases the risk of certain types of skin cancer.

supplemental type certificate (STC)   The STC is issued when an applicant receives FAA approval to modify an aircraft from its original design. The STC, which incorporates by reference the related type certificate, approves not only the modification but how that modification affects the original design of the aircraft.

swash plate   A device with which the control arms maintain contact as they spin and that changes pitch on the blade at different points in its revolution.

tail rotor   A small rotor generally located on the distal tail of the helicopter. It produces thrust to counteract the torque generated by the engine as it powers the main rotor.

thermal fatigue   Fatigue resulting from exposure to temperature extremes. As ambient temperature becomes more extreme, the body uses more energy to maintain normal temperature.

time of useful consciousness (TUC)   The period following a decrease in oxygen availability (e.g., cabin decompression) until a pilot or other crew member becomes unconscious or disoriented to the point of being unable to function.

tinnitus   A subjective sensation of persistent noise, commonly referred to as "ringing in the ears." May occur as a result of exposure to loud noise. May be a sign of temporary or permanent hearing loss.

tower (TWR)   Generally refers to a control tower in the context of contact with an air traffic controller. May also refer to a privately owned radio antennae tower that may be an obstacle to flight.

traffic   A term used by air traffic control (ATC) to refer to one or more aircraft.

transitional lift   As a helicopter leaves hover and increases airspeed, airflow across the rotor disk increases, producing increasing lift. As airspeed approaches a certain point (generally 40 to 60 knots), the aircraft begins a spontaneous climb.

tunnel vision   An actual or perceived reduction of one's field of vision. May be caused by hypoxia or anxiety.

UNICOM   A private advisory station.

urgency   A condition for which there is a safety concern and timely (but not immediate) assistance is required.

velocity to never exceed (VNE)   The maximum safe speed of an aircraft.

vestibular disorientation   Positional disorientation. Occurs when what the inner ear perceives and what the eyes perceive are dissimilar. A sensation that one's position or movement is other than what it really is.

Visual Approach Slope Indicator System (VASIS)   A series of differently colored lights located near the touchdown point on a runway, designed to aid fixed-wing pilots maintain the correct altitude and glide slope on final approach to land.

visual flight rule (VFR)   Set of conditions under which a pilot must rely on visual ground reference and dead reckoning (estimating time until reaching a desired point). VFR flight rules require a minimum horizontal and vertical visibility range. Visibility must be at least 3 statute miles during the day and 5 statute miles at night. The ceiling must also be high enough so that there is a safe distance between the clouds and the ground.

visual medical direction   A specific type of on-line medical control whereby the medical director accompanies the flight team and provides on-scene medical direction. Also referred to as medical director ride-along. May be done as a component of the quality assurance/improvement process.

visual meteorological conditions (VMC)   A Canadian term that is similar to VFR in the United States.

visual omnidirectional aid (VOR)   A radio transmission beacon. Using the transmission from this beacon, a pilot can simply and accurately navigate from point A to point B. The standard tool for navigation since the 1950s and still available in all aircraft, although GPS-based navigation is rapidly relegating the VOR to a backup role.

weathervaning   The tendency of a helicopter in flight to turn into the wind like a wind sock. The amount of weathervaning is determined by the size of the vertical stabilizer. The pilot must compensate for it in order to remain on course.

wind sock   A funnel-shaped tube of fabric attached to an upright pole and rotating freely about the pole in response to wind. Its location and movement on the pole indicate the direction in which wind is moving. Hangs loosely when no wind is blowing and is fully extended in a 10-knot wind.

ZULU   Coordinated Universal Time.

Index

Note: Page numbers followed by *f* indicate figure: those followed by *t* indicate table.

V

Ventilator, 131
Ventilator-dependent patients, 171, 179–80
Very high frequency (VHF), 79–80
Vibration, effects of, 71
Vietnam War, air medicine during, 27–28, 28f, 253–54
Violent patients, 191
Visibility issues:
  brownout, 53
  weather-related, 55
Visual flight rule (VFR), 20–21, 348

Visual medical direction, 198
Visual omnidirectional aid (VOR), 346
Vomiting, airsickness and, 185–86

W

Weather, safety issues, 55–57
  lightning, 64
  thunderstorms, 55–56
  turbulence, 56
  visibility, 55
Website, for marketing, 236–37, 243
Weight, in aircraft flight, 7, 7f

Weight limitations, flight, 101, 345–46
"Wilco," 88
World War I, military medical operations in, 250–51
World War II, military medical operations in, 26, 251–52

X

X rays, 154

Y

Yaw, in aircraft flight, 8f, 9